NCLEX-RN
Psychiatric Nursing

made

Incredibly Easy!®

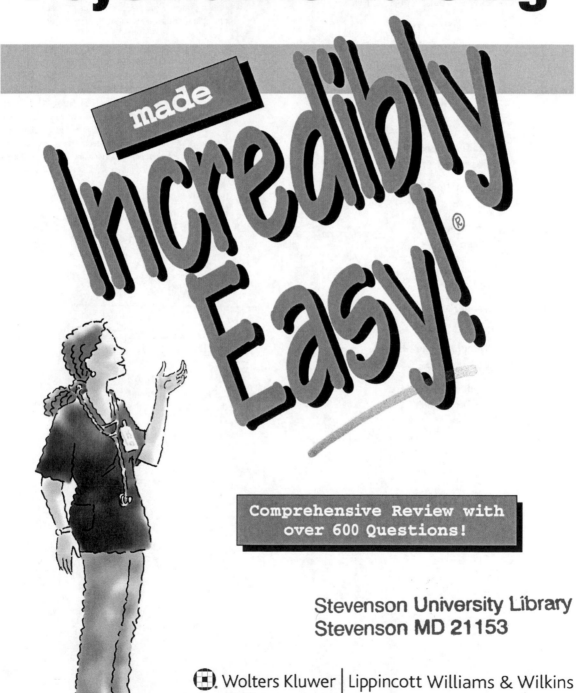

Comprehensive Review with over 600 Questions!

Wolters Kluwer | Lippincott Williams & Wilkins
Health

Philadelphia · Baltimore · New York · London
Buenos Aires · Hong Kong · Sydney · Tokyo

Staff

Publisher
Chris Burghardt

Clinical Director
Joan M. Robinson, RN, MSN

Clinical Project Manager
Beverly Ann Tscheschlog, RN, MS

Clinical Editor
Jennifer Meyering, RN, BSN, MS, CCRN

Acquisitions Editor
Bill Lamsback

Product Director
David Moreau

Product Managers
Rosanne Hallowell and Jennifer K. Forestieri

Editorial Assistants
Karen J. Kirk, Jeri O'Shea, Linda K. Ruhf

Art Director
Elaine Kasmer

Illustrator
Bot Roda

Vendor Manager
Cynthia Rudy

Manufacturing Manager
Beth J. Welsh

Production Services
SPi Technologies

RNPSYIE010810-050212

Library of Congress Cataloging-in-Publication Data

ISBN-13: 978-1-4511-0817-0
ISBN-10: 1-4511-0817-6

IBT0112

Contents

Preface

NCLEX-RN Psychiatric Nursing Made Incredibly Easy is really two books in one. The first is designed to provide you with a detailed review of essential nursing concepts, nursing diagnoses, and clinical information you need to pass the NCLEX-RN. The second provides hundreds of challenging questions, answers, and detailed rationales following the NCLEX 2010 test plan. The content review section follows the same chapter structure as the Q&A section to help you organize your study.

The content section is presented in the appealing and effective style of the *Incredibly Easy* series. Its humor encourages you to relax and have fun while learning. You will also find these valuable features in every chapter of the review:
- **Brush up on key concepts** provides an overview of anatomy and physiology.
- **Cheat sheets** provide you with a concise overview of key signs and symptoms, test results, treatments, and interventions of common diseases. Use this feature to quickly review the material you will cover in depth in the *Polish up on client care* section.
- **Keep abreast of diagnostic tests** highlights the most important tests for the disorders being discussed, including pertinent nursing actions you will need to perform to ensure client safety—a key area of NCLEX-RN testing.
- **Polish up on client care** provides a thorough review of disorders with a focus on the expected nursing care. Starting with a description of the problem, this section also covers causes, assessment findings, diagnostic test results, nursing diagnoses, treatments, and drug therapy for each disorder. Key interventions and their rationales are also provided.

In addition to your nursing knowledge, your test-taking skills can help you pass the exam. This book introduces you to the NCLEX-RN exam structure and covers techniques that will help you learn how to read test questions and understand what they are really asking—skills that are vital to NCLEX success. You also have access to study strategies, such as scheduling study time, maintaining your concentration, and finding the right study space.

Questions, Questions, and More Questions

The more you become accustomed to the styles and types of questions that may be asked, the more successful you will be on the actual exam, and that's a special strength of this book. You will find *Pump up on practice questions* at the end of each chapter, and in addition you will find an entire second section of the book featuring hundreds of additional questions. The easy-to-use format features questions on the left and answers on the right side of the same page. The questions help you assess and remember what you've just reviewed and determine areas in which you might need further review. Detailed rationales for both correct and incorrect answers are provided, and each answer provides information on the client needs category, the cognitive level of the question, and the nursing process. Helpful hints are scattered throughout the practice questions. These hints greatly increase your ability to determine the correct answer, retain important content information, and learn essential test-taking strategies. In addition, the graphics keep you focused and help build your confidence.

Be proud of your accomplishments and of your decision to prepare yourself well for the NCLEX-RN. You've worked hard to come this far. Now it's time to prepare, to practice, to build your confidence, and to succeed!

Part I   Getting ready

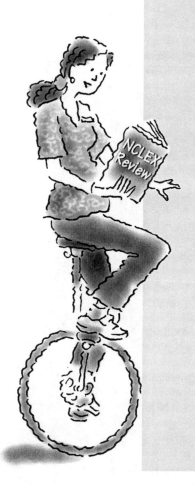

1 Preparing for the NCLEX®

NCLEX basics

Passing the National Council Licensure Examination (NCLEX®) is an important landmark in your career as a nurse. The first step on your way to passing the NCLEX is to understand what it is and how it's administered.

NCLEX structure

The *NCLEX* is a test written by nurses who, like most of your nursing instructors, have an advanced degree and clinical expertise in a particular area. Only one small difference distinguishes nurses who write NCLEX questions: They're trained to write questions in a style particular to the NCLEX.

If you've completed an accredited nursing program, you've already taken numerous tests written by nurses with backgrounds and experiences similar to those of the nurses who write for the NCLEX. The test-taking experience you've already gained will help you pass the NCLEX. So your NCLEX review should be just that — a review. (For eligibility and immigration requirements for nurses from outside of the United States, see *Guidelines for international nurses,* page 4.)

What's the point of it all?
The NCLEX is designed for one purpose: namely, to determine whether it's appropriate for you to receive a license to practice as a nurse. By passing the NCLEX, you demonstrate that you possess the minimum level of knowledge necessary to practice nursing safely.

Mix 'em up
In nursing school, you probably took courses that were separated into such subjects as pharmacology, nursing leadership, health assessment, adult health, pediatric, maternal-neonatal, and psychiatric nursing. In contrast, the NCLEX is integrated, meaning that different subjects are mixed together.

As you answer NCLEX questions, you may encounter clients in any stage of life, from neonatal to geriatric. These clients — clients, in NCLEX lingo — may be of any background, may be completely well or extremely ill, and may have any disorder.

Client needs, front and center
The NCLEX draws questions from four categories of client needs that were developed by the *National Council of State Boards of Nursing* (NCSBN), the organization that sponsors and manages the NCLEX. *Client needs categories* ensure that a wide variety of topics appear on every NCLEX examination.

The NCSBN developed client needs categories after conducting a practice analysis of new nurses. All aspects of nursing care observed in the study were broken down into four main categories, some of which were broken down further into subcategories. (See *Client needs categories,* page 5.)

The whole kit and caboodle
The categories and subcategories are used to develop the *NCLEX test plan,* the content guidelines for the distribution of test questions. Question-writers and the people who put the NCLEX together use the test plan and client needs categories to make sure that a full spectrum of nursing activities is covered in the examination. Client needs categories appear in most NCLEX review and question-and-answer books, including this one. As a test-taker, you don't have to concern yourself with client needs categories. You'll see those categories for each question and answer in this book, but they'll be invisible on the actual NCLEX.

Guidelines for international nurses

To become eligible to work as a registered nurse in the United States, you'll need to complete several steps. In addition to passing the NCLEX® examination, you may need to obtain a certificate and credentials evaluation from the Commission on Graduates of Foreign Nursing Schools (CGFNS®) and acquire a visa. Requirements vary from state to state, so it's important that you first contact the Board of Nursing in the state where you want to practice nursing.

CGFNS CERTIFICATION PROGRAM

Most states require that you obtain CGFNS certification. This certification requires:
• review and authentication of your credentials, including your nursing education, registration, and licensure
• passing score on the CGFNS Qualifying Examination of nursing knowledge
• passing score on an English language proficiency test.

To be eligible to take the CGFNS Qualifying Examination, you must complete a minimum number of classroom and clinical practice hours in medical-surgical nursing, maternal-infant nursing, pediatric nursing, and psychiatric and mental health nursing from a government-approved nursing school. You must also be registered as a first-level nurse in your country of education and currently hold a license as a registered nurse in some jurisdiction.

The CGFNS Qualifying Examination is a paper and pencil test that includes 260 multiple-choice questions and is administered under controlled testing conditions. Because the test is designed to predict your likelihood of successfully passing the NCLEX-RN examination, it's based on the NCLEX-RN test plan.

You may select from three English proficiency examinations—Test of English as a Foreign Language (TOEFL®), Test of English for International Communication (TOEIC®), or International English Language Testing System (IELTS). Each test has different passing scores, and the scores are valid for up to 2 years.

CGFNS CREDENTIALS EVALUATION SERVICE

This evaluation is a comprehensive report that analyzes and compares your education and licensure with U.S. standards. It's prepared by CGFNS for a state board of nursing, an immigration office, employer, or university. To use this service you must complete an application, submit appropriate documentation, and pay a fee.

More information about the CGFNS certification program and credentials evaluation service is available at *www.cgfns.org*.

VISA REQUIRED

You can't legally immigrate to work in the United States without an occupational visa (temporary or permanent) from the United States Citizenship and Immigration Services (USCIS). The visa process is separate from the CGFNS certification process, although some of the same steps are involved. Some visas require prior CGFNS certification and a *VisaScreen*™ Certificate from the International Commission on Healthc are Professions (ICHP). The VisaScreen program involves:
• credentials review of your nursing education and current registration or licensure
• successful completion of either the CGFNS certification program or the NCLEX-RN to provide proof of nursing knowledge
• passing score on an approved English language proficiency examination.

After you successfully complete all parts of the *VisaScreen* program, you'll receive a certificate to present to the USCIS. The visa granting process can take up to one year.

You can obtain more detailed information about visa applications at *www.uscis.gov*.

Testing by computer

Like many standardized tests today, the NCLEX is administered by computer. That means you won't be filling in empty circles, sharpening pencils, or erasing frantically. It also means that you must become familiar with computer tests, if you aren't already. Fortunately, the skills required to take the NCLEX on a computer are simple enough to

Client needs categories

Each question on the NCLEX is assigned a category based on client needs. This chart lists client needs categories and subcategories and the percentages of each type of question that appears on an NCLEX examination.

Category	Subcategories	Percentage of NCLEX questions
Safe and effective care environment	• Management of care • Safety and infection control	16% to 22% 8% to 14%
Health promotion and maintenance		6% to 12%
Psychosocial integrity		6% to 12%
Physiological integrity	• Basic care and comfort • Pharmacological and parenteral therapies • Reduction of risk potential • Physiological adaptation	6% to 12% 13% to 19% 10% to 16% 11% to 17%

allow you to focus on the questions, not the keyboard.

Q&A

When you take the test, depending on the question format, you'll be presented with a question and four or more possible answers, a blank space in which to enter your answer, a figure on which you'll identify the correct area by clicking the mouse on it, a series of charts or exhibits you'll use to select the correct response, items you must rearrange in priority order by dragging and dropping them in place, an audio recording to listen to in order to select the correct response, or a question and four graphic options.

Feeling smart? Think hard!

The NCLEX is a *computer-adaptive test*, meaning that the computer reacts to the answers you give, supplying more difficult questions if you answer correctly, and slightly easier questions if you answer incorrectly. Each test is thus uniquely adapted to the individual test-taker.

A matter of time

You have a great deal of flexibility with the amount of time you can spend on individual questions. The examination lasts a maximum of 6 hours, however, so don't waste time. If you fail to answer a set number of questions within 6 hours, the computer will determine that you lack minimum competency.

Most students have plenty of time to complete the test, so take as long as you need to get the question right without wasting time. But remember to keep moving at a decent pace to help you maintain concentration.

Difficult items = Good news

If you find as you progress through the test that the questions seem to be increasingly difficult, it's a good sign. The more questions you answer correctly, the more difficult the questions become.

Some students, though, knowing that questions get progressively harder, focus on the degree of difficulty of subsequent questions to try to figure out if they're answering questions correctly. Avoid the temptation to do this, as this may get you off track.

Free at last!

The computer test finishes when one of the following events occurs:
• You demonstrate minimum competency, according to the computer program, which

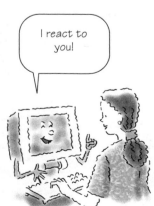

I react to you!

does so with 95% certainty that your ability exceeds the passing standard.

• You demonstrate a lack of minimum competency, according to the computer program.

• You've answered the maximum number of questions (265 total questions).

• You've used the maximum time allowed (6 hours).

Unlocking the NCLEX mystery

In April 2004, the NCSBN added alternate-format items to the examination. However, most of the questions on the NCLEX are four-option, multiple-choice items with only one correct answer. Certain strategies can help you understand and answer any type of NCLEX question.

Alternate formats

The first type of alternate-format item is the *multiple-response question*. Unlike a traditional multiple-choice question, each multiple-response question has one or more correct answers for every question, and it may contain more than four possible answer options. You'll recognize this type of question because it will ask you to select *all* answers that apply — not just the best answer (as may be requested in the more traditional multiple-choice questions).

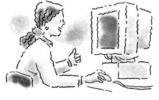

> The harder it gets, the better I'm doing.

All or nothing
Keep in mind that, for each multiple-response question, you must select at least one answer and you must select all correct answers for the item to be counted as correct. On the NCLEX, there is no partial credit in the scoring of these items.

Don't go blank!
The second type of alternate-format item is the *fill-in-the-blank* question. These questions require you to provide the answer yourself, rather than select it from a list of options. You will perform a calculation and then type your answer (a number, without any words, units of measurements, commas, or spaces) in the blank space provided after the question. Rules for rounding are included in the question stem if appropriate. A calculator button is provided so you can do your calculations electronically.

Mouse marks the spot!
The third type of alternate-format item is a question that asks you to identify an area on an illustration or graphic. For these "*hot spot*" questions, the computerized exam will ask you to place your cursor and click over the correct area on an illustration. Try to be as precise as possible when marking the location. As with the fill-in-the-blanks, the identification questions on the computerized exam may require extremely precise answers in order for them to be considered correct.

Click, choose, and prioritize
The fourth alternate-format item type is the *chart/exhibit* format. For this question type, you'll be given a problem and then a series of small screens with additional information you'll need to answer the question. By clicking on the tabs on screen, you can access each chart or exhibit item. After viewing the chart or exhibit, you select your answer from four multiple-choice options.

Drag n' drop
The fifth alternate-format item type involves prioritizing actions or placing a series of statements in correct order using a *drag-and-drop* (ordered response) technique. To move an answer option from the list of unordered options into the correct sequence, click on it using the mouse. While still holding down the mouse button, drag the option to the ordered response part of the screen. Release the mouse button to "drop" the option into place. Repeat this process until you've moved all of the available options into the correct order.

Now hear this!
The sixth alternate-format item type is the *audio item* format. You'll be given a set of headphones and you'll be asked to listen to an

audio clip and select the correct answer from four options. You'll need to select the correct answer on the computer screen as you would with the traditional multiple-choice questions.

Picture perfect

The final alternate-format item type is the *graphic option* question. This varies from the exhibit format type because in the graphic option, your answer choices will be graphics such as ECG strips. You'll have to select the appropriate graphic to answer the question presented.

The standard's still the standard

The NCSBN hasn't yet established a percentage of alternate-format items to be administered to each candidate. In fact, your exam may contain only one alternate-format item. So relax; the standard, four-option, multiple-choice format questions constitute the bulk of the test. (See *Sample NCLEX questions*, pages 8 to 10.)

Understanding the question

NCLEX questions are commonly long. As a result, it's easy to become overloaded with information. To focus on the question and avoid becoming overwhelmed, apply proven strategies for answering NCLEX questions, including:
* determining what the question is asking
* determining relevant facts about the client
* rephrasing the question in your mind
* choosing the best option or options before entering your answer.

DETERMINE WHAT THE QUESTION IS ASKING

Read the question twice. If the answer isn't apparent, rephrase the question in simpler, more personal terms. Breaking down the question into easier, less intimidating terms may help you to focus more accurately on the correct answer.

Give it a try

For example, a question might be, "A 74-year-old client with a history of heart failure is admitted to the coronary care unit with pulmonary edema. He's intubated and placed on a mechanical ventilator. Which parameters should the nurse monitor closely to assess the client's response to a bolus dose of furosemide (Lasix) I.V.?"

The options for this question — numbered from 1 to 4 — might include:
1. Daily weight
2. 24-hour intake and output
3. Serum sodium levels
4. Hourly urine output

Hocus, focus on the question

Read the question again, ignoring all details except what's being asked. Focus on the last line of the question. It asks you to select the appropriate assessment for monitoring a client who received a bolus of furosemide I.V.

DETERMINE WHAT FACTS ABOUT THE CLIENT ARE RELEVANT

Next, sort out the relevant client information. Start by asking whether any of the information provided about the client isn't relevant. For instance, do you need to know that the client has been admitted to the coronary care unit? Probably not; his reaction to I.V. furosemide won't be affected by his location in the hospital.

Determine what you do know about the client. In the example, you know that:
* he just received an I.V. bolus of furosemide, a crucial fact
* he has pulmonary edema, the most fundamental aspect of the client's underlying condition
* he's intubated and placed on a mechanical ventilator, suggesting that his pulmonary edema is serious
* he's 74 years old and has a history of heart failure, a fact that may or may not be relevant.

REPHRASE THE QUESTION

After you've determined relevant information about the client and the question being asked, consider rephrasing the question to make it more clear. Eliminate jargon and put the question in simpler, more personal terms. Here's how you might rephrase the question in the example: "My client has pulmonary edema. He requires intubation and

(Text continues on page 10.)

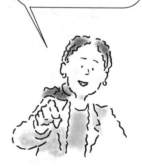

Focusing on what the question is really asking can help you choose the correct answer.

Sample NCLEX questions

Sometimes, getting used to the format is as important as knowing the material. Try your hand at these sample questions and you'll have a leg up when you take the real test!

Sample four-option, multiple-choice question

A client's arterial blood gas (ABG) results are as follows: pH, 7.16; $Paco_2$, 80 mm Hg; Pao_2, 46 mm Hg; HCO_3^-, 24 mEq/L; Sao_2, 81%. These ABG results represent which condition?

1. Metabolic acidosis
2. Metabolic alkalosis
3. Respiratory acidosis
4. Respiratory alkalosis

Correct answer: 3

Sample multiple-response question

A nurse is caring for a 45-year-old married woman who has undergone hemicolectomy for colon cancer. The woman has two children. Which concepts about families should the nurse keep in mind when providing care for this client?

Select all that apply:
1. Illness in one family member can affect all members.
2. Family roles don't change because of illness.
3. A family member may have more than one role at a time in the family.
4. Children typically aren't affected by adult illness.
5. The effects of an illness on a family depend on the stage of the family's life cycle.
6. Changes in sleeping and eating patterns may be signs of stress in a family.

Correct answer: 1, 3, 5, 6

Sample fill-in-the-blank calculation question

An infant who weighs 8 kg is to receive ampicillin 25 mg/kg I.V. every 6 hours. How many milligrams should the nurse administer per dose? Record your answer using a whole number.

_____ milligrams

Correct answer: 200

Sample hot spot question

A client has a history of aortic stenosis. Identify the area where the nurse should place the stethoscope to best hear the murmur.

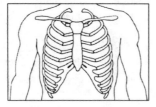

Correct answer:

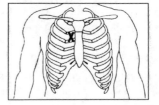

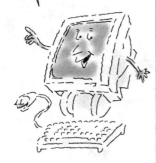

I can be ambivalent. More than one answer may be correct.

Sample NCLEX questions (continued)

Sample exhibit question

A 3-year old child is being treated for severe status asthmaticus. After reviewing the progress notes (shown below), the nurse should determine that this client is being treated for which condition?

Progress notes	
9/1/10 0600	Pt. was acutely restless, diaphoretic, and with dyspnea at 0530. Dr. T. Smith notified of findings at 0545 and ordered ABG analysis. ABG drawn from R radial artery. Stat results as follows: pH 7.28, $Paco_2$ 55 mm Hg, HCO_3^- 26 mEg/L. Dr. Smith with pt. now. ———————— J. Collins, RN.

1. Metabolic acidosis
2. Respiratory alkalosis
3. Respiratory acidosis
4. Metabolic alkalosis

Correct answer: 3

Sample drag-and-drop (ordered response) question

When teaching an antepartal client about the passage of the fetus through the birth canal during labor, the nurse describes the cardinal mechanisms of labor. Place these events in the sequence in which they occur. Use all options:

1. Flexion	
2. External rotation	
3. Descent	
4. Expulsion	
5. Internal rotation	
6. Extension	

Correct answer:

3. Descent
1. Flexion
5. Internal rotation
6. Extension
2. External rotation
4. Expulsion

(continued)

Sample NCLEX questions *(continued)*

Sample audio item question

Listen to the audio clip. What sound do you hear in the bases of this client with heart failure?

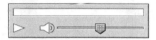

1. Crackles
2. Rhonchi
3. Wheezes
4. Pleural friction rub

Correct answer: 1

Sample graphic option question

Which electrocardiogram strip should the nurse document as sinus tachycardia?

1.

2.

3.

4.

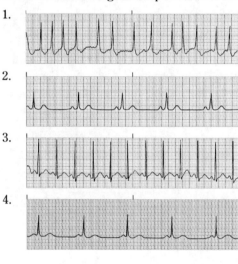

Correct answer: 1

mechanical ventilation. He's 74 years old and has a history of heart failure. He received an I.V. bolus of furosemide. What assessment parameter should I monitor?"

CHOOSE THE BEST OPTION
Armed with all the information you now have, it's time to select an option. You know that the client received an I.V. bolus of furosemide, a diuretic. You know that monitoring fluid intake and output is a key nursing intervention for a client taking a diuretic, a fact that eliminates options 1 and 3 (daily weight and serum sodium levels), narrowing the answer down to option 2 or 4 (24-hour intake and output or hourly urine output).

Can I use a lifeline?
You also know that the drug was administered by I.V. bolus, suggesting a rapid effect. (In fact, furosemide administered by I.V. bolus takes effect almost immediately.)

Monitoring the client's 24-hour intake and output would be appropriate for assessing the effects of repeated doses of furosemide. Hourly urine output, however, is most appropriate in this situation because it monitors the immediate effect of this rapid-acting drug.

Key strategies

Regardless of the type of question, four key strategies will help you determine the correct answer for each question. These strategies are:
- considering the nursing process
- referring to Maslow's hierarchy of needs
- reviewing client safety
- reflecting on principles of therapeutic communication.

Nursing process

One of the ways to answer a question is to apply the nursing process. Steps in the nursing process include:
- assessment
- diagnosis
- planning
- implementation
- evaluation.

First things first

The nursing process may provide insights that help you analyze a question. According to the nursing process, assessment comes before analysis, which comes before planning, which comes before implementation, which comes before evaluation.

You're halfway to the correct answer when you encounter a four-option, multiple-choice question that asks you to assess the situation and then provides two assessment options and two implementation options. You can immediately eliminate the implementation options, which then gives you, at worst, a 50-50 chance of selecting the correct answer. Use the following sample question to apply the nursing process:

A client returns from an endoscopic procedure during which he was sedated.

Before offering the client food, which action should the nurse take?
1. Assess the client's respiratory status.
2. Check the client's gag reflex.
3. Place the client in a side-lying position.
4. Have the client drink a few sips of water.

Assess before intervening

According to the nursing process, the nurse must assess a client before performing an intervention. Does the question indicate that the client has been properly assessed? No, it doesn't. Therefore, you can eliminate options 3 and 4 because they're both interventions.

That leaves options 1 and 2, both of which are assessments. Your nursing knowledge should tell you the correct answer — in this case, option 2. The sedation required for an endoscopic procedure may impair the client's gag reflex, so you would assess the gag reflex before giving food to the client to reduce the risk of aspiration and airway obstruction.

Final elimination

Why not select option 1, assessing the client's respiratory status? You might select this option but the question is specifically asking about offering the client food, an action that wouldn't be taken if the client's respiratory status was at all compromised. In this case, you're making a judgment based on the phrase, "Before offering the client food." If the question was trying to test your knowledge of respiratory depression following an endoscopic procedure, it probably wouldn't mention a function — such as giving food to a client — that clearly occurs only after the client's respiratory status has been stabilized.

Maslow's hierarchy

Knowledge of Maslow's hierarchy of needs can be a vital tool for establishing priorities on the NCLEX. Maslow's theory states that physiologic needs are the most basic human needs of all. Only after physiologic needs have been met can safety concerns be addressed. Only after safety concerns are met can concerns involving love and belonging be addressed, and so forth. Apply the principles of Maslow's hierarchy of needs to the following sample question:

A client complains of severe pain 2 days after surgery. Which action should the nurse perform first?

1. Offer reassurance to the client that he will feel less pain tomorrow.
2. Allow the client time to verbalize his feelings.
3. Check the client's vital signs.
4. Administer an analgesic.

Phys before psych
In this example, two of the options — 3 and 4 — address physiologic needs. Options 1 and 2 address psychosocial concerns. According to Maslow, physiologic needs must be met before psychosocial needs, so you can eliminate options 1 and 2.

Final elimination
Now, use your nursing knowledge to choose the best answer from the two remaining options. In this case, option 3 is correct because the client's vital signs should be checked before administering an analgesic (assessment before intervention). When prioritizing according to Maslow's hierarchy, remember your ABCs — airway, breathing, circulation — to help you further prioritize. Check for a patent airway before addressing breathing. Check breathing before checking the health of the cardiovascular system.

One caveat...
Just because an option appears on the NCLEX doesn't mean it's a viable choice for the client referred to in the question. Always examine your choice in light of your knowledge and experience. Ask yourself, "Does this choice make sense for this client?" Allow yourself to eliminate choices — even ones that might normally take priority — if they don't make sense for a particular client's situation.

Client safety

As you might expect, client safety takes high priority on the NCLEX. You'll encounter

many questions that can be answered by asking yourself, "Which answer will best ensure the safety of this client?" Use client safety criteria for situations involving laboratory values, drug administration, activities of daily living, or nursing care procedures.

Client first, equipment second
You may encounter a question in which some options address the client and others address the equipment. When in doubt, select an option relating to the client; never place equipment before a client.

For example, suppose a question asks what the nurse should do first when entering a client's room where an infusion pump alarm is sounding. If two options deal with the infusion pump, one with the infusion tubing, and another with the client's catheter insertion site, select the one relating to the client's catheter insertion site. Always check the client first; the equipment can wait.

Therapeutic communication

Some NCLEX questions focus on the nurse's ability to communicate effectively with the client. Therapeutic communication incorporates verbal or nonverbal responses and involves:
• listening to the client
• understanding the client's needs
• promoting clarification and insight about the client's condition.

Room for improvement
Like other NCLEX questions, those dealing with therapeutic communication commonly require choosing the best response. First, eliminate options that indicate the use of poor therapeutic communication techniques, such as those in which the nurse:
• tells the client what to do without regard to the client's feelings or desires (the "do this" response)
• asks a question that can be answered "yes" or "no," or with another one-syllable response
• seeks reasons for the client's behavior
• implies disapproval of the client's behavior
• offers false reassurances

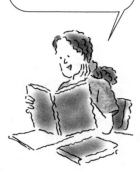

Say it 1,000 times: Studying for the exam is fun... studying for the exam is fun...

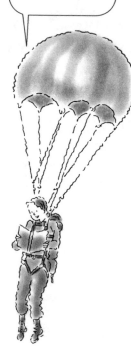

Client safety takes a high priority on the NCLEX.

- attempts to interpret the client's behavior rather than allow the client to verbalize his own feelings
- offers a response that focuses on the nurse, not the client.

Ah, that's better!

When answering NCLEX questions, look for responses that:
- allow the client time to think and reflect
- encourage the client to talk
- encourage the client to describe a particular experience
- reflect that the nurse has listened to the client, such as through paraphrasing the client's response.

Avoiding pitfalls

Even the most knowledgeable students can get tripped up on certain NCLEX questions. (See *A tricky question*, page 14.) Students commonly cite three areas that can be difficult for unwary test-takers:

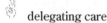 knowing the difference between the NCLEX and the "real world"

delegating care

knowing laboratory values.

NCLEX versus the real world

Some students who take the NCLEX have extensive practical experience in health care. For example, many test-takers have worked as licensed practical nurses or nursing assistants. In one of those capacities, test-takers might have been exposed to less than optimum clinical practice and may carry those experiences over to the NCLEX.

However, the NCLEX is a textbook examination — not a test of clinical skills. Take the NCLEX with the understanding that what happens in the real world may differ from what the NCLEX and your nursing school say should happen.

Don't take shortcuts

If you've had practical experience in health care, you may know a quicker way to perform a procedure or tricks to get by when you don't have the right equipment. Situations such as staff shortages may force you to improvise. On the NCLEX, such scenarios can lead to trouble. Always check your practical experiences against textbook nursing care, taking care to select the response that follows the textbook.

Delegating care

On the NCLEX, you may encounter questions that assess your ability to delegate care. Delegating care involves coordinating the efforts of other health care workers to provide effective care for your client. On the NCLEX, you may be asked to assign duties to:
- licensed practical nurses or licensed vocational nurses
- direct-care workers, such as certified nursing assistants and personal care aides
- other support staff, such as nutrition assistants and housekeepers.

In addition, you'll be asked to decide when to notify a physician, a social worker, or another hospital staff member. In each case, you'll have to decide when, where, and how to delegate.

Shoulds and shouldn'ts

As a general rule, it's okay to delegate actions that involve stable clients or standard, unchanging procedures. Bathing, feeding, dressing, and transferring clients are examples of procedures that can be delegated.

Be careful not to delegate complicated or complex activities. In addition, don't delegate activities that involve assessment, evaluation, or your own nursing judgment. On the NCLEX and in the real world, these duties fall squarely on your shoulders. Make sure that you take primary responsibility for assessing and evaluating the client and for making decisions about the client's care. Never hand off those responsibilities to someone with less training.

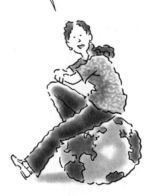

Remember, this is an exam, not the real world.

Normal laboratory values

• Blood urea nitrogen: 8 to 25 mg/dl

• Creatinine: 0.6 to 1.5 mg/dl

• Sodium: 135 to 145 mmol/L

• Potassium: 3.5 to 5.5 mEq/L

• Chloride: 97 to 110 mmol/L

• Glucose (fasting plasma): 70 to 110 mg/dl

• Hemoglobin
  Male: 13.8 to 17.2 g/dl
  Female: 12.1 to 15.1 g/dl

• Hematocrit
  Male: 40.7% to 50.3%
  Female: 36.1% to 44.3%

Advice from the experts

A tricky question

The NCLEX occasionally asks a particular kind of question called the "further teaching" question, which involves client-teaching situations. These questions can be tricky. You'll have to choose the response that suggests the client has *not* learned the correct information. Here's an example:

37. A client undergoes a total hip replacement. Which statement by the client indicates he requires further teaching?
  1. "I'll need to keep several pillows between my legs at night."
  2. "I'll need to remember not to cross my legs. It's such a bad habit."
  3. "The occupational therapist is showing me how to use a 'sock puller' to help me get dressed."
  4. "I don't know if I'll be able to get off that low toilet seat at home by myself."

The option you should choose here is 4 because it indicates that the client has a poor understanding of the precautions required after a total hip replacement and that he needs further teaching. Remember: If you see the phrase further teaching or further instruction, you're looking for a wrong answer by the client.

Calling in reinforcements

Deciding when to notify a physician, a social worker, or another hospital staff member is an important element of nursing care. On the NCLEX, however, choices that involve notifying the physician are usually incorrect. Remember that the NCLEX wants to see you, the nurse, at work.

If you're sure the correct answer is to notify the physician, though, make sure the client's safety has been addressed before notifying a physician or another staff member. On the NCLEX, the client's safety has a higher priority than notifying other health care providers.

Knowing laboratory values

Some NCLEX questions supply laboratory results without indicating normal levels. As a result, answering questions involving laboratory values requires you to have the normal range of the most common laboratory values memorized to make an informed decision (See *Normal laboratory values.*)

2 Strategies for success

In this chapter, you'll review:

✎ how to properly prepare for the NCLEX

✎ how to concentrate during difficult study times

✎ how to make more effective use of your time

✎ how creative studying strategies can enhance learning.

Study preparations

If you're like most people preparing to take the NCLEX®, you're probably feeling nervous, anxious, or concerned. Keep in mind that most test takers pass the first time around.

Passing the test won't happen by accident, though; you'll need to prepare carefully and efficiently. To help jump-start your preparations:

- determine your strengths and weaknesses
- create a study schedule
- set realistic goals
- find an effective study space
- think positively
- start studying sooner rather than later.

Strengths and weaknesses

Most students recognize that, even at the end of their nursing studies, they know more about some topics than others. Because the NCLEX covers a broad range of material, you should make some decisions about how intensively you'll review each topic.

Make a list
Base those decisions on a list. Divide a sheet of paper in half vertically. On one side, list topics you think you know well. On the other side, list topics you feel less secure about. Pay no attention if one side is longer than the other. When you're done studying, you'll feel strong in every area.

Where the list comes from
To make sure your list reflects a comprehensive view of all the areas you studied in school, look at the contents page in the front of this book. For each topic listed, place it in the "know well" column or "needs review"

column. Separating content areas this way shows immediately which topics need less study time and which need more time.

Scheduling study time

Study when you're most alert. Most people can identify a period of the day when they feel most alert. If you feel most alert and energized in the morning, for example, set aside sections of time in the morning for topics that need a lot of review. Then you can use the evening to study topics for which you just need some refreshing. The opposite is true as well; if you're more alert in the evening, study difficult topics at that time.

What you'll do, when
Set up a basic schedule for studying. Using a calendar or organizer, determine how much time remains before you'll take the NCLEX. (See *2 to 3 months before the NCLEX,* page 16.) Fill in the remaining days with specific times and topics to be studied. For example, you might schedule the respiratory system on a Tuesday morning and the GI system that afternoon. Remember to schedule difficult topics during your most alert times.

Keep in mind that you shouldn't fill each day with studying. Be realistic and set aside time for normal activities. Try to create ample study time before the NCLEX and then stick to the schedule. Allow some extra time in the schedule in case you get behind or come across a topic that requires extra review.

Set goals you can meet
Part of creating a schedule means setting goals you can accomplish. You no doubt studied a great deal in nursing school, and by now you have a sense of your own capabilities. Ask yourself, "How much can I cover in a day?" Set that amount of time aside and

To-do list

2 to 3 months before the NCLEX

With 2 to 3 months remaining before you plan to take the examination, take these steps:
• Establish a study schedule. Set aside ample time to study but also leave time for social activities, exercise, family or personal responsibilities, and other matters.
• Become knowledgeable about the NCLEX-RN, its content, the types of questions it asks, and the testing format.
• Begin studying your notes, texts, and other study materials.
• Answer some NCLEX practice questions to help you diagnose strengths and weaknesses as well as to become familiar with NCLEX-style questions.

then stay on task. You'll feel better about yourself — and your chances of passing the NCLEX — when you meet your goals regularly.

Study space

Find a space conducive to effective learning and then study there. Whatever you do, don't study with a television on in the room. Instead, find a quiet, inviting study space that:
• is located in a quiet, convenient place, away from normal traffic patterns
• contains a solid chair that encourages good posture (Avoid studying in bed; you'll be more likely to fall asleep and not accomplish your goals.)
• uses comfortable, soft lighting with which you can see clearly without eye strain
• has a temperature between 65° and 70° F
• contains flowers or green plants, familiar photos or paintings, and easy access to soft, instrumental background music.

Accentuate the positive
Consider taping positive messages around your study space. Make signs with words of encouragement, such as, "You can do it!" "Keep studying!" and "Remember the goal!" These upbeat messages can help keep you going when your attention begins to waver.

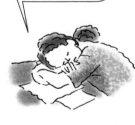

Approach your studying with enthusiasm, sincerity, and determination.

Maintaining concentration

When you're faced with reviewing the amount of information covered by the NCLEX, it's easy to become distracted and lose your concentration. When you lose concentration, you make less effective use of valuable study time. To stay focused, keep these tips in mind:
• Alternate the order of the subjects you study during the day to add variety to your study. Try alternating between topics you find most interesting and those you find least interesting.
• Approach your studying with enthusiasm, sincerity, and determination.
• Once you've decided to study, begin immediately. Don't let anything interfere with your thought processes once you've begun.
• Concentrate on accomplishing one task at a time, to the exclusion of everything else.
• Don't try to do two things at once, such as studying and watching television or conversing with friends.
• Work continuously without interruption for a while, but don't study for such a long period that the whole experience becomes grueling or boring.
• Allow time for periodic breaks to give yourself a change of pace. Use these breaks to ease your transition into studying a new topic.

• When studying in the evening, wind down from your studies slowly. Don't progress directly from studying to sleeping.

Taking care of yourself

Never neglect your physical and mental well-being in favor of longer study hours. Maintaining physical and mental health are critical for success in taking the NCLEX. (See *4 to 6 weeks before the NCLEX*.)

A few simple rules
You can increase your likelihood of passing the test by following these simple health rules:

• Get plenty of rest. You can't think deeply or concentrate for long periods when you're tired.

• Eat nutritious meals. Maintaining your energy level is impossible when you're under-nourished.

• Exercise regularly. Regular exercise, preferably 30 minutes daily, helps you work harder and think more clearly. As a result, you'll study more efficiently and increase the likelihood of success on the all-important NCLEX.

Memory powers, activate!
If you're having trouble concentrating but would rather push through than take a break, try making your studying more active by reading out loud. Active studying can renew your powers of concentration. By reading review material out loud to yourself, you're engaging your ears as well as your eyes — and making your studying a more active process. Hearing the material out loud also fosters memory and subsequent recall.

You can also rewrite in your own words a few of the more difficult concepts you're reviewing. Explaining these concepts in writing forces you to think through the material and can jump-start your memory.

Study schedule

When you were creating your schedule, you might have asked yourself, "How long should I study? One hour at a stretch? Two hours? Three?" To make the best use of your study time, you'll need to answer those questions.

Optimum study time

Consider studying in 20- to 30-minute intervals with a short break in-between. You remember the material you study at the beginning and end of a session best and tend to remember less material studied in the middle of the session. The total length of time in each study session depends on you and the amount of material you need to cover.

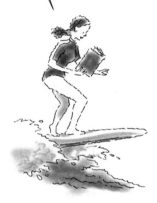

Kowabonga! Regular exercise helps you work harder and think more clearly.

To-do list

4 to 6 weeks before the NCLEX

With 4 to 6 weeks remaining before you plan to take the examination, take these steps:
• Focus on your areas of weakness. That way, you'll have time to review these areas again before the test date.
• Find a study partner or form a study group.
• Take a practice test to gauge your skill level early.
• Take time to eat, sleep, exercise, and socialize to avoid burnout.

> *To-do list*
>
> ## 1 week before the NCLEX
>
> With 1 week remaining before the NCLEX examination, take these steps:
> • Take a review test to measure your progress.
> • Record key ideas and principles on note cards or audiotapes.
> • Rest, eat well, and avoid thinking about the examination during nonstudy times.
> • Treat yourself to one special event. You've been working hard, and you deserve it!

To thine own self be true

So what's the answer? It doesn't matter as long as you determine what's best for you. At the beginning of your NCLEX study schedule, try study periods of varying lengths. Pay close attention to those that seem more successful.

Remember that you're a trained nurse who is competent at assessment. Think of yourself as a client, and assess your own progress. Then implement the strategy that works best for you.

Finding time to study

So does that mean that short sections of time are useless? Not at all. We all have spaces in our day that might otherwise be dead time. (See *1 week before the NCLEX.*) These are perfect times to review for the NCLEX but not to cover new material because, by the time you get deep into new material, your time will be over. Always keep some flash cards or a small notebook handy for situations when you have a few extra minutes.

You'll be amazed how many short sessions you can find in a day and how much reviewing you can do in 5 minutes. The following occasions offer short stretches of time you can use for studying:
• eating breakfast
• waiting for, or riding on, a train or bus

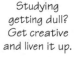

Studying getting dull? Get creative and liven it up.

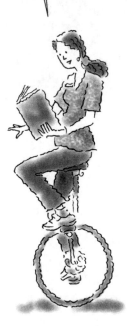

• waiting in line at the bank, post office, bookstore, or other places
• using exercise equipment, such as a treadmill.

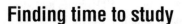

Creative studying

Even when you study in a perfect study space and concentrate better than ever, studying for the NCLEX can get a little, well, dull. Even people with terrific study habits occasionally feel bored or sluggish. That's why it's important to have some creative tricks in your study bag to liven up your studying during those down times.

Creative studying doesn't have to be hard work. It involves making efforts to alter your study habits a bit. Some techniques that might help include studying with a partner or group and creating flash cards or other audiovisual study tools.

Study partners

Studying with a partner or group of students (3 or 4 students at most) can be an excellent way to energize your studying. Working with a partner allows you to test each other on the material you've reviewed. Your partner can give you encouragement and motivation. Perhaps most important, working with a partner can provide a welcome break from solitary studying.

What to look for in a partner

Exercise some care when choosing a study partner or assembling a study group. A partner who doesn't fit your needs won't help you make the most of your study time. Look for a partner who:

• possesses similar goals to yours. For example, someone taking the NCLEX at approximately the same date who feels the same sense of urgency as you do might make an excellent partner.

• possesses about the same level of knowledge as you. Tutoring someone can sometimes help you learn, but partnering should be give-and-take so both partners can gain knowledge.

• can study without excess chatting or interruptions. Socializing is an important part of creative study but, remember, you still have to pass the NCLEX — so stay serious!

Audiovisual tools

Using flash cards and other audiovisual tools fosters retention and makes learning and reviewing fun.

Flash Gordon? No, it's Flash Card!

Flash cards can provide you with an excellent study tool. The process of writing material on a flash card will help you remember it. In addition, flash cards are small and easily portable, perfect for those 5-minute slivers of time that show up during the day.

Creating a flash card should be fun. Use magic markers, highlighters, and other colorful tools to make them visually stimulating. The more effort you put into creating your flash cards, the better you'll remember the material contained on the cards.

Other visual tools

Flowcharts, drawings, diagrams, and other image-oriented study aids can also help you learn material more effectively. Substituting images for text can be a great way to give your eyes a break and recharge your brain. Remember to use vivid colors to make your creations visually engaging.

Hear's the thing

If you learn more effectively when you hear information rather than see it, consider recording key ideas using a handheld tape recorder. Recording information helps promote memory because you say the information aloud when taping and then listen to it when playing it back. Like flash cards, tapes are portable and perfect for those short study periods during the day. (See *The day before the NCLEX*.)

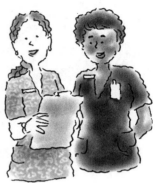

It wasn't easy finding a partner who has the same study habits I do.

To-do list

The day before the NCLEX

With 1 day before the NCLEX examination, take these steps:

• Drive to the test site, review traffic patterns, and find out where to park. If your route to the test site occurs during heavy traffic or if you're expecting bad weather, set aside extra time to ensure prompt arrival.

• Do something relaxing during the day.

• Avoid concentrating on the test.

• Eat well and avoid dwelling on the NCLEX during nonstudy periods.

• Call a supportive friend or relative for some last-minute words of encouragement.

• Get plenty of rest the night before and allow plenty of time in the morning.

To-do list

The day of the NCLEX

On the day of the NCLEX examination, take these steps:
• Get up early.
• Wear comfortable clothes, preferably with layers you can adjust to fit the room temperature.
• Leave your house early.
• Arrive at the test site early with required paperwork in hand.
• Avoid looking at your notes as you wait for your test computer.
• Listen carefully to the instructions given before entering the test room.

Good luck!

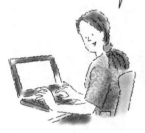

> Practice questions provide an excellent means of marking your progress.

Practice questions

Practice questions should be an important part of your NCLEX study strategy. Practice questions can improve your studying by helping you review material and familiarizing yourself with the exact style of questions you'll encounter on the NCLEX.

Practice at the beginning
Consider working through some practice questions as soon as you begin studying for the NCLEX. For example, you might try a few of the questions that appear at the end of each chapter in this book.

If you do well, you probably know the material contained in that chapter fairly well and can spend less time reviewing that particular topic. If you have trouble with the questions, spend extra study time on that topic.

I'm getting there
Practice questions can also provide an excellent means of marking your progress. Don't worry if you have trouble answering the first few practice questions you take; you'll need time to adjust to the way the questions are asked. Eventually you'll become accustomed to the question format and begin to focus more on the questions themselves.

If you make practice questions a regular part of your study regimen, you'll be able to notice areas in which you're improving. You can then adjust your study time accordingly.

Practice makes perfect
As you near the examination date, you should increase the number of NCLEX practice questions you answer at one sitting. This will enable you to approximate the experience of taking the actual NCLEX examination. Note that 75 questions is the minimum number of questions you'll be asked on the actual NCLEX examination. By gradually tackling larger practice tests, you'll increase your confidence, build test-taking endurance, and strengthen the concentration skills that enable you to succeed on the NCLEX. (See *The day of the NCLEX.*)

Part II   Review

Brush up on key concepts

Effective client care of all kinds requires consideration of both psychological and physiologic aspects of health. A client who seeks medical help for chest pain, for example, may also need to be assessed for anxiety or depression. As a nurse, you'll need a fundamental understanding of communication techniques as well as an understanding of psychiatric disorders.

At anytime, you can review the major points of the essentials of psychiatric nursing by consulting the *Cheat sheet* on pages 24 and 25.

The key to any relationship

Therapeutic communication is the foundation for developing a nurse-client relationship. It's the primary intervention in psychiatric nursing. Therapeutic communication requires awareness of both the client's verbal and nonverbal messages.

To uncover and investigate the client's inner thoughts, personal problems, and emotions, the nurse must establish trust and help the client feel safe and respected. A therapeutic relationship helps the client feel understood, become comfortable discussing problems, and find better ways to meet his emotional needs and develop satisfying relationships.

You got your ears on?

Listening intently to the client enables the nurse to hear and analyze everything the client is saying, alerting the nurse to the client's communication patterns.

Connect the dots

Succinct **rephrasing** of key client statements helps ensure the nurse's understanding and emphasizes important points in the client's message. For example, the nurse might say, "You're feeling angry and you say it's because of the way your friend treated you yesterday."

Keep the door open

Using **broad openings** and **general statements** to initiate conversations encourages the client to talk about any subject that comes to mind. These openings allow the client to focus the conversation and demonstrate the nurse's willingness to interact. An example of this technique is: "Tell me what's on your mind."

Polish the rough edges

Asking the client to **clarify** a confusing or vague message demonstrates the nurse's desire to understand what the client is saying. It can also elicit precise information crucial to the client's recovery. An example of clarifying is: "I'm not sure I understood what you said."

A sharper focus

In the technique called **focusing,** the nurse assists the client in redirecting attention toward something specific. It fosters the client's self-control and helps avoid vague generalizations, thereby enabling the client to accept responsibility for facing problems. "Let's go back to what we were just talking about," is one example of this technique.

It's golden

Refraining from comment can have several benefits. **Silence** gives the client time to talk, think, and gain insight into problems. It also permits the nurse to gather more information. The nurse must use this technique judiciously, however, to avoid giving the impression of disinterest or judgment.

Valuable assistance

When used correctly, the technique of **suggesting collaboration** gives the client the

Cheat sheet

Essentials of psychiatric nursing refresher

KEY CONCEPTS

Therapeutic communication

- Requires awareness of the client's verbal and nonverbal messages
- Involves establishing trust and helping the client feel safe and respected
- Listening intently—allows the nurse to analyze what the patient is saying and alerts the nurse to communication patterns
- Rephrasing—involves rephrasing what the client says to ensure the nurse's understanding
- Broad openings and general statements—give the client an opening to focus the conversation and demonstrate the nurse's willingness to talk
- Clarification—helps the nurse resolve confusing or vague messages and demonstrates to the client a willingness to understand
- Focusing—involves redirecting the client's attention to something specific
- Silence—gives the client time to talk, think, and gain insight into problems; gives the nurse a chance to gather more information

KEY ASSESSMENTS

Client history

- Client's chief complaint or concern
- History of the present illness
- Past psychiatric illness
- Personal or developmental history
- Family history
- Social history
- Cultural considerations

Physical examination

- General appearance
- Behavior
- Mood
- Thought processes and cognitive function
- Coping mechanisms
- Potential for self-destructive behavior

KEY PSYCHOLOGICAL TESTS

- Mini–Mental Status Examination—measures orientation, registration, recall, calculation, language, and motor skills

- Cognitive Capacity Screening Examination—measures orientation, memory, calculation, and language
- Global Deterioration Scale—assesses and stages primary degenerative dementia, based on orientation, memory, and neurologic function
- Functional Dementia Scale—measures orientation, affect, and the ability to perform activities of daily living
- Beck Depression Inventory—helps diagnose depression, determine its severity, and monitor the client's response during treatment
- Eating Attitudes Test—detects patterns that suggest an eating disorder
- Minnesota Multiphasic Personality Inventory—helps assess personality traits and ego function in adults and adolescents
- Michigan Alcoholism Screen Test—24-item timed test; score of 5 or better classifies the client as an alcoholic
- CAGE Questionnaire—four questions in which two or three positive responses indicate alcoholism
- Cocaine Addiction Severity Test and Cocaine Assessment Profile—evaluate for cocaine abuse

KEY TREATMENTS

- Individual therapy—uses three phrases to establish a structured relationship between the nurse and client in attempt to achieve change in the client
- Milieu therapy—uses the hospital environment to promote self-esteem and learning of new skills and behaviors so the client can live outside of the institutional setting
- Biological therapies—used for disturbances thought to be caused by chemical imbalances or by disease-causing organisms; includes psychoactive drugs and electroconvulsive therapy
- Cognitive behavioral therapy—employs strategies, such as role playing and thought substitution, to modify the beliefs and attitudes that influence a client's feelings and behaviors

It's okay to look at this Cheat sheet.

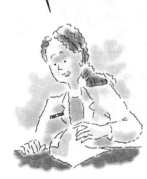

Essentials of psychiatric nursing refresher *(continued)*

KEY TREATMENTS *(CONTINUED)*

• Reality therapy—focuses on assisting the client to love and be loved and feel worthwhile and feel that others are worthwhile
• Family therapy—involves the entire family to improve family function
• Group therapy—includes an advanced practice nurse–therapist and six to eight clients and aims to increase self-awareness, change maladaptive behaviors, and improve interpersonal relationships

• Crisis intervention—short-term therapy to address an unbearable situation
• Hypnosis—induces deep relaxation by altering the client's state of consciousness; used for anxiety disorders, pain, repressed traumatic events, and addictive disorders

---

opportunity to explore the pros and cons of a suggested approach. It must be used carefully to avoid directing the client. An example of this technique is: "Perhaps we can meet with your parents to discuss the matter."

A two-way street

In the technique called **sharing impressions,** the nurse attempts to describe the client's feelings and then seeks corrective feedback from the client. This allows the client to clarify any misperceptions and gives the nurse a better understanding of the client's true feelings. For example, the nurse might say, "Tell me if my perception of what you're telling me agrees with yours."

Brush up on assessment

Because a nurse is commonly the health care provider who develops the closest long-term relationship with a client, the nurse is commonly most capable of assessing the emotional and mental health care needs of the client and identifying the appropriate interventions.

During the assessment stage, the nurse determines a client's psychological and physiologic status by assessing:
• client's history
• client's physical status (including mental status examination)
• laboratory and diagnostic tests.

Gathering data #1: Getting history

A complete **client history** provides information about:
• client's chief complaint or concern
• history of the present illness
• past psychiatric illness
• personal or developmental history
• family history
• social history
• cultural considerations that may affect the client's outcome.

Gathering data #2: Getting physical

The **physical examination** provides objective data that will help confirm or rule out assessments made during the health history interview.

In addition to the routine physical examination, the nurse should assess the client's:
• general appearance — helps indicate the client's emotional and mental status. The nurse should specifically note his dress and grooming.
• behavior — the nurse should note the client's demeanor and overall attitude as well as any extraordinary behavior.
• mood — ask the client to describe his current feelings in concrete terms and to suggest possible reasons for these feelings. Be sure to note inconsistencies between body language and mood.
• thought processes and cognitive function — the client's orientation to time, place, or person can indicate confusion or disorientation. The presence of delusions, hallucinations, obsessions, compulsions, fantasies, and day-dreams should be noted.

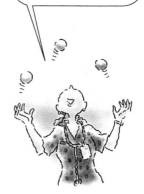

Consider all aspects of the client's functioning: biological, psychological, and social.

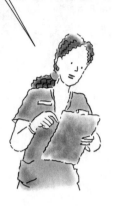

Every therapeutic relationship calls for sensitive and attentive communication.

• coping mechanisms — a client who is faced with a stressful situation may adopt excessive coping or defense mechanisms, which operate on an unconscious level to protect the ego. Examples include denial, regression, displacement, projection, reaction formation, and fantasy.

• potential for self-destructive behavior — a client who has lost touch with reality may cut or mutilate body parts to focus on physical pain, which may be less overwhelming than emotional distress.

Keep abreast of diagnostic tests

Diagnosing psychiatric disorders differs from diagnosing other medical disorders. (See *The authority*.) While many medical tests involve instrumentation and physical analyses, psychological testing focuses on questioning and observing the client.

Performing diagnostic tests on a client with a suspected psychiatric disorder may assist with accurate diagnosis, can reveal underlying physiologic disorders, establishes normal renal and hepatic function, and monitors for therapeutic medication levels.

Blood study #1

A **blood chemistry test** assesses a blood sample for potassium, sodium, calcium, phosphorus, glucose, bicarbonate, blood urea nitrogen, creatinine, protein, albumin, osmolality, amylase, lipase, alkaline phosphatase, ammonia, bilirubin, lactate dehydrogenase, aspartate aminotransferase, and alanine aminotransferase.

Nursing actions
• Explain the procedure to the client.
• Withhold food and fluids before the procedure, as directed.
• Check the venipuncture site for bleeding after the procedure.

Blood study #2

A **hematologic study** uses a blood sample to analyze red blood cells, white blood cells, prothrombin time, international normalized ratio, partial thromboplastin time, erythrocyte sedimentation rate, platelets, hemoglobin, and hematocrit.

Nursing actions
• Explain the procedure to the client.
• Note current drug therapy before the procedure.
• Check the venipuncture site for bleeding after the procedure.

Blood study #3

The **dexamethasone suppression test,** which involves administration of dexamethasone, is used to analyze a blood sample for serum cortisol.

Nursing actions
• Explain the procedure to the client.
• On the first day, give the client 1 mg of dextramethasone at 11 p.m.

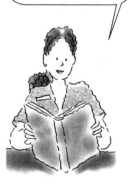

The DSM is updated regularly... make sure your information is up-to-date!

The authority

Published by the American Psychiatric Association, the *Diagnostic and Statistical Manual of Mental Disorders (DSM)* is a standard interdisciplinary psychiatric diagnostic system designed to be used by all members of the mental health care team. The manual includes a complete description of psychiatric disorders and other conditions and describes diagnostic criteria that must be met to support each diagnosis.

The current manual is the fourth edition, text revision, commonly known as *DSM-IV-TR.* The *DSM* is updated periodically, and new information regularly replaces old.

- On the next day, collect blood samples at 4 p.m. and 11 p.m.
- Monitor the venipuncture site; if hematoma develops, apply warm soaks.
- List any medications that might interfere with the test.

AIDS-related blood study #1

Enzyme-linked immunosorbent assay uses a blood sample to detect the human immunodeficiency virus (HIV)-1 antibody (acquired immunodeficiency syndrome [AIDS] can cause psychiatric complications).

Nursing actions
- Explain the procedure to the client.
- Verify that informed consent has been obtained and documented.
- Provide the client with appropriate pretest counseling.
- After the procedure, check the venipuncture site for bleeding.

AIDS-related blood study #2

A **Western blot test** uses a blood sample to detect the presence of specific viral proteins to confirm HIV infection.

Nursing actions
- Explain the procedure to the client.
- Verify that informed consent has been obtained and documented.
- After the procedure, check the venipuncture site for bleeding.

Drug detection

Toxicology screening uses a urine specimen to detect unknown drugs.

Nursing actions
- Explain the procedure to the client.
- Make sure that written, informed consent has been obtained.
- Witness the procurement of the urine specimen and process according to the facility's protocol.

Brain meter-reading

An **electroencephalogram** records the electrical activity of the brain. Using electrodes, this noninvasive test gives a graphic representation of brain activity.

Nursing actions
- Explain the procedure to the client.
- Determine the client's ability to lie still.
- Reassure the client that electrical shock won't occur.
- Warn the client that he will be subjected to stimuli, such as lights and sounds.
- Withhold medications and caffeine for 24 to 48 hours before the procedure, as directed.

Dye job

A **computed tomography (CT) scan,** used to identify brain abnormalities, produces a finely detailed image of the brain and its structures. It may be performed with or without the injection of contrast dye.

Nursing actions
- Explain the procedure to the client.
- Note the client's allergies to iodine, seafood, and radiopaque dyes.
- Allay the client's anxiety.
- Ensure that signed, informed consent has been obtained per facility policy.
- Inform the client about possible throat irritation and flushing of the face, if contrast dye is injected.

Mental picture

Magnetic resonance imaging uses electromagnetic energy to create a detailed visualization of the brain and its structures.

Nursing actions
- Explain the procedure to the client.
- Be aware that clients with pacemakers, surgical and orthopedic clips, or shrapnel shouldn't be scanned.
- Remove jewelry and metal objects from the client.
- Determine the client's ability to lie still.
- Check that informed consent or other pretesting forms are completed as required by facility policy.
- Administer sedation, as prescribed.

> Computed tomography is used to identify brain abnormalities because it produces a finely detailed image of the brain.

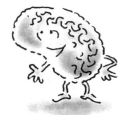

Brain metabolism test

Positron emission tomography involves injection of a radioisotope, allowing visualization of the brain's oxygen uptake, blood flow, and glucose metabolism.

Nursing actions

- Explain the procedure to the client.
- Determine the client's ability to lie still during the procedure.
- Withhold alcohol, tobacco, and caffeine for 24 hours before the procedure.
- Withhold medications, as directed, before the procedure.
- Check that informed consent or pre-testing forms are signed, as required by facility policy.
- Check the injection site for bleeding after the procedure.

Thyroid function test

A **thyroid uptake,** also called **radioactive iodine uptake** or **RAIU,** is used to measure the amount of radioactive iodine taken up by the thyroid gland in 24 hours. This measurement evaluates thyroid function.

Nursing actions

- Explain the procedure to the client.
- Instruct the client not to ingest iodine-rich foods for 24 hours before the test.
- Discontinue all thyroid and cough medications 7 to 10 days before the test.

Radiograph of the 'roid

A **thyroid scan** gives visual imaging of radioactivity distribution in the thyroid gland that helps assess size, shape, position, and anatomic function of the thyroid.

Nursing actions

- Explain the procedure to the client.
- If iodine-123 (^{123}I) or ^{131}I is to be used, tell the client to fast after midnight the night before the test. Fasting isn't required if an I.V. injection of ^{99m}Tc pertechnetate is used.
- Withhold any medications that may interfere with the procedure.
- Instruct the client to stop consuming iodized salt, iodinated salt substitutes, and seafood one week before the procedure.

- Imaging follow soral administration (^{123}I or ^{131}I) by 24 hours and I.V. injection (^{99m}Tc pertechnetate) by 20 to 30 minutes.
- Remove dentures, jewelry, and other materials that may interfere with imaging.
- After the procedure, tell the client he may resume medications that were suspended for testing.

Keep abreast of psychological tests

Psychological tests evaluate the client's mood, personality, and mental status. Here's a review of the most common psychological tests.

Pop quiz

The **Mini–Mental Status Examination** measures orientation, registration, recall, calculation, language, and motor skills.

Cognitive capacity

The **Cognitive Capacity Screening Examination** measures orientation, memory, calculation, and language.

General knowledge

The **Cognitive Assessment Scale** measures orientation, general knowledge, mental ability, and psychomotor function.

Measuring what's lost

The **Global Deterioration Scale** assesses and stages primary degenerative dementia, based on orientation, memory, and neurologic function.

Getting by

The **Functional Dementia Scale** measures orientation, affect, and the ability to perform activities of daily living.

Measuring depression

The **Beck Depression Inventory** helps diagnose depression, determine its severity, and monitor the client's response during treatment.

What's on the menu?

The **Eating Attitudes Test** detects patterns that suggest an eating disorder.

Who are you?

The **Minnesota Multiphasic Personality Inventory** helps assess personality traits and ego function in adolescents and adults. Test results include information on coping strategies, defenses, strengths, gender identification, and self-esteem. The test pattern may strongly suggest a diagnostic category, point to a suicide risk, or indicate the potential for violence.

Alcoholism test #1

The **Michigan Alcoholism Screening Test** is a 24-item timed test in which a score of 5 or better classifies the client as an alcoholic.

Alcoholism test #2

The **CAGE Questionnaire** is a four-question tool in which two or three positive responses indicate alcoholism.

Cocaine addiction tests

The **Cocaine Addiction Severity Test** and **Cocaine Assessment Profile** are used when cocaine use is suspected.

Polish up on client care

Various treatment options coexist in psychiatric and mental health care. Nurses may use one specific treatment approach or a combination of approaches to guide client care.

One on one

Individual therapy is the establishment of a structured relationship between nurse and client in an attempt to achieve change in the client. The nurse works with the client to develop an approach to resolve conflict, decrease emotional pain, and develop appropriate ways of meeting the client's needs. This relationship with the client consists of three overlapping phases:
- the orientation phase, in which the nurse builds a connection with the client by establishing rapport and a sense of trust (goals are formulated in this phase)
- the working phase, in which the client becomes increasingly involved in self-exploration (the nurse assists the client as he tries to develop self-understanding and encourages him to take risks in terms of changing dysfunctional behavior)
- the termination phase, in which the client and nurse determine that closure of the relationship is appropriate (both parties agree that the problem that initiated the relationship has been alleviated or has become manageable).

Milling around

During **milieu therapy,** the nurse uses all aspects of the hospital environment in a therapeutic manner. Clients are exposed to rules, expectations, peer pressure, and social interactions. Nurses encourage communication and decision making and provide opportunities for enhancing self-esteem and learning new skills and behaviors. The goal of therapy is to enable the client to live outside the institutional setting.

Treating disease and imbalance

Biological therapies are called for when emotional and behavioral disturbances are thought to be caused by chemical imbalances or by disease-causing organisms.

Some examples of biological therapies are:
- psychoactive drugs
- electroconvulsive therapy
- nonconvulsive electrical stimulation.

Changing ideas

Cognitive behavioral therapy employs strategies to modify the beliefs and attitudes that influence a client's feelings and behaviors.

Some basic cognitive interventions include:
- teaching thought substitution
- identifying problem-solving strategies
- finding ways to modify negative self-talk
- role playing
- modeling coping strategies.

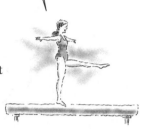

It's a balancing act! While identifying the disordered thought of a schizophrenic client, also assess for physiologic complications.

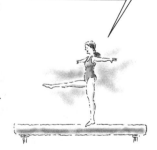

Alternatively, you may need to assess a client with a respiratory condition for depression or suicidal thoughts.

The real world

Reality therapy focuses on assisting the client meet two basic emotional needs:
- loving and being loved
- feeling worthwhile and feeling that others are worthwhile.

The nurse emphasizes personal responsibility for behavior, controlling one's own life, and fulfilling basic needs.

All in the family

During **family therapy,** the entire family is considered the treatment unit. The primary goal of therapy is to improve the functioning of the family. The types of clients that can benefit most from family therapy are those involved in marital issues, intergenerational conflicts, sibling concerns, and family crises, such as death and divorce.

The gang's all here

Group therapy includes an advanced practice nurse–therapist and six to eight people who meet regularly for the purpose of increasing self-awareness, improving interpersonal relationships, and changing maladaptive behavioral problems. Like individual therapy, group therapy goes through the orientation phase, working phase, and termination phase.

Urgent care

Crisis intervention is a systemic approach to short-term therapy in which the nurse works with a client, family, or group that's experiencing a potentially dangerous situation. The nurse initiates actions to decrease the client's sense of personal danger and facilitate the client's ability to control the situation.

Trance time

Hypnosis is used to induce deep relaxation by altering the client's state of consciousness. The result of hypnotic induction is a trancelike state during which clients use memories, mental associations, and concentration to discover experiences that are connected to their current distress. Hypnosis is effective for dealing with anxiety disorders, some types of pain, repressed traumatic events, and addictive disorders.

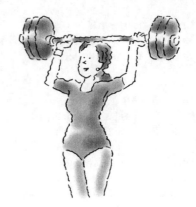

Pump up on practice questions

1. A client tells the nurse that he never disagrees with anyone and that he has loved everyone he's ever known. What would be the nurse's best response to this client?
  1. "How do you manage to do that?"
  2. "That's hard to believe. Most people couldn't do that."
  3. "What do you do with your feelings of dissatisfaction or anger?"
  4. "How did you come to adopt such a way of life?"

Answer: 4. Inquiring about the client's way of life allows for further exploration of the message he's trying to convey. Asking him how he's managed to do that has too narrow a focus and doesn't permit maximal exploration of the client's experience. Expressing disbelief is incorrect because the client could misinterpret it as a challenge and become even more defensive. Asking about feelings of dissatisfaction or anger is incorrect because the nurse shouldn't identify the client's feelings for him.

➡ **NCLEX keys**
Client needs category: Psychosocial integrity
Client needs subcategory: None
Cognitive level: Application

2. A nurse is working with a client who has just stimulated her anger by using a condescending tone of voice. Which response by the nurse is most therapeutic?
1. "I feel angry when I hear that tone of voice."
2. "You make me so angry when you talk to me that way."
3. "Are you trying to make me angry?"
4. "Why do you use that condescending tone of voice with me?"

Answer: 1. This response allows the nurse to provide feedback without making the client responsible for the nurse's reaction. Stating that the client makes you angry is accusatory and blocks communication. "Are you trying to make me angry" is a challenging remark that can lead to power struggles, lowers the client's self-esteem, and blocks opportunities for open communication. Avoid "why" questions such as "Why do you use that condescending tone of voice with me" because these questions put the client on the defensive.

➡ **NCLEX keys**
Client needs category: Psychosocial integrity
Client needs subcategory: None
Cognitive level: Application

3. A client on the unit tells the nurse that his wife's nagging really gets on his nerves. He asks the nurse if she'll talk with his wife about her nagging during their family session tomorrow afternoon. Which response is the most therapeutic?
1. "Tell me more specifically about her complaints."
2. "Can you think why she might nag you so much?"
3. "I'll help you think about how to bring this up yourself tomorrow."
4. "Why do you want me to initiate this discussion in tomorrow's session rather than you?"

Answer: 3. The client needs to learn how to communicate directly with his wife about her behavior. The nurse's assistance will enable him to practice a new skill and will communicate the nurse's confidence in his ability to confront this situation directly. Asking about the wife's specific complaints or reasons for nagging inappropriately directs attention

away from the client and toward his wife, who isn't present. Asking why you should initiate the discussion implies that there might be a legitimate reason for the nurse to assume responsibility for something that rightfully belongs to the client. Instead of focusing on his problems, he will waste time convincing the nurse why she should do his work.

➡ **NCLEX keys**
Client needs category: Psychosocial integrity
Client needs subcategory: None
Cognitive level: Application

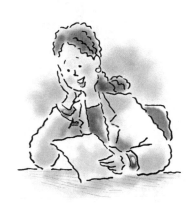

4. A nurse is caring for a client diagnosed with conversion disorder who has developed paralysis of her legs. Diagnostic tests fail to uncover a physiologic cause. During the working phase of the nurse-client relationship, the client says to her nurse, "You think I could walk if I wanted to, don't you?" Which response by the nurse would be best?
1. "Yes, if you really wanted to, you could."
2. "Tell me why you're concerned about what I think."
3. "Do you think you could walk if you wanted to?"
4. "I think you are unable to walk now, whatever the cause."

Answer: 4. This response answers the question honestly and nonjudgmentally and helps to preserve the client's self-esteem. Telling the client that she could walk if she really wanted to is an open and candid response but diminishes the client's self-esteem. Asking the client why she's concerned about what you think doesn't answer the client's question and isn't helpful. Asking her if she thought she could walk if she really wanted to would increase the client's anxiety because her inability to walk is directly related to an unconscious psychological conflict that hasn't yet been resolved.

➡ NCLEX keys
Client needs category: Psychosocial integrity
Client needs subcategory: None
Cognitive level: Application

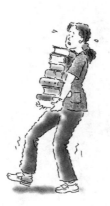

5.   A 42-year-old homemaker arrives at the emergency department with uncontrollable crying and anxiety. Her husband of 17 years has recently asked her for a divorce. The client is sitting in a chair, rocking back and forth. Which is the best response for the nurse to make?

1. "You must stop crying so that we can discuss your feelings about the divorce."
2. "Once you find a job, you'll feel much better and more secure."
3. "I can see how upset you are. Let's sit in the office so that we can talk about how you're feeling."
4. "Once you have a lawyer looking out for your interests, you will feel better."

Answer: 3. This response validates the client's distress and provides an opportunity for her to talk about her feelings. Because clients in crises have difficulty making decisions, the nurse must be directive as well as supportive. Telling the client to stop crying doesn't provide the client with adequate support. Telling her that she will feel better after she has a job or a lawyer doesn't acknowledge the client's distress. Moreover, clients in crises can't think beyond the immediate moment, so discussing long-range plans isn't helpful.

➡ NCLEX keys
Client needs category: Psychosocial integrity
Client needs subcategory: None
Cognitive level: Application

6.   A widower is hospitalized after complaining of difficulty sleeping, extreme apprehension, shortness of breath, and a sense of impending doom. Which response by the nurse would be best?

1. "You have nothing to worry about. You're in a safe place. Try to relax."
2. "Has anything happened recently or in the past that may have triggered these feelings?"
3. "We have given you a medication that will help to decrease these feelings of anxiety."
4. "Take some deep breaths and try to calm down."

Answer: 2. This question provides support, reassurance, and an opportunity to gain insight into the cause of the client's anxiety. Brushing off the client's anxiety by telling him he has nothing to worry about dismisses the client's feelings and offers false reassurance. Simply adminisering medication or instructing him to calm down doesn't allow the client to discuss his feelings, which he must do to understand and resolve the cause of his anxiety.

➡ NCLEX keys
Client needs category: Psychosocial integrity
Client needs subcategory: None
Cognitive level: Application

7. A client is admitted to an inpatient psychiatric hospital after having been picked up by the local police while walking around the neighborhood at night without shoes in the snow. He appears confused and disoriented. Which action should take priority?

1. Assess and stabilize the client's medical needs.
2. Assess and stabilize the client's psychological needs.
3. Attempt to locate the nearest family members to get an accurate history.
4. Arrange a transfer to the nearest medical facility.

Answer: 1. The possibility of frostbite must be evaluated before the other interventions. Attending to the client's psychological needs, locating family members, or arranging for transfer doesn't address the client's immediate medical needs.

➡ *NCLEX keys*
Client needs category: Physiological integrity
Client needs subcategory: Reduction of risk potential
Cognitive level: Analysis

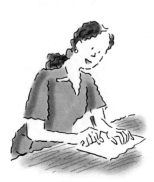

8. What occurs during the working phase of the nurse-client relationship?

1. The nurse assesses the client's needs and develops a care plan.
2. The nurse and client evaluate and modify the goals of the relationship.
3. The nurse and client discuss their feelings about terminating the relationship.
4. The nurse and client explore each other's expectations of the relationship.

Answer: 2. The therapeutic nurse-client relationship consists of three overlapping phases, the orientation, the working, and the termination. During the working phase, the nurse and the client together evaluate and refine goals established during the orientation phase. In addition, major therapeutic work takes place, and insight is integrated into a plan of action. The orientation phase involves assessing the client, formulating a contract, exploring feelings, and establishing expectations about the relationship. During the termination phase, the nurse prepares the client for separation and explores feelings about the end of the relationship.

➡ *NCLEX keys*
Client needs category: Psychosocial integrity
Client needs subcategory: None
Cognitive level: Knowledge

9. When preparing to conduct group therapy, an advanced practice nurse keeps in mind that the optimal number of clients in a group should be:

1. 3 to 5.
2. 6 to 8.
3. 10 to 12.
4. unlimited.

Answer: 2. Clinicians generally consider 6 to 8 people to be the ideal number of clients for a therapeutic group. The size allows opportunities for maximum therapeutic exchange and participation. In groups of 5 or fewer, participation commonly is inhibited by self-consciousness and insecurity. In groups larger than 8, participation and exchange among certain members may be lost.

➡ *NCLEX keys*
Client needs category: Psychosocial integrity
Client needs subcategory: None
Cognitive level: Application

10. A therapeutic nurse-client relationship begins with the nurse's:
1. sincere desire to help others.
2. acceptance of others.
3. self-awareness and understanding.
4. sound knowledge of psychiatric nursing.

Answer: 3. Although all of the options are desirable, knowledge of self is the basis for building a strong, therapeutic nurse-client relationship. Being aware of and understanding personal feelings and behavior is a prerequisite for understanding and helping clients.

➡ *NCLEX keys*
Client needs category: Safe and effective care environment
Client needs subcategory: Management of care
Cognitive level: Knowledge

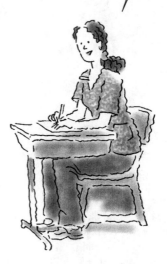

4 Somatoform & sleep disorders

Brush up on key concepts

The client with a sleep disorder commonly suffers from excessive daytime sleepiness and impaired ability to perform daily tasks safely or properly. The client with a somatoform disorder commonly suffers physical symptoms related to an inability to handle stress. These physical symptoms have no physiologic cause but are overwhelming to the client.

At any time, you can review the major points of each disorder by consulting the *Cheat sheet* on pages 36 and 37.

Somatoform disorders

The *Diagnostic and Statistical Manual of Mental Disorders,* Fourth edition, *Text Revision (DSM-IV-TR)* categorizes somatic symptoms of psychiatric origins as somatoform disorders.

The client with a somatoform disorder complains of physical symptoms and typically travels from physician to physician in search of sympathetic and enthusiastic treatment. Physical examinations and laboratory tests, however, fail to uncover an organic basis for the client's symptoms. Because the client doesn't produce the symptoms intentionally or feel a sense of control over them, he's usually unable to accept that his illness has a psychological cause.

From mind to body
Psychosomatic is a term used to describe conditions in which a psychological state contributes to the development of a physical illness.

An expression of emotional stress
Somatization is the manifestation of physical symptoms that result from psychological distress. Anyone who feels the pain of a sore throat or the ache of flu has a somatic symptom, but it isn't considered somatization unless the physical symptoms are an expression of emotional stress.

All bottled up
Internalization refers to the condition in which a client's anxiety, stress, and frustration are expressed through physical symptoms rather than confronted directly.

Sleep disorders

The client with a primary sleep disorder is unable to initiate or maintain sleep. Primary sleep disorders may be categorized as dyssomnias or parasomnias.

Too much or not enough
Dyssomnias involve excessive sleep or difficulty initiating and maintaining sleep. Examples of dyssomnias include primary insomnia, circadian rhythm sleep disorder, obstructive sleep apnea syndrome, primary hypersomnia, and narcolepsy.

Strange things in the night
Parasomnias are physiologic or behavioral reactions *during* sleep. Examples of parasomnias include nightmare disorder, sleep terror disorder, and sleepwalking disorder.

You're getting sleepy...
Sleep can be broken down into two major phases, **rapid-eye-movement** (REM) sleep and **non–rapid-eye-movement** (NREM) sleep, which alternate throughout the sleep period.

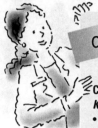

Somatoform & sleep disorders refresher

CONVERSION DISORDER
Key signs and symptoms
• La belle indifference (a lack of concern about the symptoms or limitation on functioning)

Key test results
• The absence of expected diagnostic findings can confirm the disorder.

Key treatments
• Individual therapy
• Hypnosis
• Stress management

Key interventions
• Establish a supportive relationship that communicates acceptance of the client but keeps the focus away from symptoms.
• Review all laboratory and diagnostic study results.

HYPOCHONDRIASIS
Key signs and symptoms
• Abnormal focus on bodily functions and sensations
• Anger, frustration, depression
• Frequent visits to physicians and specialists despite assurance from health care providers that the client is healthy
• Intensified physical symptoms around sympathetic people
• Rejection of the idea that the symptoms are stress related
• Use of symptoms to avoid difficult situations

Key treatments
• Individual therapy
• Cognitive behaviorial therapy
• Tricyclic antidepressants: amitriptyline (Elavil), imipramine (Tofranil), doxepin (Sinequan)
• Selective serotonin reuptake inhibitors: citalopram (Celexa), fluoxetine (Prozac), paroxetine (Paxil), sertraline (Zoloft)

Key interventions
• Assess the client's level of knowledge about how emotional issues can impact physiologic functioning.

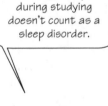

> Falling asleep during studying doesn't count as a sleep disorder.

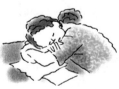

• Encourage emotional expression.
• Respond to the client's symptoms in a matter-of-fact way.

PAIN DISORDER
Key signs and symptoms
• Acute and chronic pain not associated with a psychological cause
• Frequent visits to multiple physicians to seek pain relief

Key test results
• Test results don't support client complaints.

Key treatments
• Individual therapy
• Biofeedback
• Cognitive behavioral threapy
• Tricyclic antidepressants: amitriptyline (Elavil), imipramine (Tofranil), doxepin (Sinequan)

Key interventions
• Acknowledge the client's pain.
• Encourage the client to recognize situations that precipitate pain.

DYSSOMNIAS
Key signs and symptoms
Primary insomnia
• History of light or easily disturbed sleep or difficulty falling asleep
• Insomnia
Circadian rhythm sleep disorder
• Cardiovascular and GI distubances, such as palpitations, peptic ulcer disease, and gastritis
• Fatigue
Breathing-related sleep disorder
• Abnormal breathing events during sleep including apnea, abnormally slow or shallow respirations, and hypoventilation (abnormal blood oxygen and carbon dioxide levels)
• Fatigue
• Snoring while sleeping
Primary hypersomnia
• Confusion upon awakening
• Difficulty awakening
• Poor memory

Somatoform & sleep disorders refresher *(continued)*

DYSSOMNIAS *(CONTINUED)*
Narcolepsy
- Cataplexy (bilateral loss of muscle tone triggered by strong emotion)
- Generalized daytime sleepiness
- Hypnagogic hallucination (intense dreamlike images)
- Irresistible attacks of refreshing sleep

Key test results
- Polysomnography is diagnostic for individual sleep disorder.

Key treatments
Primary insomnia or circadian rhythm sleep disorder
- Hypnotics: zolpidem (Ambien), eszopiclone (Lunesta)
- Benzodiazepines: lorazepam (Ativan), alprazolam (Xanax)
Primary hypersomnia or narcolepsy
- Stimulants: caffeine, methylphenidate (Ritalin), dextroamphetamine (Dexedrine); modafinil (Provigil)

Key interventions
Primary insomnia and circadian rhythm disturbance
- Encourage the client to discuss concerns that may be preventing sleep.
- Schedule regular sleep and awakening times.
Breathing-related sleep disorder
- Administer continuous positive nasal airway pressure.
Primary hypersomnia and narcolepsy
- Administer medication as prescribed.

- Develop strategies to manage symptoms and integrate them into their daily routine, such as taking naps during lunchtime or work breaks.

PARASOMNIAS
Key signs and symptoms
Nightmare disorder
- Dream recall
- Mild autonomic arousal upon awakening (sweating, tachycardia, tachypnea)
Sleep terror disorder
- Autonomic signs of intense anxiety (tachycardia, tachypnea, flushing, sweating, increased muscle tone, dilated pupils)
- Screaming or crying
Sleepwalking disorder
- Amnesia of the episode or limited recall
- Sitting up, talking, walking, or engaging in inappropriate behavior during episode

Key test results
- Polysomnography is diagnostic for individual sleep disorder.

Key treatments
- Relaxation techniques
- Individual counseling

Key interventions
- Lock windows and doors if sleepwalking occurs.
- Provide emotional support.

NREM sleep consists of four stages:

Stage 1 NREM sleep is a transition from wakefulness to sleep characterized by low-voltage mixed-frequency EEG and slow eye movement and occupies about 5% of time spent asleep in healthy adults.

Stage 2 NREM sleep, which is characterized by specific EEG waveforms (sleep spindles and K complexes), occupies about 50% of time spent asleep.

Stages 3 and 4 NREM sleep (also known collectively as *slow-wave sleep* or *delta sleep*) are the deepest levels of sleep and occupy about 10% to 20% of sleep time declining to 0% in the elderly.

REM sleep, during which the majority of typical storylike dreams occur, occupies about 20% to 25% of total sleep.

Light intensity can affect sleep patterns causing changes in cortisol, melatonin, and core body temperature.

Patterns after dark
Stages of sleep have a characteristic temporal organization. NREM stages 3 and 4 tend to occur in the first one-third to one-half of the night. REM sleep occurs in cycles throughout the night, alternating with NREM sleep about every 80 to 100 minutes. REM sleep periods increase in duration during the last half of the night, toward the morning.

Sparks in the night
Polysomnography is the monitoring of multiple electrophysiologic parameters during sleep and generally includes measurement of EEG activity, electro-oculographic activity (electrographic tracings made by movement

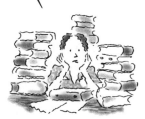

I'm sick of studying! Does that qualify as a somatoform disorder?

of the eye), and electromyographic activity (electrographic tracings made by skeletal muscles at rest).

Additional polysomnographic measures may include oral or nasal airflow, respiratory effort, chest and abdominal wall movement, oxyhemoglobin saturation, or exhaled carbon dioxide concentration. These measures are used to monitor respiration during sleep and to detect the presence and severity of sleep apnea. Measurement of peripheral electromyographic activity may be used to detect abnormal movements during sleep such as those that occur with restless leg syndrome.

You can do it during the daytime, too!

Most polysomnographic studies are performed during the client's usual sleeping hours — that is in a sleep laboratory overnight. However daytime polysomnographic studies are also used to quantify daytime sleepiness.

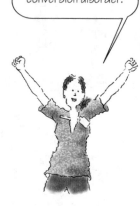

Absence means presence. The absence of expected diagnostic findings can confirm conversion disorder.

Polish up on client care

Major somatoform disorders include conversion disorder, hypochondriasis, and pain disorder. Sleep disorders include dyssomnias (primary insomnia, circadian rhythm sleep disorder, breathing-related sleep disorder, primary hypersomnia, and narcolepsy) and parasomnias (nightmare disorder, sleep terror disorder, and sleepwalking disorder).

Conversion disorder

The client with conversion disorder exhibits symptoms that suggest a physical disorder, but evaluation and observation can't determine a physiologic cause. The onset of symptoms is preceded by psychological trauma or conflict, and the physical symptoms are a manifestation of the conflict. Resolution of the symptoms usually occurs spontaneously.

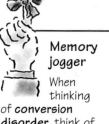

Memory jogger

When thinking of **conversion disorder,** think of the term **convert,** which means "to change from one form or function to another." Clients with conversion disorder convert stress into physical ailments.

CONTRIBUTING FACTORS
• Psychological conflict
• Overwhelming stress
• History of trauma

ASSESSMENT FINDINGS
• Aphonia (inability to produce sound)
• Laryngitis
• Blindness
• Deafness
• Dysphagia
• Impaired balance and impaired coordination
• La belle indifference (a lack of concern about the symptoms or limitation on functioning)
• Loss of touch sensation
• Lump in the throat
• Paralysis
• Seizures or pseudoseizures
• Urinary retention

DIAGNOSTIC TEST RESULTS
• Test results are inconsistent with physical findings.
• The absence of expected diagnostic findings can confirm the disorder.

NURSING DIAGNOSES
• Ineffective coping
• Anxiety
• Chronic low self-esteem

TREATMENT
• Individual therapy
• Hypnosis
• Relaxation training
• Stress management

Drug therapy
• Benzodiazepines: lorazepam (Ativan), alprazolam (Xanax), clonazepam (Klonopin)

INTERVENTIONS AND RATIONALES
• Ensure and maintain a safe environment *to protect the client.*
• Establish a supportive relationship that communicates acceptance of the client but keeps the focus away from symptoms *to help the client learn to recognize and express anxiety.*

- Review all laboratory and diagnostic study results *to ascertain whether any physical problems are present.*
- Encourage the client to identify any emotional conflicts occurring before the onset of physical symptoms *to make the relationship between the conflict and the symptoms clearer.*
- Promote social interaction *to decrease the client's level of self-involvement.*
- Identify constructive coping mechanisms *to encourage the client to use practical coping skills and relinquish the role of being sick.*
- Teach relaxation techniques and effective coping mechanisms and help the client identify areas of stress *to help decrease symptoms.*

Teaching topics
- Explanation of the disorder and treatment plan
- Medication use and possible adverse effects
- Setting limits on the client's sick role behavior while continuing to provide support (for family members)
- Stress-reduction methods

Hypochondriasis

In hypochondriasis, the client is preoccupied by fear of a serious illness, despite medical assurance of good health. The client with hypochondriasis interprets all physical sensations as indications of illness, impairing his ability to function normally.

CONTRIBUTING FACTORS
- Death of a loved one
- Family member with a serious illness
- Previous serious illness
- Marital problems
- Career changes
- History of anxiety and depression

ASSESSMENT FINDINGS
- Abnormal focus on bodily functions and sensations
- Anger, frustration, depression
- Frequent visits to physicians and specialists despite assurance from health care providers that the client is healthy

- Intensified physical symptoms around sympathetic people
- Rejection of the idea that the symptoms are stress related
- Use of symptoms to avoid difficult situations
- Vague physical symptoms

DIAGNOSTIC TEST RESULTS
- Test results are inconsistent with the client's complaints and physical findings.

NURSING DIAGNOSES
- Deficient knowledge (treatment plan)
- Ineffective coping
- Ineffective health maintenance
- Anxiety
- Disturbed sensory perception

TREATMENT
- Individual therapy
- Cognitive behavioral therapy

Drug therapy
- Benzodiazepines: lorazepam (Ativan), alprazolam (Xanax)
- Tricyclic antidepressants: amitriptyline (Elavil), imipramine (Tofranil), doxepin (Sinequan)
- Selective serotonin reuptake inhibitors (SSRIs): paroxetine (Paxil), citalopram (Celexa), fluoxetine (Prozac), sertraline (Zoloft)
- Serotonin–norepinephrine reuptake inhibitor (SNRI): venlafaxine (Effexor)

INTERVENTIONS AND RATIONALES
- Assess the client's level of knowledge about how emotional issues can impact physiologic functioning *to promote understanding of the condition.*
- Encourage emotional expression *to discourage emotional repression, which can have physical consequences.*
- Respond to the client's symptoms in a matter-of-fact way *to reduce secondary gain the client achieves from talking about symptoms.*

Teaching topics
- Explanation of the disorder and treatment plan
- Medication use and possible adverse effects

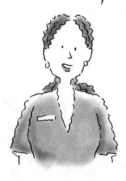

Acknowledging the client's pain helps to discourage him from striving to convince you the pain is real.

- Relaxation and assertiveness techniques
- Initiating conversations that focus on topics other than physical maladies

Pain disorder

In pain disorder, the client experiences pain in which psychological factors play a significant role in the onset, severity, exacerbation, or maintenance of the pain. The pain isn't intentionally produced or feigned by the client. The pain becomes a major focus of life, and the client is often unable to function socially or at work. The client may have a physical ailment but shouldn't be experiencing such intense pain.

CONTRIBUTING FACTORS
- Traumatic, stressful, or humiliating experience

ASSESSMENT FINDINGS
- Acute and chronic pain not associated with a physiologic cause
- Anger, frustration, depression, anxiety
- Drug-seeking behavior in an attempt to relieve pain
- Frequent visits to multiple physicians to seek pain relief
- Insomnia

DIAGNOSTIC TEST RESULTS
- Test results don't support client complaints.
- With psychotherapy, the client may recall a traumatic event.

NURSING DIAGNOSES
- Acute or chronic pain
- Ineffective coping
- Anxiety

TREATMENT
- Individual therapy
- Biofeedback
- Cognitive behavioral therapy

Drug therapy
- Anxiolytics (benzodiazepines): lorazepam (Ativan), alprazolam (Xanax)

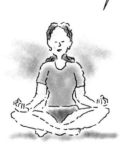

Nursing care in pain disorder may focus on pain management techniques, such as relaxation and meditation.

- Tricyclic antidepressants: amitriptyline (Elavil), imipramine (Tofranil), doxepin (Sinequan)
- SSRIs: paroxetine (Paxil), citalopram (Celexa), fluoxetine (Prozac)
- SNRI: venlafaxine (Effexor)

INTERVENTIONS AND RATIONALES
- Ensure a safe, accepting environment for the client *to promote therapeutic communication.*
- Acknowledge the client's pain *to discourage the client from striving to convince you that pain is real and to reinforce a therapeutic relationship.*
- Encourage the client to recognize situations that precipitate pain *to foster an understanding of the disorder.*

Teaching topics
- Explanation of the disorder and treatment plan
- Medication use and possible adverse effects
- Promoting social interaction
- Establishing constructive coping mechanisms
- Problem-solving techniques
- Nonpharmacologic pain management, such as guided imagery, massage, therapeutic touch, relaxation, heat, and cold

Dyssomnias

Dyssomnias are primary disorders of initiating or maintaining sleep or excessive sleepiness. These disorders are characterized by a disturbance in the amount, quality, or timing of sleep.

Primary insomnia is characterized by a subjective complaint of difficulty initiating or maintaining sleep that lasts for at least 1 month. Alternatively, the client may report that sleep isn't refreshing. A key symptom of primary insomnia is the client's intense focus and anxiety about not getting sleep, resulting in signficant distress or impairment. Commonly, the client reports being a "light sleeper."

In **circadian rhythm sleep disorder,** there's a mismatch between the internal sleep-wake circadian rhythm and timing and the duration of sleep. The client may report insomnia at particular times during the day and excessive sleepiness at other times. Causes can be intrinsic such as delays in the sleep phases or extrinsic as in jet lag or shift work.

Another class of sleep disorder identified by the *DSM-IV-TR* is **breathing-related sleep disorder.** Specific disorders in this class include central sleep apnea syndrome, central alveolar hypoventilation syndrome, and obstructive sleep apnea syndrome. Obstructive sleep apnea syndrome is the most commonly diagnosed breathing-related sleep disorder.

In breathing-related sleep disorder, a disturbance in breathing leads to a disruption in sleep that leads to excessive sleepiness or insomnia. Excessive sleepiness is the most common complaint of clients. Naps usually aren't refreshing and may be accompanied by a dull headache. These clients typically minimize the problem by bragging that they can sleep anywhere and at any time.

In **narcolepsy,** the client develops an overwhelming urge to sleep at any time of the day regardless of the amount of previous sleep. The client may fall asleep two to six times a day during inappropriate times, such as while driving the car or attending class. The client's sleepiness typically decreases after a sleep attack, only to return several hours later. The sleep attacks must occur daily over a period of 3 months to confirm the diagnosis.

In **primary hypersomnia,** the client experiences excessive sleepiness lasting at least 1 month. The client may take daytime naps or sleep extended periods at night. People with primary hypersomnia typically sleep 8 to 12 hours per night. They fall asleep easily and sleep through the night but often have trouble awakening in the morning. Some mornings they awake confused and combative. These clients have great difficulty with morning obligations.

CONTRIBUTING FACTORS
Primary insomnia
- Illness (especially pheochromocytoma or hyperthyroidism)
- Many illegal drugs
- Age older than 65

- Stress
- Life changes
- Use of certain legal drugs (see *Drugs that affect sleep*, page 42)

Circadian rhythm sleep disorder
- Delayed sleep phase
- Jet lag
- Shift work

Breathing-related sleep disorder
- Instability in the respiratory control center, which causes apnea
- Obstruction or collapse of airway, which causes apnea
- Slow or shallow breathing, which causes arterial oxygen desaturation
- Obesity; short, fat neck
- Elongated uvula

Primary hypersomnia
- Autonomic nervous system dysfunction
- Genetic predisposition
- Corticol hypoactivity

Narcolepsy
- Genetic predisposition

ASSESSMENT FINDINGS
Primary insomnia
- Anxiety related to sleep loss
- Fatigue
- Haggard appearance
- Slowed response to stimuli
- Personality changes
- History of light or easily disturbed sleep or difficulty falling asleep
- Insomnia
- Poor concentration
- Tension headache
- Poor memory

Circadian rhythm sleep disorder
- Cardiovascular and GI disturbances, such as palpitations, peptic ulcer disease, and gastritis
- Fatigue
- Haggard appearance
- Poor concentration
- Poor memory

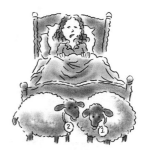

It takes more than counting sheep to cure most sleep disorders.

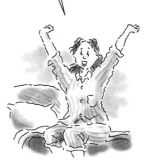

Wake up! You have more studying to do.

Management moments

Drugs that affect sleep

When caring for a client with a sleep disorder, keep in mind that medications and alcohol can affect sleep. Review the client's medication list to see if he's receiving any medications that affect sleep such as those listed here.

INCREASED TOTAL SLEEP TIME
- Barbiturates
- Benzodiazepines
- Alcohol (during the first half of the night)
- Phenothiazines

DECREASED TOTAL SLEEP TIME
- Amphetamines
- Alcohol (during the second half of the night)
- Caffeine

ALTERED DREAMING AND REM SLEEP
- Beta-adrenergic blockers: decreased rapid-eye-movement (REM) sleep, possible nightmares
- Antiparkinsonian: vivid dreams and nightmares
- Amphetamines: decreased REM sleep

- Tricyclic antidepressants and monoamine oxidase inhibitors: decreased REM sleep
- Barbiturates: decreased REM sleep
- Benzodiazepines: decreased REM sleep
- Selective serotonin reuptake inhibitors (SSRIs): decreased REM sleep, vivid dreams

INCREASED WAKING AFTER SLEEP ONSET
- Steroids
- Opioids
- Beta-adrenergic blockers
- Alcohol
- SSRIs

DECREASED WAKING AFTER SLEEP ONSET
- Benzodiazepines
- Barbiturates

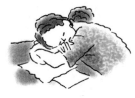

In narcolepsy, the client develops an overwhelming urge to sleep at any time of the day. Zzzz.

Breathing-related sleep disorder
- Abnormal breathing events during sleep including apnea, abnormally slow or shallow respirations, and hypoventilation (abnormal blood oxygen and carbon dioxide levels)
- Dull headache upon awakening
- Fatigue
- Gastroesophageal reflux
- Mild systemic hypertension with elevated diastolic blood pressure
- Snoring while sleeping

Primary hypersomnia
- Confusion upon awakening
- Difficulty awakening
- Poor memory

Narcolepsy
- Cataplexy (bilateral loss of muscle tone triggered by strong emotion)
- Frequent, intense, and vivid dreams may occur during nocturnal sleep
- Generalized daytime sleepiness

- Hypnagogic hallucination (intense dream-like images)
- Irresistible attacks of refreshing sleep

DIAGNOSTIC TEST RESULTS
Primary insomnia
- Polysomnography shows poor sleep continuity, increased stage 1 sleep, decreased stages 3 and 4 sleep, increased muscle tension, or increased amounts of EEG alpha activity during sleep.
- Psychophysiologic testing may show high arousal (increased muscle tension or excessive physiologic reactivity to stress).

Circadian rhythm sleep disorder
- Polysomnography shows short sleep latency (length of time it takes to fall asleep), reduced sleep duration, and sleep continuity disturbances. (Results may vary depending on the time of day testing is performed.)

Breathing-related sleep disorder
• Polysomnography measures of oral and nasal airflow are abnormal and oxyhemoglobin saturation is reduced.

Primary hypersomnia
• Polysomnography demonstrates a normal to prolonged sleep duration, short sleep latency, normal to increased sleep continuity, and normal distributions of REM and NREM sleep. Some individuals may have increased amounts of slow-wave sleep.

Narcolepsy
• Polysomnography shows sleep latencies of less than 10 minutes and frequent sleep onset REM periods, frequent transient arousals, decreased sleep efficiency, increased stage 1 sleep, increased REM sleep, and increased eye movements within the REM periods. Periodic limb movements and episodes of sleep apnea are also often noted.

NURSING DIAGNOSES
• Disturbed sleep pattern
• Fatigue
• Impaired home maintenance
• Risk for injury

TREATMENT
• Relaxation techniques
• Sleep restrictions (clients are instructed to avoid napping and to stay in bed only when sleeping)
• Regular exercise
• Light therapy

Drug therapy
Primary insomnia or circadian rhythm sleep disorder
• Antidepressant: trazodone
• Benzodiazepines: lorazepam (Ativan), alprazolam (Xanax)
• Diphenhydramine (Benadryl)
• Hypnotics: zolpidem (Ambien), eszopiclone (Lunesta)
• Melatonin
Primary hypersomnia or narcolepsy
• Stimulants: caffeine, methylphenidate (Ritalin), dextroamphetamine (Dexedrine), modafinil (Provigil)

INTERVENTIONS AND RATIONALES
• Assess the client and document symptoms of sleep disturbance *to gain information for care plan development.*

Primary insomnia and circadian rhythm disturbance
• Encourage the client to discuss concerns that may be preventing sleep. *Active listening helps elicit underlying causes of sleep disturbance such as stress.*
• Establish a sleep routine *to promote relaxation and sleep.*
• Schedule regular sleep and awakening times *to help ensure that progress is maintained after the client leaves the hospital.*
• Administer medications, as prescribed, *to induce sleep and to reduce anxiety.*
• Provide warm milk at bedtime. *L-tryptophan, found in milk, is a precursor to serotonin, a neurotransmitter necessary for sleep.*
• Plan activities that require the client to wake at a regular hour and stay out of bed during the day *to reinforce natural circadian rhythms.*
• Encourage regular exercise early in the day.
• Teach relaxation techniques *to decrease symptoms.*

Breathing-related sleep disorder
• Administer continuous positive nasal airway pressure *to treat obstructive sleep disorders.*
• Encourage weight loss, as appropriate, *to decrease incidence of apnea.*
• Suggest sleeping in reclining position *to help maintain a patent airway.*

Primary hypersomnia and narcolepsy
• Administer medications, as prescribed, *to help the client stay awake and maintain client safety.*
• Develop strategies to manage symptoms and integrate them into the client's daily routine, such as taking naps during lunch or work breaks, *to help maintain client safety and promote normal functioning.*

Teaching topics
All types
• Explanation of the disorder and treatment plan

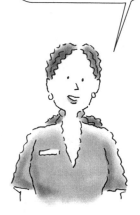

For the client with primary insomnia or circadian rhythm disturbance, plan activities that require him to wake at a regular hour and stay out of bed during the day.

• Medication use and possible adverse effects

Primary insomnia and circadian rhythm disorder
• Relaxation techniques
• Importance of limiting caffeine and alcohol
• Need to avoid exercising within 3 hours before bedtime
• Ways to identify and reduce stressors
• Healthy diet and regular exercise routine

Breathing-related sleeping disorder
• Use of home positive nasal airway pressure device
• Weight loss information

Primary hypersomnia and narcolepsy
• Integrating nap period into daily routine

Parasomnias

Parasomnias are characterized by abnormal, unpleasant motor or verbal arousals and behaviors that occur during sleep. They include nightmare disorder, sleep terror disorder, and sleepwalking disorder. The client is able to perform the behaviors but does not have conscious awareness or responsibility for them.

Nightmare disorder is characterized by the recurrence of frightening dreams that cause the client to awaken from sleep. When the client awakens, he's fully alert and experiences persistent anxiety or fear. Typically, the client can recall details of the dream involving physical danger.

Sleep terror disorder is characterized by episodes of sleep terrors that cause distress or impairment of social or occupational functioning. The client may sit up in bed screaming or crying with a frightened expression and signs of intense anxiety. During such episodes, the client is difficult to awaken and, if he does awaken, he's generally confused or disoriented. The client has no recollection of the dream content.

In **sleepwalking disorder,** the client arises from bed and walks about. The client has limited recall of the event upon awakening.

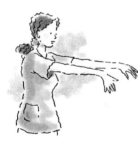

Zzzz... Sleepwalkers may also sit up, talk, or engage in inappropriate behavior with little or no recall of the incident.

CONTRIBUTING FACTORS
• Severe psychosocial stressors
• Genetic predisposition
• Sleep deprivation
• Fever

ASSESSMENT FINDINGS
Nightmare disorder
• Anxiety
• Depression
• Dream recall
• Excessive sleepiness
• Irritability
• Mild autonomic arousal upon awakening (sweating, tachycardia, tachypnea)
• Poor concentration

Sleep terror disorder
• Autonomic signs of intense anxiety (tachycardia, tachypnea, flushing, sweating, increased muscle tone, dilated pupils)
• Inability to recall dream content
• Screaming or crying

Sleepwalking disorder
• Amnesia of the episode or limited recall
• Sitting up, talking, walking, or engaging in inappropriate behavior during episode

DIAGNOSTIC TEST RESULTS
Nightmare disorder
• Polysomnography demonstrates abrupt awakenings from REM sleep that correspond to the individual's report of nightmares. These awakenings usually occur during the second half of the night. Heart rate and respiratory rate may increase or show increased variability before the awakening.

Sleep terror disorder
• Polysomnography reveals that sleep terrors begin during deep NREM sleep characterized by slow-frequency EEG activity.

Sleepwalking disorder
• Polysomnography reveals episodes of sleepwalking that begin within the first few hours of sleep, usually during NREM stage 3 or 4 sleep.

NURSING DIAGNOSES
- Disturbed sleep pattern
- Fatigue
- Ineffective role performance
- Risk for injury

TREATMENT
- Relaxation training
- Guided imagery
- Individual counseling

Drug therapy
- Rarely used

INTERVENTIONS AND RATIONALES
- Assess the client and document the symptoms of sleep disturbance *to aid in formulating a treatment plan.*
- Lock windows and doors if sleepwalking occurs *to maintain client safety.*
- Provide emotional support *to allay the client's anxiety.*
- Establish a sleep routine *to promote relaxation and sleep.*
- Schedule regular sleep and awakening times *so that the client can learn specific planning strategies for managing sleep.*
- Administer medications, as prescribed *to promote sleep.*
- Help the client identify stressors to sleep disturbance *to help reduce incidence.*

Teaching topics
- Safety measures for the client with sleepwalking disorder
- Ways to identify and reduce stressors

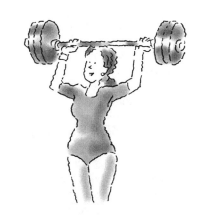

Pump up on practice questions

1. A client complains of experiencing an overwhelming urge to sleep. He states that he's been falling asleep while working at his desk. He reports that these episodes occur about five times daily. This client is most likely experiencing which sleep disorder?
1. Breathing-related sleep disorder
2. Narcolepsy
3. Primary hypersomnia
4. Circadian rhythm disorder

Answer: 2. Narcolepsy is characterized by irresistible attacks of refreshing sleep that occur two to six times per day and last for 5 to 20 minutes. The client with breathing-related sleep disorder suffers interruptions in sleep that leave the client with excess sleepiness. In hypersomnia, the client suffers excess sleepiness and reports prolonged periods of nighttime sleep or daytime napping. With circadian rhythm disorder, the client has periods of insomnia followed by periods of increased sleepiness.

➡ *NCLEX keys*
Client needs category: Psychosocial integrity
Client needs subcategory: None
Cognitive level: Application

2. A nurse is caring for a client who complains of fatigue, inability to concentrate, and palpitations. The client states that she has been experiencing these symptoms for the past 6 months. The nurse suspects that the client is experiencing circadian rhythm sleep disturbance related to which factor?

1. History of recent fever
2. Shift work
3. Hyperthyroidism
4. Pheochromocytoma

Answer: 2. The client is experiencing circadian rhythm sleep disorder (palpitations, GI disturbances, fatigue, haggard appearance, and poor concentration), which is typically caused by shift work, jet lag, or a delayed sleep phase. Fever is a contributing factor in parasomnias. Hyperthyroidism and pheochromocytoma are causative factors for primary insomnia.

➡ *NCLEX keys*

Client needs category: Psychosocial integrity
Client needs subcategory: None
Cognitive level: Analysis

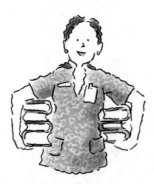

3. A client comes to the clinic complaining of the inability to sleep over the past 2 months. He states that his inability to sleep is ruining his life because "getting sleep" is all he can think about. This client is most likely experiencing which sleep disorder?

1. Circadian rhythm sleep disorder
2. Breathing-related sleep disorder
3. Primary insomnia
4. Primary hypersomnia

Answer: 3. The client with primary insomnia experiences difficulty initiating or maintaining sleep. A key symptom of primary insomnia is the client's intense focus and anxiety about not getting to sleep. The client diagnosed with circadian rhythm sleep disorder reports periods of insomnia at particular times during a 24-hour period and excessive sleepiness

at other times. Excessive sleepiness is the most common complaint of clients affected by breathing-related sleep disorder. The client experiencing primary hypersomnia typically sleeps 8 to 12 hours per night. They fall asleep easily and sleep through the night but commonly have trouble awakening in the morning.

➡ *NCLEX keys*

Client needs category: Psychosocial integrity
Client needs subcategory: None
Cognitive level: Analysis

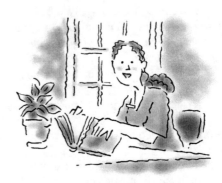

4. A nurse is preparing a teaching plan for a client diagnosed with primary insomnia. Which teaching topic should be included?

1. Eating unlimited spicy foods and limiting caffeine and alcohol
2. Exercising 1 hour before bedtime to promote sleep
3. Importance of sleeping whenever the client tires
4. Drinking warm milk before bed to induce sleep

Answer: 4. Clients diagnosed with primary insomnia should be taught that drinking warm milk before bedtime can help induce sleep. They should also be taught the importance of limiting spicy foods, alcohol, and caffeine; avoiding exercise within 3 hours before bedtime; establishing a routine bedtime; and avoiding napping.

➡ *NCLEX keys*

Client needs category: Psychosocial integrity
Client needs subcategory: None
Cognitive level: Application

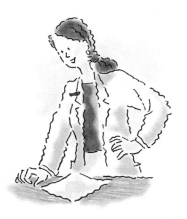

5. A nurse is caring for a client hospitalized on numerous occasions for complaints of chest pain and fainting spells, which she attributes to her deteriorating heart condition. No relatives or friends report ever actually seeing a fainting spell. After undergoing an extensive cardiac, pulmonary, GI, and neurologic work-up, she's told that all test results are completely negative. The client remains persistent in her belief that she has a serious illness. What diagnosis is appropriate for this client?

    1.   Exhibitionism
    2.   Somatoform disorder
    3.   Degenerative dementia
    4.   Echolalia

Answer: 2. Somatoform disorders are characterized by recurrent and multiple physical symptoms that have no organic or physiologic base. Exhibitionism involves public exposure of genitals. Degenerative dementia is characterized by deterioration of mental capacities. Echolalia is a repetition of words or phrases.

➡ NCLEX keys
Client needs category: Safe and effective care environment
Client needs subcategory: Management of care
Cognitive level: Analysis

6. A client is prescribed sertraline (Zoloft), a selective serotonin reuptake inhibitor. Which adverse effects about this drug should the nurse include when creating a medication teaching plan? Select all that apply.

    1.   Agitation
    2.   Agranulocytosis
    3.   Sleep disturbance
    4.   Intermittent tachycardia
    5.   Dry mouth
    6.   Seizures

Answer: 1, 3, 5. Common adverse effects of sertraline are agitation, sleep disturbance, and dry mouth. Agranulocytosis, intermittent tachycardia, and seizures are adverse effects of clonazepam (Klonopin).

➡ NCLEX keys
Client needs category: Physiological integrity
Client needs subcategory: Pharmacological and parenteral therapies
Cognitive level: Application

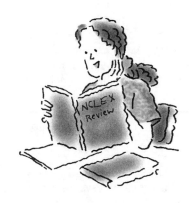

7. A nurse is caring for a client who exhibits signs of somatization. Which statement is most relevant?

    1.   Clients with somatization are cognitively impaired.
    2.   Anxiety rarely coexists with somatization.
    3.   Somatization exists when medical evidence supports the symptoms.
    4.   Clients with somatization often have lengthy medical records.

Answer: 4. Clients with somatization are prone to "physician shop" and have extensive medical records as a result of their multiple procedures and tests. Clients with somatization aren't usually cognitively impaired.

These clients have coexisting anxiety and depression and no medical evidence to support a clear-cut diagnosis.

➡ *NCLEX keys*
Client needs category: Psychosocial integrity
Client needs subcategory: None
Cognitive level: Analysis

8. A nurse is caring for a client who reveals symptoms of a sleep disorder during the admission assessment. The client also admits that he has "broken down and cried for no apparent reason." Which criterion is most important for the nurse to initially consider to gain insight into the client's patterns of sleep and feelings of depression?
1. Stressors in the client's life
2. The client's weight
3. Periods of apnea
4. Sexual activity

Answer: 1. Recognizing that sleep disturbances are often symptoms of stress, depression, and anxiety, the nurse is prudent to discuss these possible factors initially. If the client has a weight problem, suffers from sleep apnea, or reports sexual problems, these also can affect sleep; however, consideration of life stressors occurs first.

➡ *NCLEX keys*
Client needs category: Psychosocial integrity
Client needs subcategory: None
Cognitive level: Application

9. A nurse is caring for a client who displays gait disturbances, paralysis, pseudoseizures, and tremors. These symptoms may be manifestations of what psychiatric disorder?
1. Pain disorder
2. Adjustment disorder
3. Delirium
4. Conversion disorder

Answer: 4. Conversion disorders are most frequently associated with psychologically mediated neurologic deficits, such as gait disturbances, paralysis, pseudo-seizures, and tremors. Pain disorders and adjustment disorders aren't generally expressed in terms of neurologic deficits. Delirium is associated with cognitive impairment.

➡ *NCLEX keys*
Client needs category: Psychosocial integrity
Client needs subcategory: None
Cognitive level: Analysis

10. A nurse is caring for a client who complains of chronic pain. Given this complaint, why would the nurse simultaneously evaluate both general physical and psychosocial problems?
1. Depression is commonly associated with pain disorders and somatic complaints.
2. Combining evaluations will save time and allow for quicker delivery of health care.
3. Most insurance plans won't cover evaluation of both as separate entities.
4. The physician doesn't have the training to evaluate for psychosocial considerations.

Answer: 1. Psychosocial factors should be suspected when pain persists beyond the normal tissue healing time and physical causes have been investigated. The other choices may or may not be correct but certainly aren't credible in all cases.

➡ *NCLEX keys*
Client needs category: Psychosocial integrity
Client needs subcategory: None
Cognitive level: Analysis

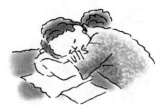

You've finished the chapter on sleep disorders. You may want to nap before the next chapter.

5 Anxiety & mood disorders

Brush up on key concepts

Anxiety disorders are characterized by anxiety and avoidant behavior. Clients are overwhelmed by feelings of impending catastrophe, guilt, shame, and worthlessness. Clients with anxiety cling to maladaptive behaviors in an attempt to alleviate their own distress, but these behaviors only increase their symptoms.

Mood disorders are characterized by depressed or elevated moods that alter the client's ability to cope with reality and to function normally.

At any time, you can review the major points of each disorder by consulting the *Cheat sheet* on pages 50 and 51.

Polish up on client care

Major mood disorders include bipolar disorder and major depression. Major anxiety disorders include generalized anxiety, obsessive-compulsive disorder, panic disorder, phobias, and posttraumatic stress disorder (PTSD).

Bipolar disorder

Bipolar disorder is a severe disturbance in affect, manifested by episodes of extreme sadness alternating with episodes of euphoria. Severity and duration of episodes vary. The exact biological basis of bipolar disorder remains unknown, although it's thought that a combination of genetic factors and stressful events contribute to the development of mania.

Two common patterns of bipolar disorder include:
• bipolar I, in which depressive episodes alternate with full manic episodes (hyperactive behavior, delusional thinking, grandiosity, and often hostility)
• bipolar II, characterized by recurrent depressive episodes and occasional manic episodes.

CONTRIBUTING FACTORS
• Concurrent major illness
• Environment
• Heredity
• History of psychiatric illnesses
• Seasons and circadian rhythms that affect mood
• Sleep deprivation
• Stressful events may produce limbic system dysfunction

ASSESSMENT FINDINGS
During episodes of mania
• Bizarre and eccentric appearance
• Cognitive manifestations, such as difficulty concentrating, flight of ideas, delusions of grandeur, impaired judgment
• Decreased sleep
• Deteriorated physical appearance
• Euphoria and hostility
• Feelings of grandiosity
• Impulsiveness
• Increased energy (feeling of being charged up)
• Increased sexual interest and activity
• Increased social contacts
• Inflated sense of self-worth
• Lack of inhibition
• Rapid, jumbled speech

(Text continues on page 52.)

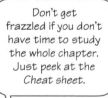

Cheat sheet

Anxiety & mood disorders refresher

BIPOLAR DISORDER

Key signs and symptoms
During episodes of mania
- Euphoria and hostility
- Feelings of grandiosity
- Substance abuse
- Increased sexual interest and activity
- Inflated sense of self-worth
- Increased energy (feeling of being charged up)

During episodes of depression
- Altered sleep patterns
- Anorexia and weight loss
- Helplessness
- Irritability
- Lack of motivation
- Low self-esteem
- Sadness and crying
- Suicidal ideation or attempts

Key test results
- EEG is abnormal during the depressive episodes of bipolar I disorder and major depression.

Key treatments
- Individual therapy
- Family therapy
- Antimanic agents: lithium carbonate (Eskalith), lithium citrate

Key interventions
During manic phase
- Decrease environmental stimuli by behaving consistently and supplying external controls.
- Ensure a safe environment.
- Define and explain acceptable behavior and then set limits.
- Monitor drug levels, especially lithium and carbamazepine.

During depressive phase
- Assess the level and intensity of the client's depression.
- Ensure a safe environment.
- Assess the risk for suicide and formulate a safety contract with the client, as appropriate.
- Observe the client for medication compliance and adverse effects.
- Encourage the client to identify current stressors and support systems.

GENERALIZED ANXIETY DISORDER

Key signs and symptoms
- Easy startle reflex
- Excessive worry and anxiety
- Diaphoresis
- Fatigue
- Fears of grave misfortune or death
- Muscle tension and aches
- Trembling and tingling of hands and feet

Key test results
- Laboratory tests exclude physiologic causes.

Key treatments
- Relaxation training
- Cognitive behavioral therapy
- Anxiolytics: alprazolam (Xanax), lorazepam (Ativan), clonazepam (Klonopin), buspirone (BuSpar)
- Serotonin norepinephrine reuptake inhibitors (SNRIs): venlafaxine (Effexor), duloxetine (Cymbalta)
- Selective serotonin reuptake inhibitors (SSRIs): fluoxetine (Prozac), paroxetine (Paxil), sertraline (Zoloft), citalopram (Celexa)

Key interventions
- Help the client identify and explore coping mechanisms used in the past.
- Observe for signs of mounting anxiety.

MAJOR DEPRESSION

Key signs and symptoms
- Altered sleep patterns
- Appetite changes resulting in weight loss or gain
- Anorexia and weight loss
- Helplessness
- Irritability
- Lack of motivation
- Low self-esteem
- Sadness and crying
- Suicidal ideation or attempts

Key test results
- Beck Depression Inventory indicates depression.

Key treatments
- SSRIs: paroxetine (Paxil), fluoxetine (Prozac), sertraline (Zoloft), citalopram (Celexa)

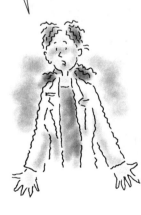

Don't get frazzled if you don't have time to study the whole chapter. Just peek at the Cheat sheet.

Anxiety & mood disorders refresher (continued)

MAJOR DEPRESSION (CONTINUED)
- Tricyclic antidepressants (TCAs): imipramine (Tofranil), desipramine (Norpramin), amitriptyline (Elavil)
- SNRIs: venlafaxine (Effexor), duloxetine (Cymbalta)

Key interventions
- Assess the level and intensity of the client's depression.
- Ensure a safe environment for the client.
- Assess the risk of suicide and formulate a safety contract with the client as appropriate.
- Observe the client for medication compliance and adverse effects.

OBSESSIVE-COMPULSIVE DISORDER
Key signs and symptoms
- Compulsive behavior (which may include repetitive touching or counting, doing and undoing small tasks, or any other repetitive activity or hoarding of certain items such as newspapers)
- Obsessive thoughts (which may include thoughts of contamination, repetitive worries about impending tragedy, repeating and counting images or words)

Key test results
- Positron emission tomography shows increased activity in the frontal lobe of the cerebral cortex.

Key treatments
- Cognitive behavioral therapy
- Individual therapy
- Benzodiazepines: alprazolam (Xanax), lorazepam (Ativan), clonazepam (Klonopin)
- SSRIs: fluoxetine (Prozac), paroxetine (Paxil), sertraline (Zoloft), fluvoxamine (Luvox)

Key interventions
- Encourage the client to express his feelings.
- Encourage the client to identify situations that produce anxiety and precipitate obsessive-compulsive behavior.

PANIC DISORDER
Key signs and symptoms
- Diminished ability to focus, even with direction from others
- Edginess, impatience
- Loss of objectivity
- Severely impaired rational thought
- Uneasiness and tension

Key test results
- Medical tests eliminate physiologic cause.

Key treatments
- Cognitive behavioral therapy
- Benzodiazepines: alprazolam (Xanax), lorazepam (Ativan), clonazepam (Klonopin)

Key interventions
During panic attacks
- Distract the client from the attack.
- Approach the client calmly and unemotionally.
- Use short, simple sentences.

PHOBIAS
Key signs and symptoms
- Panic when confronted with the feared object
- Persistent fear of specific things, places, or situations

Key test results
- No specific tests can be used to diagnose phobias.

Key treatments
- Benzodiazepines: alprazolam (Xanax), lorazepam (Ativan), clonazepam (Klonopin)
- Cognitive behavioral therapy
- Family therapy
- Supportive therapy

Key interventions
- Help the client to identify the feared object or situation.
- Assist in desensitizing the client.

POSTTRAUMATIC STRESS DISORDER
Key signs and symptoms
- Anxiety
- Flashbacks of the traumatic experience
- Nightmares about the traumatic experience
- Poor impulse control
- Social isolation
- Survivor guilt

Key test results
- No specific tests identify or confirm posttraumatic stress disorder.

Key treatments
- Cognitive behavioral therapy
- Group therapy
- Systematic desensitization
- Benzodiazepines: alprazolam (Xanax), lorazepam (Ativan), clonazepam (Klonopin)
- TCAs: imipramine (Tofranil), amitriptyline (Elavil)

Key interventions
- Help the client to identify stressors.
- Provide for client safety.
- Encourage the client to explore the traumatic event and the meaning of the event.
- Assist the client with problem solving and resolving guilt.

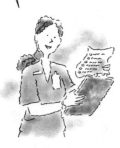

> Bipolar disorder isn't indicated by mood swings alone. It involves extreme behavior during both manic and depressive phases.

- Recklessness and poor judgment
- Substance abuse

During episodes of depression
- Altered sleep patterns
- Amenorrhea
- Anorexia and weight loss
- Confusion and indecisiveness
- Constipation
- Decreased alertness
- Delusions, hallucinations
- Difficulty thinking logically
- Guilt
- Helplessness
- Impotence and lack of interest in sex
- Inability to experience pleasure
- Irritability
- Lack of motivation
- Low self-esteem
- Pessimism
- Poor hygiene
- Poor posture
- Sadness and crying
- Suicide ideation or attempts

DIAGNOSTIC TEST RESULTS
- Abnormal dexamethasone suppression test results indicate bipolar I disorder.
- Cortisol secretion increases during manic episodes of bipolar I disorder.
- EEG is abnormal during the depressive episodes of bipolar I disorder and major depression.

NURSING DIAGNOSES
- Bathing self-care deficit
- Disturbed sleep pattern

TREATMENT
- Electroconvulsive therapy (ECT), if drug therapy fails
- Individual therapy
- Family therapy
- Interpersonal and social rhythm therapy
- Rehabilitation for substance abuse

Drug therapy
- Anticonvulsant agents: carbamazepine (Tegretol), gabapentin (Neurontin), divalproex sodium (Depakote)
- Antimanic agents: lithium carbonate (Eskalith), lithium citrate
- Selective serotonin reuptake inhibitors (SSRIs): paroxetine (Paxil), fluoxetine (Prozac), sertraline (Zoloft), citalopram (Celexa)
- Antipsychotic: aripiprazole (Abilify) for acute agitation

INTERVENTIONS AND RATIONALES
During manic phase
- Decrease environmental stimuli by behaving consistently and supplying external controls *to promote relaxation and enable sleep.*
- Ensure a safe environment *to protect the client from injuring himself.*
- Define and explain acceptable behaviors and then set limits *to begin a process in which the client will eventually define and set his own limits.*
- Monitor drug levels, especially lithium and carbamazepine, *to keep the dosage within the therapeutic range.*
- Monitor for suicidal ideations and innitiate safety measures *to prevent injury.*

During depressive phase
- Assess the level and intensity of the client's depression *because baseline information is essential for effective nursing care.*
- Ensure a safe environment *to protect the client from self-inflicted harm.*
- Assess the risk for suicide and formulate a safety contract with the client, as appropriate, *to ensure well-being and open lines of communication.*
- Observe the client for medication compliance and adverse effects; *without compliance, there's little hope of progress.*
- Encourage the client to identify current stressors and support systems *so that he can begin therapeutic treatment.*
- Promote opportunities for increased involvement in activities through a structured, daily program *to help the client feel comfortable with himself and others.*
- Select activities that ensure success and accomplishment *to increase self-esteem.*
- Help the client to modify negative expectations and think more positively; *positive thinking helps begin a healing process.*
- Spend time with the client *to enhance a therapeutic relationship.*

Teaching topics
• Explanation of the disorder and treatment plan
• Medication and possible adverse effects
• Recognizing signs of relapse
• Strategies to reduce stress
• Contacting the National Depressive and Manic Depressive association for support

Generalized anxiety disorder

A client with generalized anxiety disorder worries excessively and experiences tremendous anxiety almost daily. The worry lasts for longer than 6 months and is usually disproportionate to the situation. Both adults and children can be diagnosed with generalized anxiety disorder, though the content of the worry may differ.

CONTRIBUTING FACTORS
• Family history of anxiety
• Preexisting psychiatric problems, such as social phobia, panic disorder, and major depression

ASSESSMENT FINDINGS
• Autonomic hyperactivity
• Chest pain
• Distractibility
• Diaphoresis
• Easy startle reflex
• Excessive attention to surroundings
• Excessive worry and anxiety
• Fatigue
• Fears of grave misfortune or death
• Headaches
• Motor tension
• Muscle tension and aches
• Pounding heart
• Repetitive thoughts
• Sleep disorder
• Strained expression
• Trembling and tingling of hands and feet
• Vigilance and scanning

DIAGNOSTIC TEST RESULTS
• Laboratory tests exclude physiologic causes.

NURSING DIAGNOSES
• Anxiety
• Ineffective coping
• Deficient knowledge (disorder and treatment plan)

TREATMENT
• Relaxation training
• Cognitive behavioral therapy

Drug therapy
• Serotonin norepinephrine reuptake inhibitors (SNRIs): venlafaxine (Effexor), duloxetine (Cymbalta)
• Anxiolytics: alprazolam (Xanax), lorazepam (Ativan), clonazepam (Klonopin), buspirone (BuSpar)
• Beta-adrenergic blocker: propranolol (Inderal)
• Antihypertensive: clonidine (Catapres)
• Monoamine oxidase inhibitors (MAOIs): phenelzine (Nardil), tranylcypromine (Parnate)
• SSRIs: paroxetine (Paxil), sertraline (Zoloft), fluoxetine (Prozac), citalopram (Celexa)
• Tricyclic antidepressants (TCAs): imipramine (Tofranil), desipramine (Norpramin)

INTERVENTIONS AND RATIONALES
• Help the client identify and explore coping mechanisms used in the past. *Establishing a baseline for the level of current functioning will enable the nurse to build on the client's knowledge.*
• Observe for signs of mounting anxiety *to direct measures to moderate it.*
• Negotiate a contract to work on goals *to give the client control of his own situation.*
• Alter the environment *to reduce anxiety or meet the client's needs.*
• Monitor diet and nutrition; reduce caffeine intake *to reduce anxiety.*

Teaching topics
• Explanation of the disorder and treatment plan
• Medication use and possible adverse effects
• Recognizing signs of anxiety

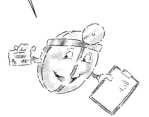

Finding the most effective drug and dosage for anxiety and mood disorders is often a process of trial and error.

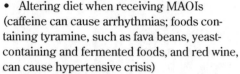

Treatment for depression usually requires collaboration with the client to find an effective program of drug therapy and psychotherapy.

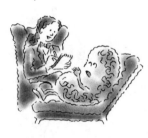

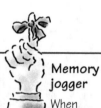

Memory jogger

When dealing with depressed clients, Think **COMPARE**.

Consult with staff.

Observe the suicidal client.

Maintain personal contact.

Provide a safe environment.

Assess for clues to suicide.

Remove dangerous objects.

Encourage expression of feelings.

• Altering diet when receiving MAOIs (caffeine can cause arrhythmias; foods containing tyramine, such as fava beans, yeast-containing and fermented foods, and red wine, can cause hypertensive crisis)
• Contact information for counseling and support groups

Major depression

Major depression is a syndrome of persistent sad, dysphoric mood accompanied by disturbances in sleep and appetite from lethargy and an inability to experience pleasure. Depression is confirmed when the client exhibits five or more classic symptoms of depression for at least 2 weeks.

Major depression can profoundly alter social functioning, but the most severe complication of major depression is the potential for suicide.

CONTRIBUTING FACTORS
• Current substance abuse
• Deficiencies in the receptor sites for some neurotransmitters: norepinephrine, serotonin, dopamine, and acetylcholine
• Family history of depressive disorders
• Hormonal imbalances
• Lack of social support
• Nutritional deficiencies
• Prior episode of depression
• Significant medical problems
• Stressful life events

ASSESSMENT FINDINGS
• Altered sleep patterns
• Amenorrhea
• Appetite changes resulting in weight loss or gain
• Confusion and indecisiveness
• Constipation
• Decreased alertness
• Delusions, hallucinations
• Difficulty thinking logically
• Guilt
• Helplessness
• Impotence or lack of interest in sex

• Inability to experience pleasure
• Irritability
• Lack of motivation
• Low self-esteem
• Pessimism
• Poor hygiene
• Poor posture
• Sadness and crying
• Suicidal ideation or attempt

DIAGNOSTIC TEST RESULTS
• Thyroid test is abnormal in major depression.
• Beck Depression Inventory indicates depression.

NURSING DIAGNOSES
• Hopelessness
• Impaired social interaction
• Chronic low self-esteem

TREATMENT
• ECT
• Individual therapy
• Family therapy
• Phototherapy

Drug therapy
• MAOI: phenelzine (Nardil)
• SSRIs: paroxetine (Paxil), fluoxetine (Prozac), sertraline (Zoloft), citalopram (Celexa)
• TCAs: imipramine (Tofranil), desipramine (Norpramin), amitriptyline (Elavil)
• SNRIs: venlofaxine (Effexor), duloxetine (Cymbalta)

INTERVENTIONS AND RATIONALES
• Assess the level and intensity of the client's depression *because baseline information is essential for effective nursing care.*
• Address issues that trigger depression, and assist the client in using effective coping skills *to minimize depressive episodes.*
• Ensure a safe environment for the client *to protect the client from self-inflicted harm.*
• Assess the risk of suicide and formulate a safety contract with the client, as appropriate,

to ensure his well-being and open lines of communication.
- Reorient the client undergoing ECT as needed. *Clients receiving ECT often have temporary memory loss.*
- Observe the client for medication compliance and adverse effects; *without compliance, there's little hope of progress.*
- Encourage the client to identify current stressors and support systems *so that he can begin therapeutic treatment.*
- Promote opportunities for increased involvement in activities through a structured, daily program *to help the client feel comfortable with himself and others.*
- Select activities that ensure success and accomplishment *to increase self-esteem.*
- Help the client to modify negative expectations and think more positively; *positive thinking helps the client begin the healing process.*
- Spend time with the client *to enhance the therapeutic relationship.*

Teaching topics
- Explanation of the disorder and treatment plan
- Medication use and possible adverse effects
- Learning relaxation and sleep methods
- Complying with therapy
- If taking MAOIs, avoiding tyramine-containing foods, such as wine, beer, cheese, fermented fruits, meats, and vegetables

Obsessive-compulsive disorder

Obsessive-compulsive disorder is characterized by recurrent obsessions (intrusive thoughts, images, and impulses) and compulsions (repetitive behaviors in response to an obsession). The obsessions and compulsions may cause intense stress and impair the client's functioning. Some clients have simultaneous symptoms of depression.

CONTRIBUTING FACTORS
- Brain lesions
- Childhood trauma
- Lack of role models to teach coping skills
- Multiple stressors

ASSESSMENT FINDINGS
- Compulsive behavior (which may include repetitive touching or counting, doing and undoing, or any other repetitive activity or hoarding of items such as newspapers)
- Obsessive thoughts (which may include thoughts of contamination, repetitive worries about impending tragedy, repeating and counting images or words)
- Social impairment

DIAGNOSTIC TEST RESULTS
- Positron emission tomography shows increased activity in the frontal lobe of the cerebral cortex and abnormal metabolic rate of basal ganglia.

NURSING DIAGNOSES
- Anxiety
- Ineffective coping
- Chronic low self-esteem

TREATMENT
- Cognitive behavioral therapy
- Individual therapy

Drug therapy
- Benzodiazepines: alprazolam (Xanax), lorazepam (Ativan), clonazepam (Klonopin)
- MAOIs: phenelzine (Nardil), tranylcypromine (Parnate)
- SSRIs: fluoxetine (Prozac), sertraline (Zoloft), paroxetine (Paxil), fluvoxamine (Luvox)
- TCAs: imipramine (Tofranil), desipramine (Norpramin)

INTERVENTIONS AND RATIONALES
- Encourage the client to express his feelings *to decrease the client's level of stress.*

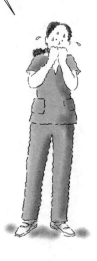

Don't worry. Dreading the exam doesn't mean you've developed panic disorder.

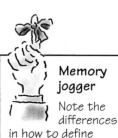

Memory jogger

Note the differences in how to define fear, anxiety, and panic:

Fear is a response to external stimuli.

Anxiety is a response to internal conflict.

Panic is an extreme level of anxiety.

• Help the client assess how his obsessions and compulsive behaviors affect his functioning. The client needs *to realistically evaluate the consequences of his behavior.*
• Encourage the client to identify situations that produce anxiety and precipitate obsessive-compulsive behavior *to help him evaluate and cope with his condition.*
• Work with the client to develop appropriate coping skills *to reduce anxiety.*

Teaching topics

• Explanation of the disorder and treatment plan
• Medication use and possible adverse effects

Panic disorder

Although everyone experiences some level of anxiety, clients with panic disorder experience a nonspecific feeling of terror and dread, accompanied by symptoms of physiologic stress. This level of anxiety makes it difficult, if not impossible, for the client to carry out the normal functions of everyday life.

CONTRIBUTING FACTORS

• Agoraphobia (fear of being alone or in public places)
• Asthma
• Cardiovascular disease
• Familial pattern
• GI disorders
• History of anxiety disorders
• History of depression
• Neurologic abnormalities: abnormal activity on the medial portion of the temporal lobe in the parahippocampal area and significant asymmetrical atrophy of the temporal lobe
• Neurotransmitter involvement
• Stressful lifestyle

ASSESSMENT FINDINGS

• Abdominal discomfort or pain, nausea, heartburn, or diarrhea
• Avoidance (the client's refusal to encounter situations that may cause anxiety)
• Chest pressure, lump in throat, or choking sensation

• Confusion
• Decreased ability to relate to others
• Diminished ability to focus, even with direction from others
• Dizziness or light-headedness
• Edginess, impatience
• Eyelid twitching
• Fidgeting or pacing
• Flushing or pallor
• Generalized weakness, tremors
• Increased or decreased blood pressure
• Insomnia
• Loss of appetite or revulsion toward food
• Loss of objectivity
• Palpitations and tachycardia
• Physical tension
• Potential for dangerous, impulsive actions
• Rapid speech
• Rapid, shallow breathing or shortness of breath
• Severely impaired rational thought
• Startle reaction
• Sudden urge and frequent urination
• Sweating, itching
• Trembling
• Uneasiness and tension

DIAGNOSTIC TEST RESULTS

• Medical tests eliminate physiologic cause.
• Urine and blood tests check for presence of psychoactive agents.

NURSING DIAGNOSES

• Anxiety
• Ineffective coping
• Powerlessness

TREATMENT

• Cognitive behavioral therapy
• Group therapy
• Relaxation training

Drug therapy

• Benzodiazepines: alprazolam (Xanax), lorazepam (Ativan), clonazepam (Klonopin)
• MAOIs: phenelzine (Nardil); in clients with severe panic disorder, tranylcypromine (Parnate)
• SSRI: paroxetine (Paxil)

- TCAs: imipramine (Tofranil), desipramine (Norpramin)

INTERVENTIONS AND RATIONALES
During panic attacks
- Distract the client from the attack *to alleviate the effects of panic.*
- Approach the client calmly and unemotionally *to reduce the risk of further stressing the client.*
- Use short, simple sentences *because the client's ability to focus and to relate to others is diminished.*
- Administer medications, as needed, *to ensure a therapeutic response.*

After panic attacks
- Attempt to identify triggers to panic attacks *to assist with treatment.*
- Discuss other methods of coping with stress *to make the client aware of alternatives.*

Teaching topics
- Explanation of the disorder and treatment plan
- Medication use and possible adverse effects
- Learning decision-making and problem-solving skills
- Learning relaxation techniques

Phobias

A phobia is an intense, irrational fear of something external. It's a fear that persists, even though the client recognizes its irrationality. Phobias are resistant to insight-oriented therapies.

CONTRIBUTING FACTORS
- Biochemical, involving neurotransmitters
- Familial patterns
- Traumatic events

ASSESSMENT FINDINGS
- Displacement (shifting of emotions from their original object) and symbolization
- Disruption in social life or work life

- Panic when confronted with the feared object
- Persistent fear of specific things, places, or situations

DIAGNOSTIC TEST RESULTS
- No specific test is used to diagnose phobias.

NURSING DIAGNOSES
- Anxiety
- Fear
- Powerlessness

TREATMENT
- Cognitive behavioral therapy
- Family therapy
- Social skills training
- Supportive therapy
- Systematic desensitization

Drug therapy
- Beta-adrenergic blocker: propranolol (Inderal) for phobia related to public speaking
- Benzodiazepines: alprazolam (Xanax), lorazepam (Ativan), clonazepam (Klonopin)
- MAOIs: phenelzine (Nardil), tranylcypromine (Parnate)
- SSRI: paroxetine (Paxil)
- TCAs: imipramine (Tofranil), desipramine (Norpramin)

INTERVENTIONS AND RATIONALES
- Help the client to identify the feared object or situation *to develop an effective treatment plan.*
- Assist in desensitizing the client *to diminish his fear.*
- Remind the client about resources and personal strengths *to build self-esteem.*

Teaching topics
- Explanation of the disorder and treatment plan
- Medication use and possible adverse effects
- Learning assertiveness techniques
- Learning relaxation techniques
- Participating in the desensitizing process

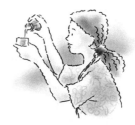

Note that depressed or anxious clients often attempt to self-medicate. Be aware of possible interactions with prescribed treatments.

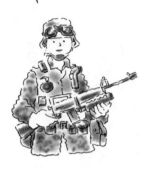

> PTSD was originally called "shell shock" because participation in active combat is a common cause of this disorder.

Posttraumatic stress disorder

PTSD is a group of symptoms that develop after a traumatic event. This traumatic event may involve death, injury, or threat to physical integrity. In PTSD, ordinary coping behaviors fail to relieve the anxiety. The client may experience reactions that are acute, chronic, or delayed.

CAUSES
• Personal experience of threatened injury or death
• Witnessing a traumatic event happen to a close friend or family member
• Extreme distress causing a profound sense of fear, terror, or helplessness

CONTRIBUTING FACTORS
• Anxiety
• Low self-esteem
• Preexisting psychopathology

ASSESSMENT FINDINGS
• Anger
• Anxiety
• Apathy
• Avoidance of people involved in the trauma
• Avoidance of places where the trauma occurred
• Chronic tension
• Detachment
• Difficulty concentrating
• Difficulty falling or staying asleep
• Emotional numbness
• Flashbacks of the traumatic experience
• Hyperalertness
• Inability to recall details of the traumatic event
• Labile affect
• Nightmares about the traumatic experience
• Poor impulse control
• Social isolation
• Survivor guilt

DIAGNOSTIC TEST RESULTS
• No specific tests identify or confirm PTSD.

NURSING DIAGNOSES
• Fear
• Posttrauma syndrome
• Powerlessness
• Situational low self-esteem

TREATMENT
• Alcohol and drug rehabilitation, when indicated
• Cognitive behavioral therapy
• Group therapy
• Relaxation training
• Systematic desensitization

Drug therapy
• Benzodiazepines: alprazolam (Xanax), lorazepam (Ativan), clonazepam (Klonopin)
• Beta-adrenergic blocker: propranolol (Inderal)
• MAOIs: phenelzine (Nardil), tranylcypromine (Parnate)
• SSRIs: fluoxetine (Prozac), paroxetine (Paxil), sertraline (Zoloft)
• TCAs: imipramine (Tofranil), amitriptyline (Elavil)

INTERVENTIONS AND RATIONALES
• Help the client to identify stressors *to initiate effective coping.*
• Provide for client safety *because the client's ineffective coping, coupled with the intensity of the reaction and poor impulse control, increases the risk of injury.*
• Encourage the client to explore the traumatic event and the meaning of the event *to promote effective coping.*
• Assist the client with problem solving and resolving guilt *to help him understand that uncontrollable factors were responsible for the trauma and the event was beyond his personal control.*

Teaching topics

• Explanation of the disorder and treatment plan
• Medication use and possible adverse effects
• Learning relaxation techniques
• Promoting social interaction
• Contact information for counseling and support groups

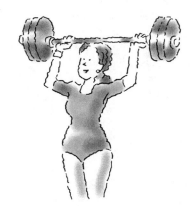

Pump up on practice questions

1.   A nurse is caring for a client who is experiencing a panic attack. Which intervention is most appropriate?
  1.   Tell the client that there's no need to panic.
  2.   Speak in short, simple sentences.
  3.   Explain that there's no need to worry.
  4.   Give the client a detailed explanation of his panic reaction.

Answer: 2. The client experiencing a panic attack is unable to focus and his ability to relate to others is diminished; therefore, short, simple sentences are the most effective means of communication. Telling the client that there's no need to panic or that he's safe, or offering detailed explanations invalidates the client's feelings of anxiety.

➡ **NCLEX keys**
Client needs category: Psychosocial integrity
Client needs subcategory: None
Cognitive level: Analysis

2.   A nurse is caring for a client who reports that she feels a choking sensation in her throat, a racing heart, and fearfulness. These symptoms have occurred almost daily for the past 3 months. Suspecting a psychological component the nurse anticipates administering:
  1.   benzodiazepines.
  2.   proton pump inhibitors.
  3.   nitroprusside.
  4.   lithium carbonate.

Answer: 1. Pharmacologic management would consist of either tricyclic antidepressants or benzodiazepines. Proton pump inhibitors are used for GI disorders. Nitroprusside is a vasodilator used for hypertensive emergencies. Lithium carbonate is an antimanic agent.

➡ **NCLEX keys**
Client needs category: Physiological integrity
Client needs subcategory: Pharmacological and parenteral therapies
Cognitive level: Application

3.   A client who experiences panic disorder states that he's frequently overwhelmed by feelings of powerlessness. In working with this client, the nurse should initiate which intervention?
  1.   Assist the client to recognize unnecessary risk-taking.
  2.   Explore with the client issues related to identity problems.
  3.   Teach the client problem-solving and decision-making skills.
  4.   Have the client discuss the things he desires in a relationship.

Answer: 3. A client with panic disorder commonly has feelings of powerlessness and helplessness, and can easily feel out of control.

Teaching the client problem-solving and decision-making skills can promote the ability to cope and to have a sense of personal control. A client who experiences panic disorder typically doesn't tend to engage in high-risk behaviors or have identity problems. A discussion about relationships is premature for this client.

➡ NCLEX keys

Client needs category: Psychosocial integrity
Client needs subcategory: None
Cognitive level: Application

4. A nurse is assessing a client who struggles with social phobia. Which assessment question does the nurse need to ask?
   1. "Do you drink alcohol or use illicit drugs?"
   2. "Do you use physical outlets to handle anger?"
   3. "Do you often struggle to control your impulses?
   4. "Do you have a history of being an underachiever?"

Answer: 1. Clients with social phobia are highly likely to consume alcohol or use or abuse other substances to control the fear they experience in specific social situations. Clients with social phobia don't tend to be angry or aggressive, struggle to control their impulses, or have a history of under-achievement.

➡ NCLEX keys

Client needs category: Psychosocial integrity
Client needs subcategory: None
Cognitive level: Application

5. After a nurse teaches a client with generalized anxiety disorder some strategies for coping with stressors, another goal for the client would be to:
   1. recognize the signs associated with an elevation in mood.
   2. learn to obtain assistance when his anxiety is increasing.
   3. develop guidelines for decreasing manipulative behavior of peers.
   4. explore ways to facilitate participation in self-care activities.

Answer: 2. It's important for a client to identify when his anxiety is escalating, when his anxiety may be getting out of control, and when seeking help is necessary. Recognizing the signs associated with an elevation in mood, developing guidelines for decreasing manipulative behavior of peers, and exploring ways to facilitate participation in self-care activities are goals appropriate for a client diagnosed with bipolar disorder, not generalized anxiety disorder.

➡ NCLEX keys

Client needs category: Psychosocial integrity
Client needs subcategory: None
Cognitive level: Application

6. A client with posttraumatic stress disorder (PTSD) is preparing for a family meeting. The nurse who's working with the client should encourage him to share which topic with family members?
   1. Struggling to stop engaging in people-pleasing behaviors
   2. Using medications to help cope with feelings of survivor guilt
   3. Difficulty being emotionally attached to people
   4. Difficulty handling the hallucinations experienced after a trauma

Answer: 3. Clients who suffer from PTSD tend to avoid emotional attachments as a way to protect themselves from the trauma they've experienced. Clients with PTSD don't tend to engage in people-pleasing behaviors or experience hallucinations after the experience of extreme trauma and loss. Although clients with PTSD may be prescribed medications to assist in symptom reduction, there aren't any drugs used specifically to help clients handle their feelings of survivor guilt.

➡ NCLEX keys
Client needs category: Psychosocial integrity
Client needs subcategory: None
Cognitive level: Application

7. A nurse is observing a client on a medical unit who's pacing the room, shaking his head from side to side, and clasping and unclasping his hands. As the nurse reviews the client's health history, she should be alert for information about which medication that could be linked to the client's behavior?
  1. Anticholinergics
  2. Vasodilators
  3. Antiemetics
  4. Steroids

Answer: 4. Clients who have taken steroids can experience a manic episode. Anticholinergic, vasodilator, and antiemetic drugs don't induce a manic episode.

➡ NCLEX keys
Client needs category: Psychosocial integrity
Client needs subcategory: None
Cognitive level: Application

8. A nurse is caring for a client who has generalized anxiety disorder. Which statement about this client is true?
  1. The client has regular obsessions.
  2. Relaxation techniques are necessary for cure.
  3. Nightmares and flashbacks are common in this client.
  4. His anxiety lasts longer than 6 months.

Answer: 4. Constant patterns of anxiety that affect the client for more than 6 months and interfere with normal activities are characteristic of generalized anxiety disorder. Pharmaceutical therapy with benzodiazepines can help. Clients having regular obsessions are probably suffering from obsessive-compulsive disorder. Nightmares and flashbacks are typical symptoms of posttraumatic stress disorder.

➡ NCLEX keys
Client needs category: Psychosocial integrity
Client needs subcategory: None
Cognitive level: Analysis

9. A client with the nursing diagnosis of *fear related to being embarrassed in the presence of others* exhibits symptoms of social phobia. What should be the goals for this client? Select all that apply.
  1. Manage his fear in group situations.
  2. Develop a plan to avoid situations that may cause stress.
  3. Verbalize feelings that occur in stressful situations.
  4. Develop a plan for responding to stressful situations.
  5. Deny feelings that may contribute to irrational fears.
  6. Use suppression to deal with underlying fears.

Answer: 1, 3, 4. Improving stress management skills, verbalizing feelings, and anticipating and planning for stressful situations should be goals for this client. Avoidance, denial, and suppression are maladaptive defense mechanisms.

➡ NCLEX keys
Client needs category: Psychosocial integrity
Client needs subcategory: None
Cognitive level: Application

10. A nurse is caring for a client who suffers from depression. She tells the client that he must avoid cheese, yogurt, preserved meats, and vegetables. Based on this information, the client is most likely receiving which drug therapy to treat his depression?
  1. Monoamine oxidase inhibitor (MAOI)
  2. Benzodiazepine
  3. Selective serotonin reuptake inhibitor (SSRI)
  4. Tricyclic antidepressant (TCA)

Answer: 1. This client is receiving an MAOI, which requires the client to avoid tyramine-rich foods, such as cheese, beer, wine, yogurt, and preserved fruits, vegetables, and meats. Benzodiazepines, SSRIs, and TCAs don't require dietary restrictions except avoiding alcoholic beverages.

➡ *NCLEX keys*
Client needs category: Psychosocial integrity
Client needs subcategory: None
Cognitive level: Analysis

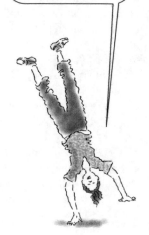

6 Cognitive disorders

Brush up on key concepts

Cognitive disorders result from any condition that alters or destroys brain tissue and, in turn, impairs cerebral functioning. Symptoms of cognitive disorders include cognitive impairment, behavioral dysfunction, and personality changes. The most common cognitive disorders described in the *Diagnostic and Statistical Manual of Mental Disorders*, Fourth edition, *Text Revision* are delirium, dementia, and amnestic disorders.

At any time, you can review the major points of each disorder by consulting the *Cheat sheet* on pages 64 and 65.

Catching up on cognitive disorders
Cognitive disorders are characterized by the disruption of cognitive functioning. Clinically, cognitive disorders are manifested as mental deficits in clients who hadn't previously exhibited such deficits.

Cognitive disorders are difficult to identify and treat. The key to diagnosis lies in the discovery of an organic problem with the brain's tissue.

Cognitive disorders may result from:
• a primary brain disease
• the brain's response to a systemic disturbance such as a medical condition
• the brain tissue's reaction to a toxic substance as in substance abuse.

Brain disruptions
Delirium is commonly caused by the disruption of brain homeostasis. When the source of the disturbance is eliminated, cognitive deficits generally resolve.

Common causes of delirium include postoperative conditions or metabolic disorders, withdrawal from alcohol and drugs, and toxic substances. Toxic substances are especially difficult to deal with because they can have residual effects. Drugs present another problem—a medication may be innocuous by itself but deadly when taken with another medication or food. Elderly clients are especially susceptible to the toxic effects of medication.

Brain defects
Unlike delirium, **dementia** is caused by primary brain pathology. Consequently, reversal of cognitive defects is less likely. Dementia can easily be mistaken for delirium, so the cause needs to be thoroughly investigated.

Polish up on client care

Major cognitive disorders include Alzheimer's-type dementia, amnesic disorder, delirium, and vascular dementia.

Alzheimer's-type dementia

A client with Alzheimer's-type dementia suffers from a global impairment of cognitive functioning, memory, and personality. The dementia occurs gradually but with continuous decline. Damage from Alzheimer's-type dementia is irreversible. Because of the difficulty of obtaining direct pathological evidence of Alzheimer's disease, the diagnosis can be made only when the etiologies for the dementia have been eliminated.

Researchers have developed different scales to measure the progression of symptoms. The Clinical Dementia Rating delineates five stages in the disease. Another, the Global Deterioration Scale, delineates seven.

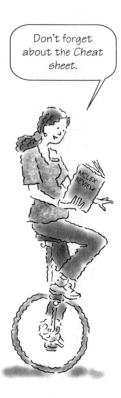

Cheat sheet

Cognitive disorders refresher

ALZHEIMER'S-TYPE DEMENTIA

Key signs and symptoms

Stage 1 (mild symptoms)
- Confusion and memory loss
- Disorientation to time and place
- Difficulty performing routine tasks
- Changes in personality and judgment
- Sleep disturbances

Stage 2 (moderate symptoms)
- Difficulty performing activities of daily living
- Anxiety
- Suspiciousness
- Agitation
- Wandering
- Pacing
- Repetitive behaviors
- Sleep disturbances
- Difficulty recognizing family members

Stage 3 (severe symptoms)
- Loss of speech
- Loss of appetite
- Weight loss
- Loss of bowel and bladder control
- Total dependence on caregiver

Key test results
- Cognitive assessment scale demonstrates cognitive impairment.
- Functional dementia scale shows degree of dementia.
- Magnetic resonance imaging shows apparent structural and neuralgic changes.
- Mini–Mental Status Examination reveals disorientation and cognitive impairment.

Key treatments
- Group therapy
- Anticholinesterase agents: tacrine (Cognex), donepezil (Aricept), rivastigmine (Exelon), galantamine (Razadyne)

Key interventions
- Remove hazardous items or potential obstacles from the client's environment.
- Provide verbal and nonverbal communication that's consistent and structured.
- Increase social interaction.
- Encourage the use of community resources; make appropriate referrals as necessary

> Don't forget about the Cheat sheet.

AMNESIC DISORDER

Key signs and symptoms
- Confusion, disorientation, and lack of insight
- Inability to learn and retain new information
- Tendency to remember remote past better than more recent events

Key test results
- Mini–Mental Status Examination shows disorientation and lack of recall.

Key treatments
- Correction of the underlying medical cause
- Group therapy

Key interventions
- Ensure the client's safety.
- Encourage exploration of feelings.
- Provide simple, clear medical information.

DELIRIUM

Key signs and symptoms
- Altered psychomotor activity, such as apathy, withdrawal, and agitation
- Bizarre, destructive behavior that worsens at night
- Disorganized thinking
- Distractibility
- Impaired decision making
- Inability to complete tasks
- Insomnia or daytime sleepiness
- Poor impulse control
- Rambling, bizarre, or incoherent speech

Key test results
- Laboratory results indicate delirium is a result of a physiologic condition, intoxication, substance withdrawal, toxic exposure, prescribed medicines, or a combination of these factors.

Key treatments
- Correction of underlying physiologic problem
- Cholinesterase inhibitor: physostigmine (Antilirium)
- Antipsychotic agent: risperidone (Risperdal)

Key interventions
- Determine the degree of cognitive impairment.
- Create a structured and safe environment.
- Keep the client's room lit.

Cognitive disorders refresher *(continued)*

VASCULAR DEMENTIA
Key signs and symptoms
- Depression
- Difficulty following instructions
- Emotional lability
- Inappropriate emotional reactions
- Memory loss
- Wandering and getting lost in familiar places

Key test results
- Cognitive Assessment Scale shows deterioration in cognitive ability.
- Global Deterioration Scale signifies degenerative dementia.
- Mini–Mental Status Examination reveals disorientation and recall difficulty.

Key treatments
- Carotid endarterectomy to remove blockages in the carotid artery
- Treatment of underlying condition (hypertension, high cholesterol, or diabetes)
- Aspirin to decrease platelet aggregation and prevent clots

Key interventions
- Orient the client to his surroundings.
- Monitor the environment.
- Encourage the client to express feelings of sadness and loss.

However, most health care providers categorize the disease in only three stages: mild, moderate, and severe. These three stages may overlap, and the appearance and progression of symptoms may vary from one individual to the next.

CONTRIBUTING FACTORS
- Alterations in acetylcholine (a neurotransmitter)
- Altered immune function, with autoantibody production in the brain
- Familial history, such as a first-degree relative with Alzheimer's disease or Down syndrome
- Increased brain atrophy with wider sulci and cerebral ventricles than seen in normal aging
- Neurofibrillary tangles and beta amyloid neuritic plaques, mainly in the cerebral cortex and hippocampus (early) and later in the frontal, parietal, and temporal lobes

ASSESSMENT FINDINGS
Stage 1 (mild symptoms)
- Confusion and memory loss
- Disorientation to time and place
- Difficulty performing routine tasks
- Changes in personality and judgment
- Sleep disturbances

Stage 2 (moderate symptoms)
- Difficulty performing activities of daily living, such as feeding and bathing

- Anxiety
- Suspiciousness
- Agitation
- Wandering
- Pacing
- Repetitive behaviors
- Sleep disturbances
- Difficulty recognizing family members

Stage 3 (severe symptoms)
- Loss of speech
- Loss of appetite
- Weight loss
- Loss of bowel and bladder control
- Total dependence on caregiver

DIAGNOSTIC TEST RESULTS
- Cognitive assessment scale demonstrates cognitive impairment.
- Functional dementia scale shows degree of dementia.
- Magnetic resonance imaging (MRI) shows apparent structural and neurologic changes.
- Mini–Mental Status Examination reveals disorientation and cognitive impairment.
- Spinal fluid contains increased beta amyloid.

NURSING DIAGNOSES
- Bathing self-care deficit
- Impaired memory
- Caregiver role strain

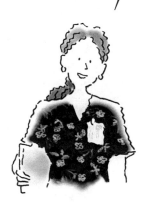

To recall symptoms, it may help to remember that people with Alzheimer's used to be described as "going senile."

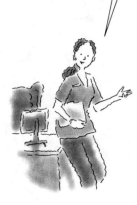

TREATMENT
- Group therapy
- Palliative medical treatment
- Diet adequate in folic acid

Drug therapy
- Anticholinesterase agents: tacrine (Cognex), donepezil (Aricept), rivastigmine (Exelon), galantamine (Razadyne)
- Antipsychotic agents: haloperidol (Haldol), risperidone (Risperdal) in low doses, olanzapine (Zyprexa)
- Benzodiazepines: alprazolam (Xanax), lorazepam (Ativan), oxazepam
- Vitamin E supplements
- Antidepressants: citalopram (Celexa), fluoxetine (Prozac), paroxetine (Paxil), sertraline (Zoloft)

INTERVENTIONS AND RATIONALES
- Remove any hazardous items or potential obstacles from the client's environment *to maintain a safe environment.*
- Monitor food and fluid intake *to ensure adequate nutrition.*
- Identify triggers to agitation (typically, changes in the client's environment) *to maintain client and caregiver safety.*
- When the client is agitated, redirect the client's focus, *to prevent worsening agitation.*

- Simplify the client's environmental tasks and routines *to prevent agitation.*
- Encourage the consumption of foods containing folic acid, such as green, leafy vegetables, citrus fruits and juices, whole wheat bread, and dry beans *to help decrease symptoms of diagnosis.*
- Encourage the client and his caregiver to initiate health care directives and decisions while the client still has the capacity to do so *to ease the burden on the caregiver as the disease progresses.*
- Provide verbal and nonverbal communication that's consistent and structured *to prevent added confusion.*
- State expectations simply and completely *to orient the client.*
- Increase social interaction *to provide stimuli for the client.*
- Encourage the use of community resources; make appropriate referrals as necessary *to find outside support for caregivers.*
- Promote physical activity and sensory stimulation *to alleviate symptoms of the disorder.*

Teaching topics
- Explanation of the disorder and treatment plan
- Medication use and possible adverse effects

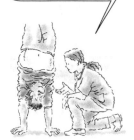

Management moments

Caring for the caregiver

Caring for a family member or friend with Alzheimer's disease can place considerable strain on the caregiver. Therefore, encourage the caregiver to express his feelings. In many cases, caregivers feel confused, fearful, guilty, and grief stricken when a family member is diagnosed with Alzheimer's disease. Help the caregiver cope by:
- discussing situations that are typically stressful, such as dealing with the client's hostility, anxiety, and suspicion
- discussing resources needed to provide adequate, safe care (caring for a client with

Alzheimer's disease can place financial strain on the family)
- developing a plan for the caregiver to obtain assistance from other family members, neighbors, friends, and community resources
- reinforcing the importance of the caregiver establishing a plan for maintaining personal well-being, including recreation, rest, and exercise (the stress of caring for a client with Alzheimer's disease can leave the caregiver susceptible to illness).

- Finding support and education (for caregivers) (see *Caring for the caregiver*)
- Learning stress-relief techniques (for caregivers)
- Contacting the Alzheimer's Association and local support services

Amnesic disorder

In amnesic disorder, the client experiences a loss of both short-term and long-term memory. He can't recall some or many past events. The client's abstract thinking, judgment, and personality usually remain intact. Symptoms may have a sudden or gradual onset and may be transient or long-lasting.

Amnesic disorder differs from dissociative amnesia in that it results from an identifiable physical cause, rather than psychosocial stressors.

CONTRIBUTING FACTORS
- Adverse effects of certain medications
- Brain surgery
- Cerebrovascular events
- Encephalitis
- Exposure to a toxin
- Poorly controlled type 1 diabetes
- Substance abuse
- Sustained nutritional deficiency
- Traumatic brain injury

ASSESSMENT FINDINGS
- Apathy, emotional blandness
- Confabulation in early stages
- Confusion, disorientation, and lack of insight
- Inability to learn and retain new information
- Tendency to remember remote past better than more recent events

DIAGNOSTIC TEST RESULTS
- Medical tests (electrolyte levels, MRI, and computed tomography [CT] scan) confirm a physical basis.
- Mini–Mental Status Examination shows disorientation and lack of recall.
- Neuropsychological testing demonstrates memory deficits.

NURSING DIAGNOSES
- Dressing self-care deficit
- Impaired memory
- Deficient knowledge (disease process and treatment plan)

TREATMENT
- Correction of the underlying medical cause
- Group therapy

Drug therapy
- Anticholinisterase agents: tacrine (Cognex), donepezil (Aricept), rivastigmine (Exelon)

INTERVENTIONS AND RATIONALES
- Ensure the client's safety *because the client may be unable to maintain a safe environment.*
- Use environmental cues—for example, post the client's name and schedule in his room—*to promote orientation.*
- Spend time with the client and talk about the client's health and self-care needs *to encourage greater self-understanding.*
- Identify realistic short-term goals *so the client doesn't become overwhelmed.*
- Encourage exploration of feelings, *which can spark memory.*
- Provide simple, clear medical information *to help the client understand the condition.*

Teaching topics
- Understanding the underlying illness and its relationship to amnestic disorder

Delirium

Delirium is a disturbance of consciousness accompanied by a change in cognition that can't be attributed to preexisting dementia. Delirium is characterized by an acute onset and may last from several hours to several days. It's potentially reversible but can be life-threatening if not treated.

CONTRIBUTING FACTORS
- Cerebral hypoxia
- Effects of medication
- Fever
- Fluid and electrolyte imbalances

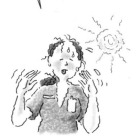

Dehydration is a common cause of delirium, especially in older clients.

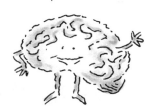

Treatment of delirium focuses on the underlying cause.

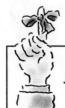

Memory jogger

To help remember the difference between delirium and dementia, think DR. DID (delirium reversible; dementia irreversible damage):

Delirium is reversible (though serious if not treated).

Dementia stems from irreversible damage.

- Infection (especially of the urinary tract and upper respiratory system)
- Metabolic disorders
- Neurotransmitter imbalance
- Pain
- Polypharmacy, especially anticholinergics
- Sensory overload or deprivation
- Sleep deprivation
- Stress
- Substance intoxication or withdrawal

ASSESSMENT FINDINGS
- Altered psychomotor activity, such as apathy, withdrawal, and agitation
- Altered respiratory depth or rhythm
- Bizarre, destructive behavior that worsens at night
- Disorganized thinking
- Disorientation (especially to time and place)
- Distractibility
- Impaired decision making
- Inability to complete tasks
- Insomnia or daytime sleepiness
- Picking at bed linen and clothes
- Poor impulse control
- Rambling, bizarre, or incoherent speech
- Tremors, generalized seizures
- Visual and auditory illusions

DIAGNOSTIC TEST RESULTS
- Laboratory test results indicate delirium is a result of a physiologic condition, intoxication, substance withdrawal, toxic exposure, prescribed medicines, or a combination of these factors.

NURSING DIAGNOSES
- Risk for injury
- Impaired memory
- Disturbed sensory perception (visual)

TREATMENT
- Correction of underlying physiologic problem
- Individual therapy

Drug therapy
- Tranquilizer: droperidol (Inapsine)
- Benzodiazepine: low-dose lorazepam (Ativan)

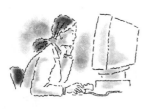

Hmmm... Slurred speech and wandering, along with stroke symptoms? That sounds like vascular dementia.

- Antipsychotic agent: risperidone (Risperdal)
- B vitamins (if related to alcohol)

INTERVENTIONS AND RATIONALES
- Determine the degree of cognitive impairment *to understand and treat the client.*
- Create a structured and safe environment *to prevent the client from harming himself.*
- Institute measures to help the client relax and fall asleep *to comfort him.*
- Keep the client's room lit *to allay his fears and prevent visual hallucinations.*
- Monitor the effects of medications *to prevent exacerbating symptoms.*

Teaching topics
- Explanation of the disorder and treatment plan (to the client's family)
- Medication use and possible adverse effects (to family)
- Contacting community resources
- Managing the client's basic needs

Vascular dementia

Also called *multi-infarct dementia,* vascular dementia impairs the client's cognitive functioning, memory, and personality but doesn't affect the client's level of consciousness. It's caused by an irreversible alteration in brain function that damages or destroys brain tissue.

CONTRIBUTING FACTORS
- Cerebral emboli or thrombosis
- Diabetes
- Heart disease
- High cholesterol level
- Hypertension (leading to stroke)
- Transient ischemic attacks

ASSESSMENT FINDINGS
- Depression
- Difficulty following instructions
- Dizziness
- Emotional lability
- Inappropriate emotional reactions
- Memory loss
- Neurologic symptoms that last only a few days

- Rapid onset of symptoms
- Slurred speech
- Wandering and getting lost in familiar places
- Weakness in an extremity

DIAGNOSTIC TEST RESULTS
- Cognitive Assessment Scale shows deterioration in cognitive ability.
- Global Deterioration Scale signifies degenerative dementia.
- Mini–Mental Status Examination reveals disorientation and recall difficulty.
- Structural and neurologic changes can be seen on MRI or CT scans.

NURSING DIAGNOSES
- Impaired memory
- Risk for injury

TREATMENT
- Carotid endarterectomy to remove blockages in the carotid artery
- Low-fat diet
- Smoking cessation
- Treatment of underlying condition (hypertension, high cholesterol, or diabetes)

Drug therapy
- Aspirin to decrease platelet aggregation and prevent clots

INTERVENTIONS AND RATIONALES
- Orient the client to his surroundings *to alleviate client anxiety.*
- Monitor the environment *to prevent overstimulation.*
- Encourage the client to express feelings of sadness and loss *to foster a healthy therapeutic environment.*

Teaching topics
- Explanation of the disorder and treatment plan (to the client's family)
- Medication use and possible adverse effects (to family)
- Controlling weight and diet
- Exercising to decrease cardiovascular risk factors

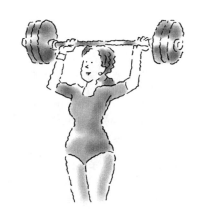

Pump up on practice questions

1. A client is experiencing acute confusion due to poisoning from an accidental exposure to toxic chemicals in the workplace. What type of behavior should the nurse expect this client to demonstrate upon admission to the nursing unit?
 1. Inability to eat without experiencing nausea
 2. Frequently verbalizing ambivalent feelings
 3. Difficulty expressing ideas and needs
 4. Despondency in the presence of family members

Answer: 3. A client with delirium has disorganized thinking and has difficulty expressing his ideas and needs to the nurse. A client in a state of confusion can usually eat without experiencing nausea, doesn't tend to verbalize feelings of ambivalence, and doesn't demonstrate irritability in the presence of others.

➡ *NCLEX keys*
Client needs category: Physiological integrity
Client needs subcategory: Reduction of risk potential
Cognitive level: Application

2. A nurse is caring for a 78-year-old client hospitalized with bilateral pneumonia. Shortly after admission, he became extremely belligerent, confused, and hypotensive, and he developed tachypnea. The nurse prepares the client for intubation, administers anti-infectives stat, and requests that the computed tomography (CT) scan of his head be delayed. Why?

1. His change in mental status was related to hypoxia, metabolic encephalopathy, and sepsis.
2. Taking this client to the radiology department would jeopardize his condition.
3. The client exhibited no signs of focal neurologic impairment.
4. His prognosis was poor and didn't justify a CT scan.

Answer: 1. Severe functional abnormalities and confusion are commonly caused by nonneurologic diseases, especially in elderly clients. Encephalopathies such as these are reversible if the underlying cause is treated. An unstable condition, absence of signs of focal neurologic impairment, and poor prognosis aren't appropriate justifications for delaying a diagnostic CT scan.

➡ *NCLEX keys*

Client needs category: Physiological integrity
Client needs subcategory: Reduction of risk potential
Cognitive level: Analysis

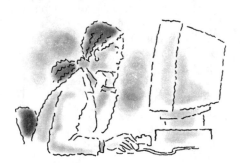

3. A client with dementia suffers from sundown syndrome. Which nursing action should be included in this client's care plan?

1. Integrate the client's cultural preferences into the care provided.
2. Maintain a consistent schedule and sequence of daily activities.
3. Provide opportunities for the client to learn and practice new skills.
4. Serve a warm beverage and snacks in the early evening.

Answer: 2. A client with dementia benefits from a consistent schedule of activities; routine is reassuring and can promote comfort. Cultural preferences don't tend to influence the client's agitation. Providing opportunities to learn and practice new skills could upset the routine and cause additional agitation. Although serving a beverage and snack is a thoughtful strategy to implement, it won't decrease the potential for agitation associated with sundown syndrome.

➡ *NCLEX keys*

Client needs category: Physiological integrity
Client needs subcategory: Reduction of risk potential
Cognitive level: Application

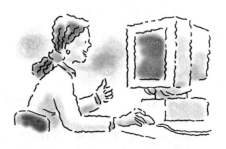

4. A nurse is teaching the wife of a client who has mild symptoms of dementia how to more effectively communicate with her spouse. The teaching would be considered successful if the nurse observed the wife:

1. having a face-to-face conversation with her husband.
2. talking quietly into her husband's ear.
3. discussing only events related to their past.
4. speaking loudly and enunciating each word.

Answer: 1. Speaking face-to-face is the most effective strategy to use when communicating with a cognitively impaired client because it allows the client to pick up visual cues to assist him in understanding his wife. Talking directly into the client's ear prohibits the client from having access to the reinforcement of non-verbal communication. It isn't good practice to assume that all recent memory is gone; it is better to stay current, explain things, and orient as necessary. There's no need to speak loudly and enunciate each word to a client with mild dementia unless he has a hearing impairment.

➥ NCLEX keys
Client needs category: Physiological integrity
Client needs subcategory: Reduction of risk potential
Cognitive level: Application

5. A nurse is assessing a client for vascular dementia. Which finding helps confirm the diagnosis?
1. Positive drug screen for toxicology
2. Findings upon autopsy
3. Magnetic resonance imaging (MRI)
4. Response to electroconvulsive therapy
Answer: 3. Vascular dementia is commonly caused by cerebrovascular disease and small infarctions, which can be detected with MRI. A positive drug screen wouldn't be helpful in diagnosing dementia caused by vascular problems. Attempts to diagnosis vascular dementia wouldn't be delayed until autopsy. Electroconvulsive therapy is occasionally used in the treatment for selected psychiatric disorders but isn't a diagnostic tool for dementia.

➥ NCLEX keys
Client needs category: Physiological integrity
Client needs subcategory: Reduction of risk potential
Cognitive level: Comprehension

6. A nurse is caring for a client with vascular dementia. When planning activities for this client, the nurse should select which activity?
1. Simple crafts
2. Memory games
3. Playing cards
4. Chair exercising
Answer: 4. A client with vascular dementia can benefit from exercising, even chair exercising. Doing simple crafts, playing memory games, and playing cards are inappropriate because a client with vascular dementia manifests memory loss and has difficulty following directions.

➥ NCLEX keys
Client needs category: Physiological integrity
Client needs subcategory: Reduction of risk potential
Cognitive level: Application

7. A nurse is planning care for a client with substance abuse delirium. When the nurse implements care that addresses the client's hygiene needs, which action should be taken?
1. Provide an electric shaver instead of a razor.
2. Administer medication before starting care.
3. Set limits for staff involvement in the client's daily care.
4. Bathe the client, but permit the client's family to dress him.
Answer: 1. For a client with delirium, using an electric shaver is preferable because the client may be predisposed to injury if a standard razor is used. Medication is administered to promote comfort and address illness issues, not to promote the client's participation in self-hygiene. The client requires assistance during the recovery process, not limits for staff involvement. Bathing the client facilitates dependency; the goal is to provide optimal functioning and self-care ability.

➥ NCLEX keys
Client needs category: Physiological integrity
Client needs subcategory: Reduction of risk potential
Cognitive level: Application

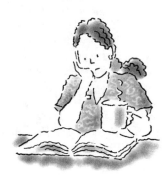

8. A nurse is caring for a client who is diagnosed with delirium. What must the nurse provide for the client?
1. A safe environment
2. An opportunity to release frustration
3. Prescribed medications
4. Medications, as needed, judiciously

Answer: 1. Keeping the client with delirium safe is the most important aspect of care. All other choices are logical and appropriate, but safety issues and meeting the client's basic physiologic needs are of primary importance.

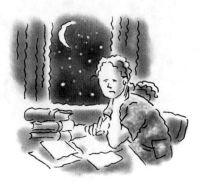

➡ *NCLEX keys*

Client needs category: Safe and effective care environment
Client needs subcategory: Safety and infection control
Cognitive level: Application

9. An elderly male client develops symptoms of delirium after a surgical procedure. To effectively minimize the client's agitation, which action should the nurse take?
1. Discuss the behavior change with the client.
2. Maintain continuous staff-client contact.
3. Introduce appropriate sensory stimulation.
4. Limit unnecessary interactions with the client.

Answer: 2. A client with delirium will benefit from the reassuring presence of familiar staff monitoring his condition and maintaining a consistent environment. A client suffering from delirium can't discuss his behavior change with the nurse. An agitated client must not have additional stimulation. Interactions are necessary to promote calmness, reinforce reality, build trust, and provide support during this stressful period.

➡ *NCLEX keys*

Client needs category: Physiological integrity
Client needs subcategory: Reduction of risk potential
Cognitive level: Application

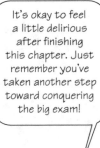

It's okay to feel a little delirious after finishing this chapter. Just remember you've taken another step toward conquering the big exam!

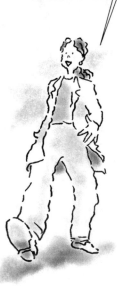

10. A 76-year-old client is admitted to a long-term-care facility with a diagnosis of Alzheimer's-type dementia. The client has been wearing the same dirty clothes for several days and the nurse contacts the family to bring in clean clothing. Which intervention would best prevent further regression in the client's personal hygiene?
1. Encouraging the client to perform as much self-care as possible
2. Making the client assume responsibility for physical care
3. Assigning a staff member to take over the client's physical care
4. Accepting the client's desire to go without bathing

Answer: 1. Clients with Alzheimer's-type dementia tend to fluctuate in their capabilities. Encouraging self-care to the extent possible will help increase the client's orientation and promote a trusting relationship with the nurse. Making the client assume responsibility for physical care is unreasonable. Assigning a staff member to take over restricts the client's independence. Accepting the client's desire to go without bathing promotes bad hygiene.

➡ *NCLEX keys*

Client needs category: Physiological integrity
Client needs subcategory: Reduction of risk potential
Cognitive level: Application

Brush up on key concepts

Personality traits are patterns of behavior that reflect how people perceive and relate to others and themselves. Personality disorders occur when these traits become **rigid** and **maladaptive.** According to the *Diagnostic and Statistical Manual of Mental Disorders*, Fourth edition, *Text Revision,* a personality disorder is a problematic pattern occurring in two of the following four areas: cognition, affectivity, interpersonal functioning, and impulse control. A person with a personality disorder uses maladaptive behavior to relate to others and fulfill basic emotional needs.

At any time, you can review the major points of each disorder by consulting the *Cheat sheet* on pages 74 and 75.

Polish up on client care

Major personality disorders include antisocial personality disorder, borderline personality disorder, dependent personality disorder, and paranoid personality disorder.

Antisocial personality disorder

Antisocial personality disorder leads the client to have a total disregard for the rights of others. Antisocial personality disorder can begin in early childhood and continue into adulthood, but the actual diagnosis requires that the client be at least 18 years old and that the client has displayed some symptoms of the disorder before age 15.

CONTRIBUTING FACTORS
- Childhood trauma
- Genetic predisposition
- Physical abuse
- Sexual abuse
- Social isolation
- Transient friendships
- Unstable or erratic parenting

ASSESSMENT FINDINGS
- Destructive tendencies
- Excessively opinionated nature
- General disregard for the rights and feelings of others
- Impulsive actions
- Inability to learn from past experiences
- Inability to maintain close personal or sexual relationships
- Inflated and arrogant self-appraisal
- Lack of remorse
- Possible concurrent psychiatric disorders
- Power-seeking behavior
- Previous violations of societal norms or rules
- Substance abuse
- Sudden or frequent changes in job, residence, or relationships
- Superficial charm (manipulative)

DIAGNOSTIC TEST RESULTS
- Minnesota Multiphasic Personality Inventory reveals antisocial personality disorder.

NURSING DIAGNOSES
- Social isolation
- Risk for other-directed violence
- Chronic low self-esteem

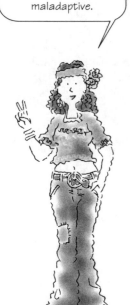

Cheat sheet

Personality disorders refresher

ANTISOCIAL PERSONALITY DISORDER

Key signs and symptoms
• Destructive tendencies
• General disregard for the rights and feelings of others
• Lack of remorse
• Sudden or frequent changes in job, residence, or relationships

Key test results
• Minnesota Multiphasic Personality Inventory reveals antisocial personality disorder.

Key treatments
• Cognitive behavioral therapy
• Antipsychotic: lithium (Eskalith)
• Anxiolitics: alprazolam (Xanax), lorazepam (Ativan) for severe anxiety, insomnia, or agitation
• Beta-adrenergic blocker: propranolol (Inderal) for controlling aggressive outbursts
• Selective serotonin reuptake inhibitors (SSRIs): paroxetine (Paxil), sertraline (Zoloft)

Key interventions
• Help the client to identify manipulative behaviors.
• Establish a behavioral contract.
• Hold the client responsible for his behavior.

BORDERLINE PERSONALITY DISORDER

Key signs and symptoms
• Destructive behavior
• Impulsive behavior
• Inability to develop a sense of self
• Inability to maintain relationships
• Moodiness
• Self-mutilation

Key test results
• Standard psychological tests reveal a high degree of dissociation.

Key treatments
• Milieu therapy
• Individual therapy
• Antimanic medications: carbamazepine (Tegretol), lithium (Eskalith)
• Anxiolytic: buspirone (BuSpar)
• SSRIs: paroxetine (Paxil), fluoxetine (Prozac), sertraline (Zoloft), citalopram (Celexa)

> Loosen up. Personality disorders occur when traits become rigid and maladaptive.

Key interventions
• Recognize behaviors that the client uses to manipulate others.
• Set appropriate expectations for social interaction, and make sure these expectations are met.

DEPENDENT PERSONALITY DISORDER

Key signs and symptoms
• Clinging, demanding behavior
• Fear and anxiety about losing the people they're dependent upon
• Hypersensitivity to potential rejection and decision making
• Low self-esteem

Key test results
• Laboratory tests rule out an underlying medical condition.

Key treatments
• Behavior modification through assertiveness training
• Individual therapy
• Benzodiazepines: alprazolam (Xanax), lorazepam (Ativan), clonazepam (Klonopin)
• SSRIs: paroxetine (Paxil), citalopram (Celexa)
• Tricyclic antidepressants: imipramine (Tofranil), desipramine (Norpramin)

Key interventions
• Encourage activities that require decision making (balancing a checkbook, planning meals, paying bills).
• Help the client to identify manipulative behaviors, focusing on specific examples.

PARANOID PERSONALITY DISORDER

Key signs and symptoms
• Feelings of being deceived
• Hostility
• Major distortions of reality
• Social isolation
• Suspiciousness, mistrusting friends and relatives

Personality disorders refresher *(continued)*

PARANOID PERSONALITY DISORDER *(CONTINUED)*

Key treatments
- Possible drug-free treatment to reduce the chance of causing increased paranoia
- Individual therapy
- Antipsychotic agents: olanzapine (Zyprexa), risperidone (Risperdal), chlorpromazine, thioridazine, fluphenazine, haloperidol (Haldol) in low doses
- SSRIs: paroxetine (Paxil), citalopram (Celexa), sertraline (Zoloft)

Key interventions
- Establish a therapeutic relationship by listening and responding to the client.
- Instruct the client in and help him practice strategies that facilitate the development of social skills

TREATMENT
- Alcohol or drug rehabilitation (if appropriate)
- Cognitive behavioral therapy
- Group therapy
- Individual therapy

Drug therapy
- Antipsychotic agent: lithium (Eskalith)
- Anxiolytics: alprazolam (Xanax), lorazepam (Ativan) for severe anxiety, insomnia, or agitation
- Beta-adrenergic blocker: propranolol (Inderal) for controlling aggressive outbursts
- Selective serotonin reuptake inhibitors (SSRIs): paroxetine (Paxil), sertraline (Zoloft)

INTERVENTIONS AND RATIONALES
- Help the client to identify manipulative behaviors *to help counteract the perception that others are extensions of himself.*
- Establish a behavioral contract *to communicate to the client that other behavior options are available.*
- Avoid confrontations and power struggles *to maintain the opportunity for therapeutic communication.* (See *Dealing with antisocial personality disorder,* page 76.)
- Hold the client responsible for his behavior *to promote development of a collaborative relationship.*
- Help the client to manage anger and observe for physical and verbal signs of agitation *to maintain a healthy therapeutic environment.*

Teaching topics
- Explanation of the disorder and treatment plan
- Medication use and possible adverse effects
- Learning appropriate behaviors
- Continuing treatments after discharge

Borderline personality disorder

Borderline personality disorder results in a pattern of instability in a person's mood, interpersonal relationships, self-esteem, self-identity, behavior, and cognition. Impulsiveness is its most prominent characteristic. Borderline personality disorder appears to originate in early childhood.

CONTRIBUTING FACTORS
- Brain dysfunction in the limbic system or frontal lobe
- Decreased serotonin activity
- Early parental loss or separation
- Increased activity in alpha$_2$-noradrenergic receptors
- Major losses early in life
- Physical abuse
- Sexual abuse
- Substance abuse

ASSESSMENT FINDINGS
- Compulsive behavior
- Destructive behavior
- Dissociation (separating objects from their emotional significance)
- Dysfunctional lifestyle
- Emotional reactions, with few coping skills
- Extreme fear of abandonment
- High self-expectations
- Impulsive behavior
- Inability to develop a healthy sense of self

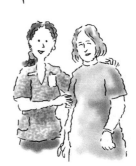

Be prepared for defensiveness. Clients suffering from a personality disorder aren't likely to recognize it in themselves.

Management moments

Dealing with antisocial personality disorder

Aggressive behavior makes caring for the client with antisocial personality disorder a challenge. Clients with this disorder are typically impulsive. They tend to lash out at those who interfere with their need for immediate gratification. Therefore, helping these clients express their anger in a nonviolent manner takes priority. Taking the following precautions may be helpful:
• Maintain a safe environment.
• Encourage the client to verbalize aggressive feelings.
• Talk with the client about appropriate ways to handle anger such as channeling energy into socially acceptable activities.
• Teach the client coping strategies, such as negotiation skills, stress reduction techniques, and ways to communicate anger effectively.

> Be careful! Clients receiving drug therapy for borderline personality disorder should take medications only for targeted symptoms and only for a short period.

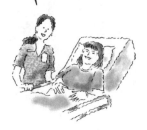

• Inability to maintain relationships
• Moodiness
• Paranoid ideation
• Self-directed anger
• Self-mutilation
• Shame
• Suicidal behavior
• View of others as either extremely good or bad

DIAGNOSTIC TEST RESULTS
• Standard psychological tests reveal a high degree of dissociation.

NURSING DIAGNOSES
• Impaired social interaction
• Risk for self-directed violence
• Chronic low self-esteem

TREATMENT
• Alcohol and drug rehabilitation, as indicated
• Milieu therapy
• Group therapy
• Family therapy
• Individual therapy

Drug therapy
• Antimanic medications: carbamazepine (Tegretol), lithium (Eskalith)
• Anxiolytic: buspirone (BuSpar)
• Monoamine oxidase inhibitor: phenelzine (Nardil)
• Opioid detoxification adjunct agent: naltrexone (ReVia)

• SSRIs: paroxetine (Paxil), fluoxetine (Prozac), sertraline (Zoloft), citalopram (Celexa)

INTERVENTIONS AND RATIONALES
• Recognize behaviors that the client uses to manipulate others *to avoid unconsciously reinforcing these behaviors.*
• Set appropriate expectations for social interaction, and praise the client when these expectations are met *to create a healthy therapeutic environment.*
• Respect the client's sense of personal space *to increase trust.*
• Provide a safe environment. Observe the client frequently *to prevent self-injury.*

Teaching topics
• Explanation of the disorder and treatment plan
• Medication use and possible adverse effects
• Developing problem-solving skills
• Developing therapeutic communication skills
• Implementing relaxation techniques

Dependent personality disorder

The client with dependent personality disorder experiences an extreme need to be taken care of that leads to submissive, clinging behavior and fear of separation. This pattern begins by early adulthood, when behaviors designed to elicit caring from others become predominant. These behaviors arise from the client's perception that he's unable to function adequately without others.

CONTRIBUTING FACTORS
• Childhood traumas
• Closed family system that discourages relationships with others
• Genetic predisposition
• Physical abuse
• Sexual abuse
• Social isolation

ASSESSMENT FINDINGS
• Clinging, demanding behavior
• Exaggerated fear of losing support and approval
• Fear and anxiety about losing the people they're dependent upon
• Hypersensitivity to potential rejection and decision making
• Indirect resistance to occupational and social performance
• Low self-esteem
• Over-reliance on family members
• Tendency to be passive

DIAGNOSTIC TEST RESULTS
• Laboratory tests rule out underlying medical condition.

NURSING DIAGNOSES
• Interrupted family processes
• Ineffective coping
• Chronic low self-esteem

TREATMENT
• Behavior modification through assertiveness training
• Individual therapy
• Group therapy

Drug therapy
• Benzodiazepines: alprazolam (Xanax), lorazepam (Ativan), clonazepam (Klonopin)
• SSRIs: paroxetine (Paxil), citalopram (Celexa)
• Tricyclic antidepressants: imipramine (Tofranil), desipramine (Norpramin)

INTERVENTIONS AND RATIONALES
• Encourage activities that require decision making (balancing a checkbook, planning meals, paying bills) *to promote independence.*
• Help the client establish and work toward goals *to foster a sense of independence.*
• Help the client identify manipulative behaviors, focusing on specific examples, *to decrease the perception that others are an extension of the self.*
• Limit interactions with the client to a few consistent staff members *to increase the client's sense of security.*

Teaching topics
• Explanation of the disorder and treatment plan
• Medication use and possible adverse effects
• Expressing ideas and feelings assertively
• Improving social skills and promoting social interaction

Paranoid personality disorder

Paranoid personality disorder is characterized by extreme distrust of others. Paranoid people avoid relationships in which they aren't in control or have the potential of losing control.

CONTRIBUTING FACTORS
• Genetic predisposition
• Neurochemical alteration
• Parental antagonism

ASSESSMENT FINDINGS
• Bad temper
• Delusional thinking
• Emotional reactions, including nervousness, jealousy, anger, or envy
• Feelings of being deceived
• Hostility
• Hyperactivity
• Hypervigilance
• Irritability
• Lack of humor
• Lack of social support systems
• Major distortions of reality
• Need to be in control
• Refusal to confide in others

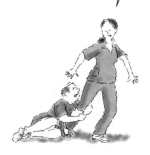

Client stuck on you? Help the client with dependent personality disorder feel secure but maintain appropriate boundaries.

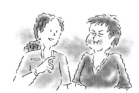

Avoid supporting the paranoid client's delusions but don't attack the delusions directly because this only increases anxiety.

- Self-righteousness
- Social isolation
- Sullen attitude
- Suspiciousness (mistrust of friends and relatives)

DIAGNOSTIC TEST RESULTS
- There are no specific tests for paranoid personality disorder.

NURSING DIAGNOSES
- Ineffective coping
- Chronic low self-esteem
- Social isolation

TREATMENT
- Possible drug-free treatment to reduce the chance of causing increased paranoia
- Individual therapy

Drug therapy
- Antipsychotic agents: olanzapine (Zyprexa), risperidone (Risperdal), chlorpromazine, thioridazine, fluphenazine, haloperidol (Haldol) in low doses
- SSRIs: paroxetine (Paxil), citalopram (Celexa), sertraline (Zoloft)

INTERVENTIONS AND RATIONALES
- Establish a therapeutic relationship by listening and responding to the client *to initiate therapeutic communication.*
- Encourage the client to take part in social interactions *to introduce other people's perceptions and realities to him.*
- Help the client identify negative behaviors that interfere with relationships *so the client can see how his behavior impacts others.*
- Instruct the client in and help him to practice strategies that facilitate the development of social skills *so the client can gain confidence and practice interacting with others.*

Teaching topics
- Explanation of the disorder and treatment plan
- Medication use and possible adverse effects
- Learning coping strategies
- Understanding the disorder (for family and client)

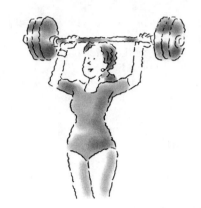

Pump up on practice questions

1. A client with a personality disorder is on a general medical-surgical unit after a recent surgery. The nurse deliberately interacts with this client more than she interacts with another client, who had the same surgery. Both clients are recovering equally well. Why would the nurse do this?
1. Other caregivers commonly minimize contact with such clients.
2. The nurse feels sorry for the client.
3. One client has health insurance; the other client doesn't.
4. The nurse suspects that the first client isn't recovering as well as reported.

Answer: 1. Because clients with personality disorders tend to be demanding and difficult, health care providers with little psychiatric experience commonly try to limit their contact with them. This approch tends to perpetuate behavioral problems, not improve them. This nurse is acting to balance that trend. Sympathy for a client, lack of health insurance, and unfounded suspicions aren't relevant considerations.

➡ *NCLEX keys*
Client needs category: Safe and effective care environment
Client needs subcategory: Management of care
Cognitive level: Application

2. A nurse is caring for a client diagnosed with paranoid personality disorder in an acute care facility. Which intervention should the nurse use to control the client's suspiciousness?

1. Keeping messages clear and consistent, while avoiding deception
2. Providing pharmacologic therapy
3. Providing social interactions with others on the unit
4. Attending to basic daily needs of the client on a consistent basis

Answer: 1. Keeping messages consistent, fostering trust, and avoiding deception will help to decrease suspiciousness. Encouraging social interactions, attending to basic daily needs, and providing pharmacologic therapy are general nursing interventions that are appropriate for any psychiatric disorder.

➡ *NCLEX keys*

Client needs category: Safe and effective care environment
Client needs subcategory: Management of care
Cognitive level: Analysis

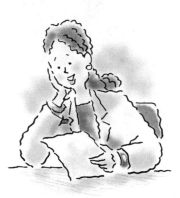

3. A client arrived on the psychiatric unit from the emergency department. His diagnosis is personality disorder, and he exhibits manipulative behavior. As the nurse reviews the unit rules with him, the client asks "Can I go to the snack shop just one time and then I will answer whatever you ask?" What is the nurse's most appropriate response?

1. "Yes, but hurry, because I need to finish your assessment."
2. "Okay but be back in 5 minutes."

3. "No, you can't go."
4. "No, you can't go. The rules here apply to everyone."

Answer: 4. This response sets limits with an appropriate explanation. Allowing the client to go gives in to his manipulative behavior. Simply saying no doesn't explain the purpose of the refusal.

➡ *NCLEX keys*

Client needs category: Psychosocial integrity
Client needs subcategory: None
Cognitive level: Application

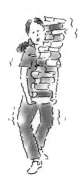

4. During group therapy on the addiction disorder unit, one client says to another client, "That's a stupid thing to be worried about." Which statement by the nurse group facilitator would address the client's unacceptable comment?

1. "It's important to let a person speak about the things that he finds bothersome."
2. "There are alternative social behaviors that you must demonstrate in this group."
3. "Think before you speak or others in the group will act disrespectful to you."
4. "Restate in a positive way what you want to share with your colleague."

Answer: 4. Clients with personality disorders, especially antisocial personality disorder, are typically insensitive to the feelings and rights of others. A nursing response that encourages the client to identify and practice appropriate behavior and provides the opportunity to perform in socially acceptable ways is considered therapeutic care. Telling the client that others should be able to say what they want doesn't address the client's unacceptable behavior. Telling the client that he must demonstrate alternate behaviors helps correct his behavior but doesn't help him correct the situation. Telling the client that others in the group may act disrespectful to him has the potential to come across as threatening or punitive and doesn't assist the client in addressing the issue.

➥ *NCLEX keys*

Client needs category: Physiological integrity
Client needs subcategory: None
Cognitive level: Application

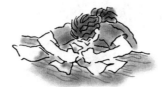

5. A client with a borderline personality has a history of unsuccessful suicidal behavior. After creating a safe environment for this client, the nurse should implement which intervention?

1. Direct the client to make a personal inventory of his resentful situations.
2. Have the client work on addressing the source of his pain and anger.
3. Address with the client how to document problematic conditions as they arise.
4. Tell the client to verbalize disturbing and disorganized thoughts as they occur.

Answer: 2. After securing a safe environment for a client with borderline personality disorder who has a history of incomplete suicide attempts, the nurse should work with the client to discover the origin of his pain and anger. Often, these clients displace their anger and hurt themselves rather than recognize actual painful situations. If the client takes a personal inventory of resentful situations, he won't

learn how to work on his hurtful feelings. Documenting problematic conditions only identifies negative events; it doesn't address how to handle them. Telling the client to verbalize disturbing thoughts as they occur contributes to promoting impulsive and reckless behavior.

➥ *NCLEX keys*

Client needs category: Physiological integrity
Client needs subcategory: None
Cognitive level: Application

6. A nurse is teaching a client about healthy interpersonal relationships. Which characteristic should the nurse include?

1. Minimal self-revelation
2. Willingness to risk self-revelation
3. Ego-dystonic behavior
4. Intimacy and merging of identities

Answer: 2. Willingness to risk self-revelation is a characteristic of a healthy interpersonal relationship. Minimal self-revelation is holding back on the relationship. Ego-dystonic behavior refers to thoughts, impulses, attitudes and behavior that the client feels are distressing, repugnant, or inconsistent with the rest of his personality. Intimacy while maintaining separate (rather than merging) identities is a characteristic of a healthy relationship.

➥ *NCLEX keys*

Client needs category: Psychosocial integrity
Client needs subcategory: None
Cognitive level: Analysis

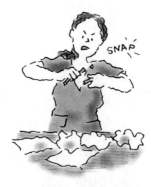

7. A client is court mandated to attend an anger management course. The client uses an aggressive tone to ask the nurse who's teaching the educational session, "Why can't I talk the way I want?" Which is the best therapeutic response from the nurse?

1. "Sometimes our words don't adequately express the point we want to make."
2. "There's often a problem when an attitude of superiority is shown to others."
3. "Tomorrow you may feel differently and you can't change the way you spoke today."
4. "The way a person speaks can be a way of acting out intense feelings."

Answer: 4. The nurse should respond in a way that helps the client recognize that the way a person speaks can escalate anger and arouse anxiety and aggressive responses in others. Although the other responses spoken could be true for some clients, they don't address the client's acting out verbally and attempting to use aggressive words to intimidate others.

➡ *NCLEX keys*

Client needs category: Physiological integrity
Client needs subcategory: None
Cognitive level: Application

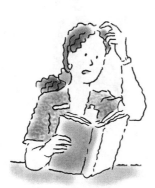

8. The nurse is assisting a client with a dependent personality disorder to work on the goal of developing healthy relationships with family members. Which nursing intervention should the nurse initiate to help the client develop healthy relationships?

1. Determine a structure for each part of the day spent alone.
2. Establish a nurse-client contract based on mutual cooperation.
3. Practice disagreeing with statements verbalized by the nurse.
4. Talk about self while participating in outside activities.

Answer: 3. A client with a dependent personality disorder can become incapacitated by a family member's criticism or disagreement. It is beneficial for the client to practice respectfully refuting or disagreeing with a person (the nurse) who will still remain in the relationship. Determining a structure for time spent alone, establishing a nurse-client contract, and talking about oneself during outside activities won't help a client with dependent personality disorder develop healthy relationships.

➡ *NCLEX keys*

Client needs category: Physiological integrity
Client needs subcategory: None
Cognitive level: Application

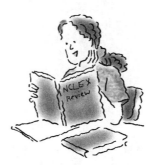

9. A nurse notices that a client with paranoid personality disorder demonstrates some instances of spying behaviors on other clients on the unit. Which nursing intervention should the nurse institute?

1. Address the client's actions that interfere with creating social relationships.
2. Talk with the client about the need to follow the rules established for the unit.

3. Encourage the client to evaluate and change personal thinking patterns.
4. Tell the client that his negative feelings are causing personality changes.

Answer: 1. By addressing the client's actions that interfere with creating social relationships, the nurse can assist the client in becoming aware of the impact of inappropriate behaviors on others and begin to work on how to prevent them. Talking with the client about following unit rules, encouraging him to change thinking patterns, and telling him that his negative feelings are causing personality changes don't address how his spying behavior influences other clients and isolates him from effectively interacting with peers.

➡ *NCLEX keys*

Client needs category: Physiological integrity
Client needs subcategory: None
Cognitive level: Application

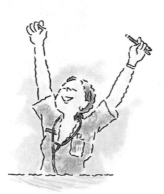

10. A nurse is caring for a client with borderline personality disorder. Which interventions should the nurse perform?
1. Setting limits on manipulative behavior
2. Allowing the client to set limits
3. Using restraints judiciously
4. Encouraging acting out behavior

Answer: 1. Setting limits on manipulative behavior provides the structure that the client needs. Encouraging acting out behavior and allowing the client to set limits would be contraindicated. The need for restraints in a client with borderline personality disorder would be rare, unless coexisting disorders exist.

➡ *NCLEX keys*

Client needs category: Psychosocial integrity
Client needs subcategory: None
Cognitive level: Application

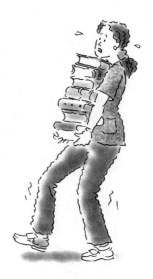

I think I'm getting a borderline anti-NCLEX disorder!

8 Schizophrenic & delusional disorders

Brush up on key concepts

Schizophrenic and delusional disorders fall under the diagnostic umbrella **psychosis.** A psychotic illness is a brain disorder characterized by an impaired perception of reality, commonly coupled with mood disturbances. Psychosis can be either progressive or episodic.

Schizophrenia is characterized by disturbances (for at least 6 months) in thought content and form, perception, affect, sense of self, volition, interpersonal relationships, work and self-care, and psychomotor behavior. Schizophrenia is usually a chronic disorder, equally prevalent in men and women. It begins in young adulthood. It's more common in African and Asian Americans.

Delusional disorders are marked by false beliefs with a plausible basis in reality. Once referred to as *paranoid disorders,* delusional disorders affect less than 1% of the population.

At any time, you can review the major points of each disorder by consulting the *Cheat sheet* on pages 84 and 85.

Positive or negative

Symptoms of schizophrenia may be characterized as positive or negative. **Positive symptoms** focus on a distortion of normal functions; **negative symptoms** focus on a loss of normal functions. Examples of positive symptoms are delusions, hallucinations, disorganized speech, and grossly disorganized or catatonic behavior. Examples of negative symptoms include flat affect, alogia (poverty of speech), avolition (lack of self-initiated behaviors), and anhedonia (minimal enjoyment of activities).

Thought broadcasting

Delusions are false, fixed beliefs that aren't shared by other members of the client's social, cultural, or religious background. Delusions may occur in the form of thought broadcasting, in which the client believes that his personal thoughts are broadcast to the external world. Many times, he believes that his feelings, thoughts, or actions aren't his own.

Look for a theme

Common themes characterize delusions. Delusional themes are described as **persecutory, somatic, erotomanic, jealous,** or **grandiose.** An example of a persecutory delusion is the idea that one is being followed, tricked, tormented, or made the subject of ridicule. The client with erotomanic delusions falsely believes he shares an idealized relationship with another person, usually someone of higher status such as a celebrity. An example of a somatic delusion is a client who believes his body is deteriorating from within. An example of a jealous delusion is the client's feeling that his or her spouse or partner is unfaithful. The client with grandiose delusions has an exaggerated sense of self-importance.

Hearing voices

Most commonly, schizophrenics experience **auditory hallucinations.** When the client hears voices, he perceives these voices as being separate from his own thoughts. The content of the voices is usually threatening and derogatory. Many times, the voices tell the client to commit an act of violence against himself or others.

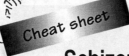

Schizophrenic & delusional disorders refresher

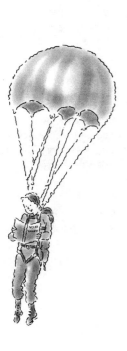

CATATONIC SCHIZOPHRENIA

Key signs and symptoms
• Bizarre postures, waxy flexibility (posture held in odd or unusual fixed positions for extended periods), and resistance to being moved
• Excessive motor activity
• Extreme negativism (resistance to instruction or movement)
• Displacement (switching emotions from their original object to a more acceptable substitute)
• Dissociation (separation of things from their emotional significance)
• Echolalia (repetition of another's words)
• Echopraxia (involuntary imitation of another person's movements and gestures)

Key test results
• Magnetic resonance imaging (MRI) shows possible enlargement of lateral ventricles, an enlarged third ventricle, enlarged sulci, cortical atrophy, and decreased cerebral blood flow.
• Clients show impaired performance on neuro-psychological and cognitive tests.

Key treatments
• Milieu therapy
• Supportive psychotherapy
• Antipsychotics: chlorpromazine, risperidone (Risperdal), olanzapine (Zyprexa)

Key interventions
• Provide skin care and reposition the client every 2 hours.
• Monitor for adverse effects of antipsychotic drugs, such as akathesia, akinesia, parkinson-ism, neuroleptic malignant syndrome, dystonic reactions, and tardive dyskinesia.
• Be aware of the client's personal space; use gestures and touch judiciously.
• Provide appropriate measures to ensure safety and explain to the client why you're doing so.
• Collaborate with the client to identify anxious behavior as well as probable causes.

DISORGANIZED SCHIZOPHRENIA

Key signs and symptoms
• Cognitive impairment
• Fantasy

• Hallucinations
• Loose associations
• Word salad
• Disorganized behavior
• Flat or inappropriate affect

Key test results
• Neuropsychological and cognitive tests indi-cate impaired performance.

Key treatments
• Milieu therapy
• Social skills training
• Supportive psychotherapy
• Antipsychotics (traditional): chlorpromazine, fluphenazine, haloperidol (Haldol), olanzapine (Zyprexa), thioridazine, thiothixene (Navane)
• Antipsychotics (atypical): clozapine (Clozaril), aripiprazole (Abilify), quetiapine (Seroquel), risperidone (Risperdal), ziprasidone (Geodon)

Key interventions
• Help the client meet basic needs for food, com-fort, and a sense of safety.
• During an acute psychotic episode, remove potentially hazardous items from the environ-ment.
• If the client experiences hallucinations, don't attempt to reason with him or challenge his perception of the hallucinations. Instead, ensure safety and provide comfort and support.
• Encourage the client with auditory hallucina-tions to reveal what voices are telling him.
• Encourage the client to participate in one-on-one interactions, and then progress to small groups.
• Provide positive reinforcement for socially acceptable behavior such as efforts to improve hygiene and table manners.
• Encourage the client to express feelings related to experiencing hallucinations.

Schizophrenic & delusional disorders refresher *(continued)*

PARANOID SCHIZOPHRENIA

Key signs and symptoms
- Delusions and auditory hallucinations
- Dissociation
- Inability to trust

Key test results
- MRI shows possible enlargement of ventricles and enlarged sulci. The presence of the enlarged sulci suggests cortical loss, particularly in the frontal lobe.

Key treatments
- Milieu therapy
- Supportive psychotherapy
- Antipsychotics (traditional): chlorpromazine, fluphenazine, haloperidol (Haldol), olanzapine (Zyprexa), thioridazine, thiothixene (Navane)
- Antipsychotics (atypical): clozapine (Clozaril), aripiprazole (Abilify), quetiapine (Seroquel), risperidone (Risperdal), ziprasidone (Geodon)

Key interventions
- Inform the client that you will help him control his behavior.
- Set limits on aggressive behavior and communicate your expectations to the client.
- Use nonphysical techniques, such as redirecting the client's focus and verbal deescalation.
- Maintain a low level of stimuli.
- Provide reality-based diversional activities.
- Provide a safe environment.
- Reorient the client to time and place, as appropriate.

DELUSIONAL DISORDER

Key signs and symptoms
- Hallucinations that are visual, auditory, or tactile
- Inability to trust
- Projection
- Delusions that are erotomanic, grandiose, jealous, persecutory, or somatic

Key test results
- Blood and urine tests eliminate an organic or chemical cause.
- Endocrine function tests rule out hyperadrenalism, pernicious anemia, and thyroid disorders.
- Neurologic evaluations rule out an organic cause.

Key treatments
- Milieu therapy
- Supportive psychotherapy
- Antipsychotics (traditional): chlorpromazine, fluphenazine, haloperidol (Haldol), olanzapine (Zyprexa), thioridazine, thiothixene (Navane)
- Antipsychotics (atypical): clozapine (Clozaril), aripiprazole (Abilify), quetiapine (Seroquel), risperidone (Risperdal), ziprasidone (Geodon)

Key interventions
- Explore events that trigger delusions.
- Don't directly attack the client's delusion.
- When the dynamics of the delusions are understood, discourage repetitious talk about delusions and refocus the conversation on the client's underlying feelings.
- Recognize delusion as the client's perception of the environment.

All over the place

Disorganized thinking or **looseness of associations** is where speech shifts randomly from one topic to another, with only a vague connection between topics. The client may digress to unrelated topics, make up new words (neologisms), repeat words involuntarily (perseveration), or repeat words or phrases similar in sound only (clang association).

Loss of self

The client may demonstrate a blunted, flat, or inappropriate affect manifested by poor eye contact; a distant, unresponsive facial expression; and very limited body language. The sense of self is disturbed, an experience referred to as **loss of ego boundaries**. This loss of a coherent sense of self causes the client to experience difficulty in maintaining an ongoing sense of identity. This may make

it impossible for the client to maintain interpersonal relationships or function at work and in other life roles.

Polish up on client care

Major psychotic disorders include catatonic schizophrenia, disorganized schizophrenia, paranoid schizophrenia, and delusional disorder.

Catatonic schizophrenia

Clients with catatonic schizophrenia show little reaction to their environments. Catatonic

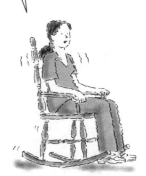

Some catatonic clients may repeat the same motion continuously for hours.

behavior involves remaining completely motionless or continuously repeating one motion. This behavior can last for hours at a time. Catatonic schizophrenia is the least common type of schizophrenia.

CONTRIBUTING FACTORS
- A fragile ego that can't withstand the demands of reality
- Brain abnormalities
- Developmental abnormalities
- Genetic factors
- Hyperactivity of the neurotransmitter dopamine
- An infectious agent or autoimmune response (unproven cause)
- Social or environmental stress, interacting with the person's inherited biological makeup

ASSESSMENT FINDINGS
- Agitation that may be unexpected and dangerous
- Bizarre postures, waxy flexibility (posture held in odd or unusual fixed positions for extended periods), and resistance to being moved
- Excessive motor activity
- Extreme negativism (resistance to instruction or movement)
- Childlike, regressed behavior
- Clang association
- Displacement (switching emotions from their original object to a more acceptable substitute)

- Dissociation (separation of things from their emotional significance)
- Echolalia (repetition of another's words)
- Echopraxia (involuntary imitation of another person's movements and gestures)
- Episodes of impulsiveness
- Fantasy
- Inability to trust
- Little reaction to environment
- Mutism
- Neologism
- Projection
- Purposeless overactivity or underactivity
- Ritualistic mannerisms
- Social isolation
- Speech resembling a word salad (string of words that aren't connected in any way)

DIAGNOSTIC TEST RESULTS
- Magnetic resonance imaging (MRI) shows possible enlargement of lateral ventricles, an enlarged third ventricle, enlarged sulci, cortical atrophy, and decreased cerebral blood flow.
- Clients show impaired performance on neuropsychological and cognitive tests.

NURSING DIAGNOSES
- Risk for impaired skin integrity
- Imbalanced nutrition: Less than body requirements
- Ineffective coping
- Dressing self-care deficit

TREATMENT
- Electroconvulsive therapy (if client isn't responsive to medication)
- Family therapy
- Milieu therapy
- Outpatient group therapy
- Psychoeducational programs
- Social skills training
- Stress management
- Supportive psychotherapy

Drug therapy
- Antiparkinsonian agents: benztropine (Cogentin) for adverse effects of antipsychotics

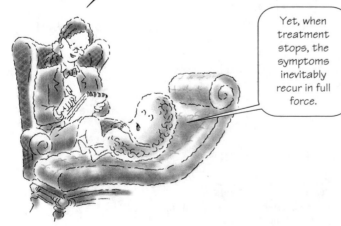

Here's a major difficulty in treating schizophrenia: After clients' more troubling symptoms recede, they believe they can discontinue therapy and medication.

Yet, when treatment stops, the symptoms inevitably recur in full force.

Understanding antipsychotics

Antipsychotic medications act against the symptoms of schizophrenia and other psychoses and are first-line therapy for schizophrenia. These medications can't "cure" the illness, but they alleviate and eliminate symptoms. In some cases, they can shorten the course of the illness.

TRADITIONAL NEUROLEPTICS

There are several antipsychotic (neuroleptic) medications available. The main differences among the medications is in their potency, their therapeutic effects, and their adverse effects. Physicians consider several factors when prescribing an antipsychotic medication, including:
- degree and type of illness
- client's age
- client's body weight
- client's medical history.

TARDIVE DYSKINESIA

Although maintenance treatment is helpful for many people, a drawback is the possibility of developing long-term adverse effects from long-term treatment with antipsychotics. In particular, a condition called tardive dyskinesia, characterized by involuntary movements (usually of the facial muscles), can occur. The disorder may range from mild to severe and can be irreversible.

ATYPICAL NEUROLEPTICS

In 1990, clozapine (Clozaril), an "atypical neuroleptic," was introduced in the United States. This medication is a more effective tool for treating individuals with treatment-resistant schizophrenia, and the risk of tardive dyskinesia is lower. However, because of the potential adverse effect of a serious blood disorder, agranulocytosis, clients who are on clozapine must have weekly blood tests. The expense involved in this monitoring, together with the cost of the medication, has made maintenance on clozapine difficult for many persons with schizophrenia.

Since clozapine was approved in the United States, other atypical neuroleptics have been introduced. Risperidone (Risperdal) was released in 1994, olanzapine (Zyprexa) in 1996, and quetiapine (Seroquel) in 1997. These agents help relieve positive and negative symptoms of schizophrenia. Although they have some adverse effects, these newer medications are generally better tolerated than clozapine or traditional antipsychotics, such as chlorpromazine (Thorazine), and they don't cause agranulocytosis. Disadvantages of atypical neuroleptics include higher cost and a tendency to cause weight gain. They also show a higher incidence of metabolic syndrome, which includes type 2 diabetes mellitus, hypertension, obesity, hyperlipidemia, and coagulation abnormalities.

- Antipsychotics: chlorpromazine, risperidone (Risperdal), olanzapine (Zyprexa) (see *Understanding antipsychotics*)

INTERVENTIONS AND RATIONALES
- Provide skin care and reposition the client every 2 hours *to prevent skin breakdown.*
- Monitor intake and output. *Body weight may decrease as a result of inadequate intake.*
- Monitor for adverse effects of antipsychotic drugs, such as akathesia, akinesia, parkinsonism, neuroleptic malignant syndrome, dystonic reactions, and tardive dyskinesia. *Early identification of extrapyramidal effects can help diminish or eliminate the client's anxiety about these symptoms.*
- Be aware of the client's personal space; use gestures and touch judiciously. *Invading the client's personal space can increase his anxiety.*
- When discussing care, give short, simple explanations at the client's level of understanding *to increase cooperation.*

- Provide appropriate measures to ensure safety and explain to the client why you're doing so. *Implementing and explaining safety measures can promote trust and decrease anxiety while increasing the client's sense of security.*
- Promote a trusting relationship *to create a safe environment in which the client can prepare for social interaction.*
- Briefly explain procedures, routines, and tests *to allay the client's anxiety.*
- Collaborate with the client to identify anxious behavior as well as probable causes. *Involving the client in examination of behavior can increase his sense of control.*
- Provide opportunities for the client to learn adaptive social skills in a nonthreatening environment. *Learning new social skills can enhance the client's adjustment after discharge.*

Memory jogger

To remember the major needs of schizophrenic clients, think **SDS**.

Structure — because they tend to have too little in their lives

Diversion — to distract them from disturbing thoughts

Stress reduction — to minimize the severity of the disorder

Teaching topics
• Explanation of the disorder and treatment plan
• Medication use and possible adverse effects
• Importance of continuing medications as prescribed
• Preventing photosensitivity reactions to drugs by avoiding exposure to sunlight

Disorganized schizophrenia

Disorganized schizophrenics have a flat or inappropriate affect and incoherent thoughts. Clients with this disorder exhibit loose associations and disorganized speech and behaviors.

CONTRIBUTING FACTORS
• A fragile ego that can't withstand the demands of external reality
• Brain abnormalities
• Developmental involvement
• Genetic factors
• Neurotransmitter abnormalities
• Social or environmental stress, interacting with the person's inherited biological makeup

ASSESSMENT FINDINGS
• Cognitive impairment
• Disorganized behavior
• Displacement
• Fantasy
• Flat or inappropriate affect
• Grimacing
• Hallucinations
• Lack of coherence
• Loose associations
• Magical thinking (client believes his thoughts can control others)
• Word salad

DIAGNOSTIC TEST RESULTS
• MRI shows possible enlargement of the ventricles and prominent cortical sulci.
• Neuropsychological and cognitive tests indicate impaired performance.

NURSING DIAGNOSES
• Social isolation
• Dressing self-care deficit
• Ineffective role performance

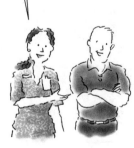

Forming a trusting relationship is a key intervention for schizophrenic clients.

TREATMENT
• Family therapy
• Milieu therapy
• Psychoeducational programs
• Social skills training
• Stress management
• Supportive psychotherapy

Drug therapy
• Antiparkinsonian agents: benztropine (Cogentin) for adverse effects of antipsychotic medications
• Antipsychotics (traditional): chlorpromazine, fluphenazine, haloperidol (Haldol), olanzapine (Zyprexa), thioridazine, thiothixene (Navane)
• Antipsychotics (atypical): clozapine (Clozaril), aripiprazole (Abilify), quetiapine (Seroquel), risperidone (Risperdal), ziprasidone (Geodon)

INTERVENTIONS AND RATIONALES
• Help the client meet basic needs for food, comfort, and a sense of safety *to ensure the client's well-being and to build trust.*
• During an acute psychotic episode, remove potentially hazardous items from the client's environment *to promote safety.*
• Briefly explain procedures, routines, and tests *to decrease the client's anxiety.*
• Protect the client from self-destructive tendencies or aggressive impulses *to ensure safety.*
• Convey sincerity and understanding when communicating *to promote a trusting relationship.*
• Formulate realistic goals with the client. *Including the client in formulating goals can help diminish suspicion while increasing self-esteem and a sense of control.*
• If the client experiences hallucinations, don't attempt to reason with him or challenge his perception of the hallucinations. Instead, ensure the client's safety and provide comfort and support. *Attempts to reason with the client increase anxiety, possibly making hallucinations worse.*
• Encourage the client with auditory hallucinations to reveal what voices are telling him *to help prevent harm to the client and others.*

- Encourage the client to participate in one-on-one interactions, and then progress to small groups *to enable the client to practice newly acquired social skills.*
- Provide positive reinforcement for socially acceptable behavior, such as efforts to improve hygiene and table manners, *to foster improved social relationships and acceptance from others.*
- Encourage the client to express feelings related to experiencing hallucinations *to promote better understanding of the client's experiences and to allow him to vent emotions, thereby reducing anxiety.*

Teaching topics
- Explanation of the disorder and treatment plan
- Medication use and possible adverse effects
- Learning to use distraction techniques

Paranoid schizophrenia

Clients with paranoid schizophrenia have delusions or frequent auditory hallucinations unrelated to reality. They commonly display bizarre behavior, are easily angered, and are at high risk for violence. The prognosis for independent functioning is usually better than for other types of schizophrenia.

CONTRIBUTING FACTORS
- A fragile ego that can't withstand the demands of external reality
- Brain abnormalities
- Developmental involvement
- Genetic factors
- Neurotransmitter abnormalities
- Social or environmental stress, interacting with the person's inherited biological makeup

ASSESSMENT FINDINGS
- Anxiety
- Argumentativeness
- Delusions and auditory hallucinations
- Displacement
- Dissociation
- Easily angered
- Inability to trust
- Potential for violence
- Projection
- Withdrawal or aloofness

DIAGNOSTIC TEST RESULTS
- MRI shows possible enlargement of ventricles and enlarged sulci. The presence of the enlarged sulci suggests cortical loss, particularly in the frontal lobe.
- Neuropsychological and cognitive tests indicate impaired performance.

NURSING DIAGNOSES
- Social isolation
- Ineffective coping
- Risk for other-directed violence
- Anxiety

TREATMENT
- Family therapy
- Group therapy
- Behavior management techniques
- Milieu therapy
- Psychoeducational programs
- Social skills training
- Stress management
- Supportive psychotherapy

Drug therapy
- Antiparkinsonian agents: benztropine (Cogentin) for adverse effects of antipsychotic drugs
- Antipsychotics (traditional): chlorpromazine, fluphenazine, haloperidol (Haldol), olanzapine (Zyprexa), thioridazine, thiothixene (Navane)
- Antipsychotics (atypical): clozapine (Clozaril), aripiprazole (Abilify), quetiapine (Seroquel), risperidone (Risperdal), ziprasidone (Geodon)

INTERVENTIONS AND RATIONALES
- Inform the client that you will help him control his behavior *to promote feelings of safety.*
- Set limits on aggressive behavior and communicate your expectations to the client *to prevent injury to the client and others.*
- Use behavior management techniques *to promote adaptive behavior.*

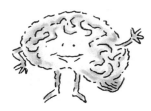

Distraction techniques such as singing along with music can alleviate hallucinations, helping to bring the client back to reality.

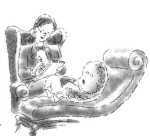

Treatment for a client with paranoid schizophrenia usually combines drug therapy with talk therapy.

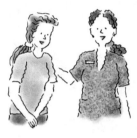

Interventions for schizophrenia promote the client's safety, meet physical needs, and help the client deal with reality.

- Use nonphysical techniques, such as redirecting the client's focus or verbal deescalation *to help the client become calm.*
- Enforce "time-outs" *to prohibit threatening or intimidating behavior.*
- Utilize seclusion and restraints only when nonphysical interventions are ineffective and there's an imminent threat of injury *to protect the client and caregivers from harm.*
- Designate one nurse to communicate with the client and to direct other staff members who care for the client *to foster trust and a stable environment and to minimize opportunities for the client to exhibit hostility.*
- Maintain a low level of stimuli *to minimize the client's anxiety, agitation, and suspiciousness.*
- Provide reality-based diversional activities *to maintain the client's focus and help him stay in touch with reality.*
- Provide a safe environment *to protect the client and others from harm.*
- Reorient the client to time and place as appropriate *to help him cope with his hallucinations and maintain orientation.*
- Be flexible — allow the client to have some control. Approach him in a calm and unhurried manner. Let him talk about anything he wishes, but keep the conversation light and social *to avoid entering into power struggles.*
- Don't take the client's remarks personally. If he tells you to leave him alone, do leave but return soon. *Brief contacts with the client may be most useful at first.*
- Don't make attempts to combat the client's delusions with logic. Instead, respond to feelings, themes, or underlying needs. *Combatting delusions may increase feelings of persecution or hostility.*
- If the client is taking clozapine, stress the importance of returning weekly to the facility or an outpatient setting to have his blood checked *to monitor for adverse effects and prevent toxicity.*
- Teach the client the importance of complying with the medication regimen. Tell him to report adverse reactions instead of discontinuing the drug *to maintain therapeutic drug levels.*

- If the client takes a slow-release formula, make sure that he understands when to return for his next dose *to promote compliance.*

Teaching topics
- Explanation of the disorder and treatment plan
- Medication use and possible adverse effects
- Avoiding exposure to sunlight (to prevent photosensitive reactions to antipsychotics)
- Reporting adverse affects of antipsychotic medications
- Visiting the hospital weekly to monitor blood chemistry

Delusional disorder

Clients with delusional disorder hold firmly to false belief despite contradictory information. They tend to be intelligent and can have a high level of competence but have impaired social and personal relationships. One indication of delusional disorder is an absence of hallucinations.

CONTRIBUTING FACTORS
- Brain abnormalities
- Developmental involvement
- Family history of schizophrenic, avoidant, and paranoid personality disorders
- Lower socioeconomic status
- Neurotransmitter abnormalities
- Social or environmental stress, interacting with the person's inherited biological makeup

ASSESSMENT FINDINGS
- Antagonism
- Brushes with the law
- Delusions that are erotomanic, grandiose, jealous, persecutory, or somatic
- Denial
- Hallucinations that are visual, auditory, or tactile
- Ideas of reference (everything in the environment takes on a personal significance)
- Inability to trust
- Irritable or depressed mood
- Marked anger and violence
- Projection

• Stalking behavior (as in erotomania [the belief that the client is loved by a prominent person])

DIAGNOSTIC TEST RESULTS
• Blood and urine tests eliminate an organic or chemical cause.
• Endocrine function tests rule out hyperadrenalism, pernicious anemia, and thyroid disorders.
• Neurologic evaluations rule out an organic cause.

NURSING DIAGNOSES
• Impaired social interaction
• Ineffective coping
• Risk for other-directed violence

TREATMENT
• Family therapy
• Group therapy
• Milieu therapy
• Psychoeducational programs
• Stress management
• Supportive psychotherapy

Drug therapy
• Antiparkinsonian agent: benztropine (Cogentin) for adverse effects of antipsychotic medications
• Antipsychotics (traditional): chlorpromazine, fluphenazine, haloperidol (Haldol), olanzapine (Zyprexa), thioridazine, thiothixene (Navane)
• Antipsychotics (atypical): clozapine (Clozaril), aripiprazole (Abilify), quetiapine (Seroquel), risperidone (Risperdal), ziprasidone (Geodon)

INTERVENTIONS AND RATIONALES
• Formulate realistic, modest goals with the client. *Including the client when setting goals may help diminish suspicion while increasing the client's self-esteem and sense of control.*
• Establish a therapeutic relationship *to foster trust.*
• Designate one nurse to communicate with the client and to supervise other staff members with regard to the client's care *to build trust and to minimize opportunities for the client to exhibit hostility.*

• Explore events that trigger delusions. Discuss anxiety associated with triggering events. *Exploring triggers will help you understand the dynamics of the client's delusional system.*
• Don't directly attack the client's delusion. *Doing so will increase the client's anxiety.* Instead, be patient in formulating a trusting relationship.
• When the dynamics of the delusions are understood, discourage repetitious talk about delusions and refocus the conversation on the client's underlying feelings. *As the client identifies and explores his feelings, he will decrease reliance on delusional thought.*
• Recognize delusion as the client's perception of the environment. Avoid getting into arguments with the client regarding the content of delusions *to foster trust.*

Teaching topics
• Explanation of the disorder and treatment plan
• Medication use and possible adverse effects
• Learning decision-making, problem-solving, and negotiating skills

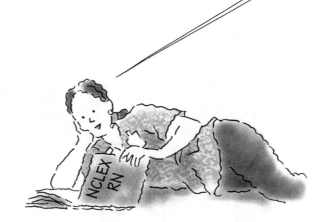

Differentiating delusional disorder from schizophrenia can be tricky. Delusions reflect reality in a somewhat distorted way. Schizophrenia is indicated by scattered and incoherent thoughts unrelated to reality.

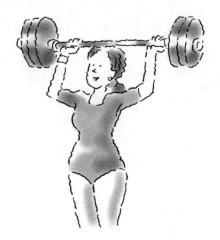

Pump up on practice questions

1. The family of a client with schizoaffective disorder tells the nurse that they haven't been successful in meeting their goal for home management of their son. They report that he's posing a threat to their safety. What primary recommendation should the nurse make based on this information?

    1. Have the client evaluated for a voluntary admission to a mental health facility.
    2. Discuss what the family can do to chemically restrain the client at home.
    3. Tell the family that the client's behavior releases them from the duty of care.
    4. Arrange for respite care because the family could be aggravating the client's condition.

Answer: 1. A voluntary admission is the preferred approach because it involves having the client recognize the problems being experienced and facilitates the client's involvement in treatment. The client's rights would be violated by the use of chemical restraints because the client has the right to freedom from the use of restraints and seclusion. The duty of care is a legal relationship that applies only to the nurse-client relationship—not to the family relationship. Respite care isn't an appropriate recommendation at this time because the safety issue must be addressed and effective treatment and care instituted. It would be prudent to talk to the family about caregiver burden and the option of using respite care after the safety issue is resolved.

➡ NCLEX keys

Client needs category: Safe and effective care environment
Client needs subcategory: Management of care
Cognitive level: Application

2. A nurse is caring for a client who was found huddled in her apartment by the police. The client stares toward one corner of the room and seems to be responding to something not visible to others. She appears hyperalert and scared. How should the nurse assess the situation?

    1. The client may be hallucinating.
    2. The client is suicidal.
    3. Nothing is wrong because the client isn't a threat to society.
    4. The client is malingering.

Answer: 1. The scenario is typical of a client who's hallucinating. Not enough information is available to suggest that she's a threat to society or to herself. Malingering refers to a medically unproven symptom that's consciously motivated.

➡ NCLEX keys

Client needs category: Psychosocial integrity
Client needs subcategory: None
Cognitive level: Analysis

3. A nurse is caring for a client whom she suspects is paranoid. How should the nurse confirm this assessment?

1. Indirect questioning
2. Direct questioning
3. Lead-in sentences
4. Open-ended sentences

Answer: 2. Direct questions (such as "Do you hear voices?" or "Do you feel safe right now?") are the most appropriate technique for eliciting verifiable responses from a psychotic client. The other options may not elicit helpful responses.

➡ NCLEX keys
Client needs category: Psychosocial integrity
Client needs subcategory: None
Cognitive level: Application

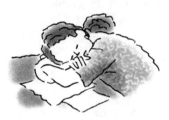

4. A nurse is caring for a client who's experiencing auditory hallucinations. What should be most crucial for the nurse to assess?

1. Possible hearing impairment
2. Family history of psychosis
3. Content of the hallucinations
4. Possible sella turcica tumors

Answer: 3. To prevent the client from harming himself or others, the nurse should encourage him to reveal the content of auditory hallucinations. Assessing for hearing impairment would be inappropriate. Family history, although important because of a possible genetic component, isn't an immediate concern. Olfactory hallucinations, not auditory hallucinations, are associated with sella turcica tumors.

➡ NCLEX keys
Client needs category: Safe and effective care environment
Client needs subcategory: Management of care
Cognitive level: Application

5. A client with schizophrenia is being prepared for discharge. He tells the nurse that he has no home or family and has been living on the street. Which response by the nurse is most appropriate?

1. Offer the name and phone numbers of various homeless shelters in the community.
2. Ask him to further explain how he feels living in such desperate conditions.
3. Contact the physician for a referral to social services for further evaluation.
4. Document the client's response and inform the charge nurse of the situation.

Answer: 3. A person who's homeless may have complex underlying needs and issues that need to be further explored by a trained social service worker to provide the most appropriate interventions. Offering the name and number of shelters may be helpful, but the nurse isn't in a position to follow up on the client's care after discharge. Having the client discuss his feelings may be therapeutic, but at this point, there's a need for direct intervention to ensure the client's safety and well-being. Documenting and informing the charge nurse is useful, but doesn't ensure that there will be appropriate intervention.

➡ NCLEX keys
Client needs category: Safe and effective care environment
Client needs subcategory: Management of care
Cognitive level: Analysis

6. A nurse is preparing to care for a client diagnosed with catatonic schizophrenia. In anticipation of this client's arrival, what should the nurse do?

1. Notify security.
2. Prepare a magnesium sulfate drip.
3. Place a specialty mattress overlay on the bed.
4. Communicate the client's nothing-by-mouth status to the dietary department.

Answer: 3. The nurse should first focus on meeting the client's immediate physical needs and preventing complications related to the catatonic state. The need for intervention from security personnel is unlikely. A magnesium sulfate drip isn't indicated. Nutritional status should be addressed after the client is fully assessed and admitted.

➡ *NCLEX keys*

Client needs category: Physiological integrity
Client needs subcategory: Basic care and comfort
Cognitive level: Application

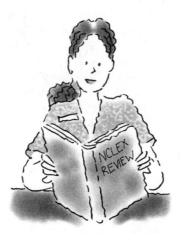

7. A nurse is caring for a client with disorganized schizophrenia. The client is responding well to therapy but has had limited social contact with others. Which of the following interventions is most appropriate?

1. Discourage the client from interacting with others because, if his efforts fail, it will be too traumatic for him.
2. Encourage the client to attend a party thrown for the residents of the facility.
3. Encourage the client to participate in one-on-one interactions.
4. Encourage the client to place a personal advertisement in the local newspaper but not to reveal his mental disability.

Answer: 3. First, encourage the client to participate in one-on-one interactions, and then progress to small groups to enable the client to practice newly acquired social skills.

➡ *NCLEX keys*

Client needs category: Psychosocial integrity
Client needs subcategory: None
Cognitive level: Application

8. A nurse is caring for a schizophrenic client who's well managed on medications. He reveals that he's doing so well, he doesn't think he needs to take medication anymore. What response indicates the nurse best understands the client's diagnosis?

1. "The medications are helping you and if you stop suddenly you could get sick again."
2. "I'll pass this information on to your doctor to see if he feels this might be wise."

3. "You should take the medication for several months after you go home."
4. "You have to take your pills because the doctor has ordered them for you."

Answer: 1. Many schizophrenic clients feel that they can stop taking their medication when their symptoms decrease. The nurse needs to plan client education to reinforce to the client that the medication is what is keeping the symptoms under control. The client will have to take the medication for life, not for a few months after discharge. Telling the client that he has to take the medications doesn't address the client's diagnosis.

➡ *NCLEX keys*

Client needs category: Safe and effective care environment
Client needs subcategory: Management of care
Cognitive level: Analysis

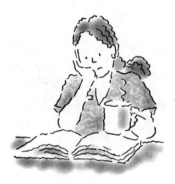

9. A client with schizophrenia is taking the atypical antipsychotic medication clozapine (Clozaril). Which signs and symptoms indicate the presence of adverse effects associated with this medication? Select all that apply.

1. Sore throat
2. Pill-rolling movements
3. Polyuria
4. Fever
5. Flulike symptoms
6. Orthostatic hypotension

Answer: 1, 4, 5. Sore throat, fever, and a sudden onset of other flulike symptoms are signs of agranulocytosis. The condition is caused by a lack of sufficient granulocytes (a type of white blood cell [WBC]), which causes the individual to be susceptible to infection. The client's WBC count should be monitored at least weekly throughout the course of treatment. Pill-rolling movements can occur in those experiencing extrapyramidal adverse effects associated with antipsychotic medication that has been prescribed for much longer than a medication such as clozapine. Polyuria (increased urine) is a common adverse effect of lithium. Orthostatic hypotension is an adverse effect of tricyclic antidepressants.

➡ *NCLEX keys*

Client needs category: Physiological integrity
Client needs subcategory: Pharmacological and parenteral therapies
Cognitive level: Application

10. A nurse is caring for a client who has schizophrenia. What's the first-line treatment for this client?

1. Group therapy
2 Thyroid replacement therapy in selected individuals
3. Milieu therapy
4. Antipsychotics

Answer: 4. Antipsychotics are used as the first-line treatment for schizophrenia. Although thyroid disorders can be a cause of psychotic-like symptoms, they aren't a cause of schizophrenia. Milieu therapy may be helpful but isn't a first-line treatment. Group therapy also wouldn't be a first-line treatment.

➡ *NCLEX keys*
Client needs category: Physiological integrity
Client needs subcategory: Pharmacological and parenteral therapies
Cognitive level: Application

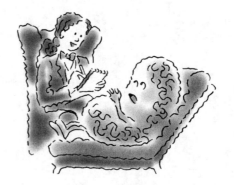

If you can't get enough of psych disorders, you're in luck. There are more coming up in the next chapter.

9 Substance-related disorders

Brush up on key concepts

The relationship between mental illness and substance use and abuse is complex. Alcohol and psychoactive drugs alter a person's perceptions, feelings, and behavior. People may use substances for just that reason. Many people who suffer from emotional disorders or mental illness turn to drugs and alcohol to self-medicate as a way of tolerating feelings. Yet, this method of self-treating doesn't work and commonly makes matters worse.

Nursing care for a substance abuser begins with a thorough assessment to determine which substance is being abused. During the acute phase, care focuses on maintaining the client's vital functions and safety. Rehabilitation involves helping the client to recognize his substance abuse problem and find alternative methods of dealing with stress. The nurse helps the client to achieve recovery and stay drug-free.

At any time, you can review the major points of each disorder by consulting the *Cheat sheet* on page 98.

Social use?
Substance intoxication is the development of a reversible substance-specific syndrome due to ingestion of or exposure to a substance. The clinically significant maladaptive behavior or psychological changes vary from substance to substance.

It's a problem
The essential feature of **substance abuse** is a maladaptive pattern of substance use coupled with recurrent and significant adverse consequences.

The monkey ON the back
Substance dependence is characterized by physical, behavioral, and cognitive changes resulting from persistent substance use. Persistent drug use can result in tolerance and withdrawal.

Just can't get enough
Tolerance is defined as an increased need for a substance or a need for an increased amount of the substance to achieve an effect.

The monkey OFF the back
Withdrawal occurs when the tissue and blood levels of the substance decrease in a person who has engaged in prolonged, heavy use of the substance.

When uncomfortable withdrawal symptoms persist, the person usually takes the drug to relieve the symptoms. Withdrawal symptoms vary from substance to substance.

Classes of controlled substances

Each class of a controlled substance has a different effect on the body and thus produces different reactions. Common classes of controlled substances include:
- cannabis
- depressants
- designer drugs
- hallucinogens
- inhalants
- opiates
- phencyclidine (PCP)
- stimulants.

CANNABIS
Tetrahydrocannabinol, the active ingredient in hashish and marijuana, produces a type

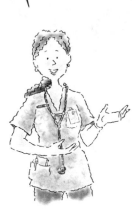

Cheat sheet

Substance-related disorders refresher

ALCOHOL DISORDER

Key signs and symptoms
- Blackouts
- Liver damage
- Pathologic intoxication

Key test results
- CAGE questionnaire indicates alcoholism.
- Michigan Alcoholism Screening test indicates alcoholism.

Key treatments
- Alcoholics Anonymous
- Individual and group therapy
- Medical detoxification and rehabilitation
- Benzodiazepines: chlordiazepoxide (Librium), diazepam (Valium), lorazepam (Ativan)
- Disulfiram (Antabuse) to prevent relapse into alcohol abuse (the client must be alcohol-free for 12 hours before administering this drug)
- Naltrexone (Revia) to prevent relapse into alcohol abuse
- Selective serotonin reuptake inhibitors (SSRIs): fluoxetine (Prozac), paroxetine (Paxil)

Key interventions
- Assess the client's use of denial as a coping mechanism.
- Set limits on denial and rationalization.
- Monitor for signs and symptoms of withdrawal, such as elevated blood pressure, tachycardia, nausea, vomiting, anxiety, agitation, and seizures.
- Have the client formulate goals for maintaining a drug-free lifestyle.

COCAINE-USE DISORDER

Key signs and symptoms
- Elevated energy and mood
- Grandiose thinking
- Impaired judgment

Key test results
- Drug screening is positive for cocaine.

Key treatments
- Detoxification
- Rehabilitation (inpatient or outpatient)

- Narcotics Anonymous
- Individual therapy
- Anxiolytics: lorazepam (Ativan), alprazolam (Xanax)
- Dopamine agent: bromocriptine (Parlodel)
- SSRIs: fluoxetine (Prozac), paroxetine (Paxil)

Key interventions
- Establish a trusting relationship with the client.
- Provide the client with well-balanced meals.
- Set limits on the client's attempts to rationalize behavior.

OTHER SUBSTANCE ABUSE DISORDERS

Key signs and symptoms
- Blaming others for problems
- Development of biological or psychological need for a substance
- Dysfunctional anger
- Feelings of grandiosity
- Impulsiveness
- Use of denial and rationalization to explain consequences of behavior

Key test results
- Drug screening is positive for the abused substance.

Key treatments
- Individual therapy
- Clonidine (Catapres) for opiate withdrawal symptoms
- Methadone maintenance for opiate addiction detoxification
- Levo-alpha-acetylmethadol to treat heroin addiction

Key interventions
- Ensure a safe, quiet environment free from stimuli.
- Monitor for withdrawal symptoms, such as tremors, seizures, anxiety, elevated blood pressure, nausea, and vomiting.
- Help the client understand the consequences of substance abuse.
- Encourage the client to vent fear and anger.

Remember, you can always refer to the Cheat sheet for a quick review of a chapter.

of euphoria, increased appetite, sensory alterations, tachycardia, lack of coordination, and impaired judgment and memory.

DEPRESSANTS

These substances slow down central nervous system (CNS) functioning, causing slurred speech, impaired judgment, and mood swings and can cause respiratory distress when taken in overdose. Common depressants include:
- alcohol
- barbiturates
- benzodiazepines.

DESIGNER DRUGS

These substances are similar to other classes of drugs but they're manufactured with chemical changes that, in some cases, make them more dangerous. The most common designer drugs are:
- adam (ecstasy)
- china white (synthetic type of heroin).

HALLUCINOGENS

These substances produce euphoria, sympathetic and parasympathetic stimulation, and hallucinations, dissociative states, and bizarre, maniclike behavior. They include:
- lysergic acid diethylamide (LSD)
- mushrooms (psilocybin)
- mescaline (from peyote cactus).

INHALANTS

Use of inhalants is called *huffing*. These substances aren't drugs, but some people have found that they can "catch a buzz" from inhaling the fumes. The following products are commonly used:
- glue
- cleaning solutions
- nail polish remover
- aerosols
- petroleum products
- paint thinners.

OPIATES AND RELATED ANALGESICS

These substances, which dull the senses, resulting in sedation and a dreamlike state, can cause respiratory depression and cardiac arrest:
- heroin
- morphine
- codeine

- opium
- methadone
- meperidine (Demerol).

PHENCYCLIDINE

PCP, also known as *angel dust*, heightens CNS function, distorts perception, and causes agitation and aggressive behavior and physiological symptoms, such as hypertension and tachycardia.

STIMULANTS

These substances stimulate the CNS:
- methamphetamines
- cocaine (including crack cocaine)
- caffeine
- nicotine.

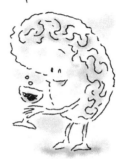

Note that alcohol is a depressant.

Polish up on client care

Almost any controlled substance can potentially become addictive. Although specific circumstances may vary, causes and treatments remain similar for each substance. Common disorders include alcohol disorder, cocaine-use disorder, and other substance abuse disorders.

Alcohol disorder

Although alcohol abuse and dependence are considered substance-related abuse disorders, assessment findings and treatment differ somewhat from that for other substances. Alcohol is a sedative but it creates a feeling of euphoria. Sedation increases with the amount ingested. Respiratory depression and coma can occur with excessive intake.

CAUSES
- Interaction of hereditary, biological, psychological, and environmental factors

CONTRIBUTING FACTORS
- Familial tendency
- Gender (males have increased likelihood of addiction)

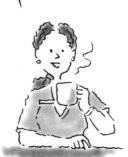

Caffeine and nicotine are classified as stimulants because of the effect they have on the body.

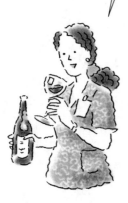

> Because alcohol use is widely accepted, therapeutic communication may involve dealing with a client's rationalizations.

- History of abuse, depression, or anxiety
- Influence of nationality and ethnicity
- Personality disorders

ASSESSMENT FINDINGS
- Adrenocortical insufficiency
- Alcoholic cardiomyopathy
- Alcoholic cirrhosis
- Alcoholic hepatitis
- Alcoholic paranoia
- Blackouts
- Erection problems
- Esophageal varices
- Gastritis or gastric ulcers
- Hallucinations
- Korsakoff's syndrome
- Liver damage
- Muscular myopathy
- Pancreatitis
- Pathologic intoxication
- Peripheral neuropathy
- Wernicke's encephalopathy

DIAGNOSTIC TEST RESULTS
- Drug screening is positive for alcohol.
- CAGE questionnaire indicates alcoholism. (See *The CAGE questionnaire*.)
- Michigan Alcoholism Screening test indicates alcoholism.

NURSING DIAGNOSES
- Ineffective denial
- Ineffective coping
- Risk for injury
- Dysfunctional family processes
- Risk for impaired liver function

TREATMENT
- Alcoholics Anonymous
- Individual and group therapy
- Medical detoxification and rehabilitation

Drug therapy
- Antidepressant: bupropion (Wellbutrin)
- Benzodiazepines: chlordiazepoxide (Librium), diazepam (Valium), lorazepam (Ativan) to treat withdrawal symptoms
- Disulfiram (Antabuse) to prevent relapse into alcohol abuse (the client must be alcohol-free for 12 hours before administering this drug)

- Naltrexone (Revia) to prevent relapse into alcohol abuse
- Selective serotonin reuptake inhibitors (SSRIs): fluoxetine (Prozac), paroxetine (Paxil)

INTERVENTIONS AND RATIONALES
- Monitor for signs and symptoms of withdrawal, such as elevated blood pressure, tachycardia, nausea, vomiting, anxiety, agitation, and seizures. The client may also experience hallucinations, tremors, and delirium tremens. *Monitoring these effects helps identify complications and promotes rapid treatment.*
- Assess the client's use of denial as a coping mechanism *to begin a therapeutic relationship.*
- Encourage the verbalization of anger, fear, inadequacy, grief, and guilt *to promote healthy coping behaviors.*
- Set limits on denial and rationalization *to help the client gain control and perspective.*
- Have the client formulate goals for maintaining of a drug-free lifestyle *to help avoid relapses.*

Teaching topics
- Explanation of the disorder and treatment plan
- Medication use and possible adverse effects
- Understanding substance abuse and relapse prevention
- Maintaining good nutrition
- Available rehabilitation and support groups

Cocaine-use disorder

Cocaine-use disorder results from the potent euphoric effects of the drug. Individuals exposed to cocaine develop dependence after a very short period. Maladaptive behavior follows, resulting in social dysfunction. Cocaine use can also cause serious physical complications, such as cardiac arrhythmias, myocardial infarction, seizures, and stroke.

CONTRIBUTING FACTORS
- Genetic predisposition
- History of abuse, depression, or anxiety
- Personality disorder

ASSESSMENT FINDINGS
- Assault or violent behavior
- Elevated energy and mood
- Grandiose thinking
- Impaired judgment
- Impaired social functioning
- Paranoia
- Weight loss

DIAGNOSTIC TEST RESULTS
- Drug screening is positive for cocaine.

NURSING DIAGNOSES
- Ineffective health maintenance
- Imbalanced nutrition: Less than body requirements
- Risk for other-directed violence

TREATMENT
- Detoxification
- Rehabilitation (inpatient or outpatient)
- Narcotics Anonymous
- Individual therapy

Drug therapy
- Anxiolytics: lorazepam (Ativan), alprazolam (Xanax)
- Dopamine agent: bromocriptine (Parlodel)
- SSRIs: fluoxetine (Prozac), paroxetine (Paxil)
- Propranolol (Inderal)
- Modanafil (Provigil)

INTERVENTIONS AND RATIONALES
- Establish a trusting relationship with the client *to alleviate anxiety or paranoia.*
- Provide the client with well-balanced meals *to compensate for nutritional deficits.*
- Provide a safe environment during withdrawal. *The client may pose a risk to himself or others.*
- Set limits on the client's attempts to rationalize behavior *to reduce inappropriate behavior.*

Teaching topics
- Explanation of the disorder and treatment plan
- Medication use and possible adverse effects
- Contacting Narcotics Anonymous
- Coping strategies
- Managing stress

Other substance abuse disorders

Other substance abuse disorders include all patterns of abuse excluding alcohol and cocaine. These disorders have a great deal in common; however, symptoms vary depending upon the abused substance.

CONTRIBUTING FACTORS
- Familial tendency
- Gender (females have increased likelihood of abusing prescription drugs; males have generally increased likelihood of addiction)
- History of abuse, depression, or anxiety
- Influence of nationality and ethnicity
- Personality disorders

ASSESSMENT FINDINGS
- Attempts to avoid anxiety and other emotions
- Attempts to avoid conscious feelings of guilt and anger
- Attempts to meet needs by influencing others
- Blaming others for problems
- Development of biological or psychological need for a substance
- Dysfunctional anger
- Feelings of grandiosity
- Impulsiveness
- Manipulation and deceit
- Need for immediate gratification
- Pattern of negative interactions
- Possible malnutrition
- Symptoms of withdrawal
- Use of denial and rationalization to explain consequences of behavior

DIAGNOSTIC TEST RESULTS
- Drug screening is positive for the abused substance.

NURSING DIAGNOSES
- Ineffective health maintenance
- Imbalanced nutrition: Less than body requirements
- Risk for other-directed violence

The CAGE questionnaire

This questionnaire is a brief, unscored examination meant to provide a standard for assessing alcohol addiction. Any two positive responses to these four yes-or-no questions strongly suggest alcohol dependence.

1. Have you ever felt you should **C**ut down on your drinking?

2. Have people **A**nnoyed you by criticizing your drinking?

3. Have you ever felt bad or **G**uilty about your drinking?

4. Have you ever had an **E**ye-opener first thing in the morning because of a hangover, or just to get the day started?

During a psychiatric evaluation, always rule out drug or alcohol use; these substances produce symptoms that mimic those of mental illness.

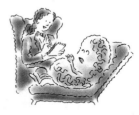

TREATMENT
- Behavior modification
- Employee assistance programs
- Family counseling
- Group therapy
- Halfway houses
- Individual therapy
- Informal social support
- Self-help groups

Drug therapy
- Clonidine (Catapres) for opiate withdrawal symptoms
- Methadone maintenance for opiate addiction detoxification
- Levo-alpha-acetylmethadol to treat heroin addiction
- Buprenorphine (Suleoxone) for opiate withdrawal

INTERVENTIONS AND RATIONALES
- Ensure a safe, quiet environment free from stimuli *to provide a therapeutic setting and to alleviate withdrawal symptoms.*
- Monitor for withdrawal symptoms, such as tremors, seizures, anxiety, elevated blood pressure, nausea, and vomiting *to provide the most comfortable environment possible.*
- Assess the client for polysubstance abuse *to plan appropriate interventions.*
- Help the client understand the consequences of substance abuse *to assist recovery.*
- Provide measures to induce sleep *to help the client manage the discomfort of withdrawal.*
- Encourage the client to vent fear and anger *so that he can begin the healing process.*
- Help the client identify appropriate lifestyle changes *to promote health and prevent complications.*

Teaching topics
- Explanation of the disorder and treatment plan
- Medication use and possible adverse reactions
- Contacting addiction support agencies
- Learning healthy coping mechanisms

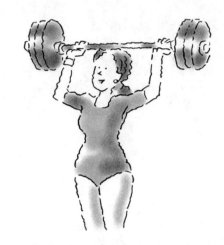

Pump up on practice questions

1. A depressed client states that her daughter uses amphetamines, then asks the nurse, "What will happen when my daughter can't get them and goes into withdrawal from them?" Which response by the nurse would be helpful information for the client?
1. "Your daughter will become very tired and may experience depression."
2. "It's hard to say because she may not have any problems except mild nausea."
3. "Sometimes it can cause people to become agitated and act aggressively toward others."
4. "There's a high risk of seizures and other neurological problems."

Answer: 1. A person withdrawing from amphetamines will become very lethargic and can experience depression or even suicidal tendencies. Telling the client that her daughter may only experience nausea, agitation, or neurological problems wouldn't be providing the client with accurate information about amphetamine withdrawal.

➡ *NCLEX keys*
Client needs category: Physiological integrity
Client needs subcategory: Reduction of risk potential
Cognitive level: Application

2. A nurse is caring for a client who has a history of alcohol abuse. Why would the client act as if he didn't have a problem?

1. The client has never taken the CAGE questionnaire.
2. Denial is a defense mechanism commonly used by alcoholics.
3. Thought processes are distorted.
4. Alcohol is inexpensive.

Answer: 2. Denial is a defense mechanism commonly used by alcoholics. The CAGE questionnaire is a direct method of discovering whether the client is a substance abuser, but the client is likely to deny the problem regardless of whether he's familiar with this assessment tool. Distorted thought processes and the cost of alcohol are less likely to influence the client's use of denial.

➡ NCLEX keys

Client needs category: Psychosocial integrity
Client needs subcategory: None
Cognitive level: Analysis

3. A nurse is caring for a client who exhibits pinpoint pupils as well as decreased blood pressure, pulse, respirations, and temperature. These symptoms may be a sign of intoxication with which substance?

1. Opiate
2. Amphetamine
3. Cannabis
4. Alcohol

Answer: 1. Opiates, such as morphine or heroin, cause these changes. Amphetamines dilate pupils. Cannabis intoxication causes tachycardia, dry mouth, and increased appetite. Alcohol intoxication causes unsteady gait, incoordination, nystagmus, and flushed face.

➡ NCLEX keys

Client needs category: Physiological integrity
Client needs subcategory: Physiological adaptation
Cognitive level: Application

4. A nurse is caring for a client in a substance abuse clinic. The client tells the nurse he needs more heroin to produce the same effect that he experienced a few weeks ago. How should the nurse describe this condition?

1. Tolerance
2. Dependence
3. Withdrawal delirium
4. Compulsion

Answer: 1. Tolerance occurs when more drug is required to produce the same effect. Dependence is a physiologic dependence on a substance. Withdrawal delirium occurs when cessation of a substance produces physiologic symptoms. Compulsion refers to an unwanted repetitive act.

➡ NCLEX keys

Client needs category: Physiological integrity
Client needs subcategory: Physiological adaptation
Cognitive level: Application

5. A nurse is interviewing a client who's currently under the influence of a controlled substance and shows signs of becoming agitated. What should the nurse do?

1. Use confrontation.
2. Express disgust with the client's behavior.
3. Be aware of hospital security.
4. Communicate a scolding attitude to intimidate the client.

Answer: 3. The nurse, for her own protection, should be aware of hospital security and other assisting personnel. The other options may cause a relatively docile client to become belligerent.

➡ NCLEX keys

Client needs category: Safe and effective care environment
Client needs subcategory: Management of care
Cognitive level: Application

6. A nurse is assessing a client who's manifesting the long-term effects of using illicit inhalant drugs. Which laboratory finding should alert the nurse to the need for further assessment and diagnostic testing?

1. Blood dyscrasia
2. Renal dysfunction
3. Thyroid abnormality
4. Muscle atrophy

Answer: 2. A client with a history of using illicit inhalant drugs will have laboratory values that indicate renal problems, and these problems should be addressed immediately by additional assessment and diagnostic testing. Blood dyscrasia, thyroid abnormality, and muscle atrophy aren't typical physiological problems that occur in clients who use illicit inhalant drugs.

➡ NCLEX keys

Client needs category: Physiological integrity
Client needs subcategory: Reduction of risk potential
Cognitive level: Application

7. A nurse is caring for a client with a history of substance abuse. Depending on the substance abused, what might treatment include?

1. Antabuse or methadone
2. Morphine
3. Demerol
4. Lithium

Answer: 1. Antabuse assists in recovery from alcoholism; methadone maintenance is used for opiate abusers. Morphine and Demerol are controlled substances and aren't used in substance abuse treatment. Lithium is used to treat bipolar disorder.

➡ NCLEX keys

Client needs category: Physiological integrity
Client needs subcategory: Pharmacological and parenteral therapies
Cognitive level: Application

8. A nurse is using the CAGE questionnaire as a screening tool for alcohol problems. What do these initials represent?

1. Cut down, Annoyed, Guilty, Eye-opener
2. Consumed, Angry, Gastritis, Esophageal varices
3. Cancer, Alcoholic liver, Gastric ulcer, Erosive gastritis
4. Cunning, Anger, Guilt, Excess

Answer: 1. CAGE stands for "Have you felt the need to **C**ut down on your drinking? Have you ever been **A**nnoyed by criticism of your drinking? Have you felt **G**uilty about your drinking? Have you felt the need for an **E**ye-opener in the morning?"

➡ NCLEX keys

Client needs category: Psychosocial integrity
Client needs subcategory: None
Cognitive level: Analysis

9. A nurse is administering disulfiram (Antabuse) to a client with a history of alcohol abuse. Before receiving therapy, which of the following is required of the client?

1. Be committed to attending AA meetings weekly
2. Admit to himself and another person that he's an alcoholic
3. Remain alcohol-free for 6 hours
4. Remain alcohol-free for 12 hours

Answer: 4. The client must be alcohol-free for 12 hours before initiating disulfiram therapy. Attending AA and acknowledging alcoholism aren't necessary before therapy.

➡ NCLEX keys

Client needs category: Physiological integrity
Client needs subcategory: Pharmacological and parenteral therapies
Cognitive level: Application

10. A client with a history of alcoholism returns to the hospital 3 hours later than the time specified on his day pass. His breath smells of alcohol and his gait is unsteady. What should the nurse say?

1. "Why are you 3 hours late?"
2. "How much did you drink tonight? Drinking is against the rules."
3. "I'm disappointed that you weren't responsible with your day pass."
4. "Please go to bed now. We'll talk in the morning."

Answer: 4. The client can best discuss his behavior when he's no longer under the influence of alcohol. Asking why he's late encourages the client to invent excuses. Being judgmental by admonishing the client or expressing disappointment discourages open communication.

➡ NCLEX keys

Client needs category: Psychosocial integrity
Client needs subcategory: None
Cognitive level: Analysis

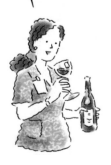

You finished another chapter. Reward yourself—but remember, moderation in all things.

10 Dissociative disorders

Brush up on key concepts

A client with a **dissociative disorder** experiences a disruption in the usual relationship among memory, identity, consciousness, and perceptions. This disturbance may occur suddenly or appear gradually. It's more common in women. Typically, dissociation is a mechanism used to protect the self and gain relief from overwhelming anxiety.

At any time, you can review the major points of each disorder by consulting the *Cheat sheet* on pages 106 and 107.

Polish up on client care

Common dissociative disorders include depersonalization disorder, dissociative amnesia, dissociative fugue, and dissociative identity disorder.

Depersonalization disorder

In depersonalization disorder, the client may feel like a detached observer, passively watching his mental or physical activity as if in a dream. Reality testing remains intact. The onset of depersonalization is sudden and the progression of the disorder may be chronic, characterized by remissions and exacerbations.

CONTRIBUTING FACTORS
- History of physical and emotional abuse
- History of substance abuse
- Neurophysiologic predisposition
- Obsessive-compulsive disorder
- Sensory deprivation
- Severe stress, such as military combat, violent crime, or other traumatic events

ASSESSMENT FINDINGS
- Anxiety symptoms
- Depressive symptoms
- Disturbance in sense of time
- Fear of going insane
- Impaired occupational functioning
- Impaired social functioning
- Low self-esteem
- Persistent or recurring feelings of detachment from mind and body

DIAGNOSTIC TEST RESULTS
- Standard dissociative disorder tests demonstrate a high degree of dissociation. These tests include:
  - diagnostic drawing series
  - dissociative experience scale
  - dissociative interview schedule
  - structured clinical interview for dissociative disorders.

NURSING DIAGNOSES
- Anxiety
- Posttrauma syndrome
- Ineffective role performance
- Ineffective coping

Establishing a support system is a key intervention for depersonalization disorder.

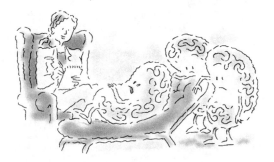

Cheat sheet

Dissociative disorders refresher

DEPERSONALIZATION DISORDER

Key signs and symptoms
- Fear of going insane
- Impaired occupational functioning
- Impaired social functioning
- Persistent or recurring feelings of detachment from mind and body

Key test results
- Standard dissociative disorder tests demonstrate a degree of dissociation. These tests include:
  - dissociative experience scale
  - dissociative interview schedule.

Key treatments
- Individual psychotherapy
- Benzodiazepines: alprazolam (Xanax), lorazepam (Ativan), clonazepam (Klonopin)
- Nonbenzodiazipine: buspirone (Buspar)
- Selective serotonin reuptake inhibitors (SSRIs): fluoxetine (Prozac), citalopram (Celexa), sertraline (Zoloft), paroxetine (Paxil)

Key interventions
- Encourage the client to recognize that depersonalization is a defense mechanism used to deal with anxiety and trauma.
- Assist the client in establishing supportive relationships.

DISSOCIATIVE AMNESIA AND DISSOCIATIVE FUGUE

Key signs and symptoms
Dissociative amnesia
- Altered memory
- Low self-esteem
- No conscious recollection of a traumatic event, yet colors, sounds, sites, or odors of the event may trigger distress or depression
- Sudden onset of amnesia and inability to recall personal information
Dissociative fugue
- Sudden, unplanned travel away from home or place of work
- Confusion about personal identity or taking on a new identity

Key test results
- Standard dissociative disorder tests demonstrate a degree of dissociation. These tests include:
  - diagnostic drawing series
  - dissociative experience scale
  - dissociative interview schedule
  - structured clinical interview for dissociative disorders.

Key treatments
- Individual therapy
- Benzodiazepines: alprazolam (Xanax), lorazepam (Ativan)
- Nonbenzodiazepine: buspirone (BuSpar)
- SSRIs: paroxetine (Paxil), citalopram (Celexa)

Key interventions
- Encourage the client to verbalize feelings of distress.
- Encourage the client to recognize that memory loss is a defense mechanism used to deal with anxiety and trauma.

DISSOCIATIVE IDENTITY DISORDER

Key signs and symptoms
- Guilt and shame
- Lack of recall (beyond ordinary forgetfulness)
- Presence of two or more distinct identities or personality states
- Disturbances not due to direct physiologic effects of a substance

Key test results
- Standard dissociative disorder tests demonstrate a degree of dissociation. These tests include:
  - diagnostic drawing series
  - dissociative experience scale
  - dissociative interview schedule
  - structured clinical interview for dissociative disorders.
- EEG readings may vary markedly among the different identities.

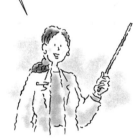

Don't forget to review the highlights of each disorder in the Cheat sheet.

Dissociative disorders refresher *(continued)*

DISSOCIATIVE IDENTITY DISORDER *(CONTINUED)*
Key treatments
- Long-term reconstructive psychotherapy
- Benzodiazepines: alprazolam (Xanax), lorazepam (Ativan), clonazepam (Klonopin)
- Nonbenzodiazepine: buspirone (BuSpar)
- SSRIs: paroxetine (Paxil), escitalopram (Lexapro)
- Tricyclic antidepressants: imipramine (Tofranil), desipramine (Norpramin)

Key interventions
- Assist the client in identifying each personality.
- Encourage the client to identify emotions that occur under duress.
- Monitor risk of self-harm.

TREATMENT
- Individual psychotherapy

Drug therapy
- Benzodiazepines: alprazolam (Xanax), lorazepam (Ativan), clonazepam (Klonopin)
- Nonbenzodiazepine: buspirone (BuSpar)
- Selective serotonin reuptake inhibitors (SSRIs): fluoxetine (Prozac), citalopram (Celcxa), sertraline (Zoloft), paroxetine (Paxil)

INTERVENTIONS AND RATIONALES
- Establish a trusting relationship by conveying acceptance and respect *to provide a safe environment for the client to express distressing feelings.*
- Encourage the client to recognize that depersonalization is a defense mechanism used to deal with anxiety and trauma *because the client needs to first recognize how depersonalization works.*
- Assist the client in establishing supportive relationships *because social interaction reduces the tendency toward depersonalization.*

Teaching topics
- Explanation of the disorder and treatment plan
- Medication use and possible adverse effects
- Effective stress management

Dissociative amnesia and dissociative fugue

In dissociative amnesia, acute memory loss is triggered by severe psychological stress. The client may repress disturbing memories or dissociate from anxiety-laden experiences.

The client may not recall important life events in an attempt to avoid traumatic memories. Recovery from dissociative amnesia is common and recurrences are rare.

With dissociative fugue, the client may travel from home or work and become suddenly confused about personal identity. The client may take on a new identity and can't recall the past.

CONTRIBUTING FACTORS
- Emotional abuse
- Low self-esteem
- Past traumatic event
- Physical abuse
- Sexual abuse

ASSESSMENT FINDINGS
Dissociative amnesia
- Altered memory
- Clinically significant distress or impairment in social or occupational functioning
- Depression
- Emotional numbness
- Low self-esteem
- No conscious recollection of a traumatic event, yet colors, sounds, sites, or odors of the event may trigger distress or depression
- Self-mutilation, suicidal or aggressive urges
- Sudden onset of amnesia and inability to recall personal information

Dissociative fugue
- Sudden unplanned travel away from home or place of work
- Confusion about personal identity or taking on a new identity

NURSING DIAGNOSES
- Anxiety
- Impaired memory

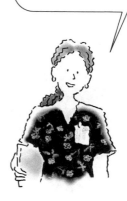

Remember, when working with clients who have dissociative disorders, keep the focus on the client, not on the symptoms.

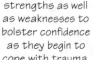

Help psychiatric clients recognize strengths as well as weaknesses to bolster confidence as they begin to cope with trauma.

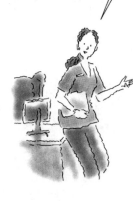

- Social isolation
- Ineffective coping

DIAGNOSTIC TEST RESULTS
- Standard dissociative disorder tests demonstrate a degree of dissociation. These tests include:
    - diagnostic drawing series
    - dissociative experience scale
    - dissociative interview schedule
    - structured clinical interview for dissociative disorders.

TREATMENT
- Hypnosis
- Individual therapy

Drug therapy
- Benzodiazepines: alprazolam (Xanax), lorazepam (Ativan)
- Nonbenzodiazepine: buspirone (BuSpar)
- SSRIs: paroxetine (Paxil), citalopram (Celexa)
- Tricyclic antidepressants (TCAs): imipramine (Tofranil), desipramine (Norpramin)

INTERVENTIONS AND RATIONALES
- Encourage the client to verbalize feelings of distress *to help him deal with anxiety before it escalates.*
- Encourage the client to recognize that memory loss is a defense mechanism used to deal with anxiety and trauma *to help him understand his condition.*

Teaching topics
- Explanation of the disorder and treatment plan
- Medication use and possible adverse effects
- Promoting positive coping skills
- Utilizing relaxation techniques

Dissociative identity disorder

In dissociative identity disorder, formerly known as *multiple personality disorder,* the client has at least two unique identities. Each identity can have unique behavior patterns and unique memories, though usually one

primary identity is associated with the client's name. The client may also have traumatic memories that intrude into his awareness. This disorder tends to be chronic and recurrent.

CONTRIBUTING FACTORS
- Emotional, physical, or sexual abuse
- Genetic predisposition
- Lack of nurturing experiences to assist in recovery from abuse
- Low self-esteem
- Traumatic experience before age 15

ASSESSMENT FINDINGS
- Eating disorders
- Guilt and shame
- Hallucinations (auditory and visual)
- Lack of recall (beyond ordinary forgetfulness)
- Low self-esteem
- Posttraumatic symptoms (flashbacks, startle responses, nightmares)
- Presence of two or more distinct identities or personality states
- Recurrent depression
- Sexual dysfunction and difficulty forming intimate relationships
- Sleep disorders
- Somatic pain syndromes
- Substance abuse
- Suicidal tendencies
- Disturbances not due to direct physiological effects of a substance

DIAGNOSTIC TEST RESULTS
- Standard dissociative disorder tests demonstrate a degree of dissociation. These tests include:
    - diagnostic drawing series
    - dissociative experience scale
    - dissociative interview schedule
    - structured clinical interview for dissociative disorders.
- EEG readings may vary markedly among the different identities.

NURSING DIAGNOSES
- Risk for self-mutilation
- Disturbed personal identity
- Chronic low self-esteem
- Ineffective coping

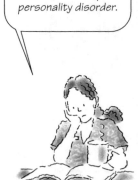

Until recently, dissociative identity disorder was known as *multiple personality disorder.*

TREATMENT
- Hypnosis to revisit the trauma
- Implementation of suicide precautions, if necessary
- Long-term reconstructive psychotherapy
- Treatment for eating disorders, sleeping disorders, and sexual dysfunction

Drug therapy
- Benzodiazepines: alprazolam (Xanax), lorazepam (Ativan), clonazepam (Klonopin)
- Nonbenzodiazepine: buspirone (BuSpar)
- Monoamine oxidase inhibitors: phenelzine (Nardil), tranylcypromine (Parnate)
- SSRIs: paroxetine (Paxil), escitalopram (Lexapro)
- TCAs: imipramine (Tofranil), desipramine (Norpramin)

INTERVENTIONS AND RATIONALES
- Establish a trusting relationship. *Because of a history of abuse, the client will have trouble developing a trusting relationship.*
- Assist the client in identifying each personality *to work toward integration.*
- Encourage the client to identify emotions that occur under duress *to demonstrate that extreme emotions are a normal result of stress.*
- Monitor risk of self-harm *to help maintain client safety.*

Teaching topics
- Explanation of the disorder and treatment plan
- Medication use and possible adverse effects
- Coping techniques to maintain safety

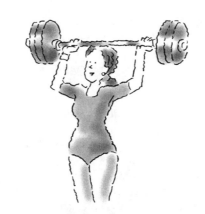

Pump up on practice questions

1. A client who was diagnosed with intermittent explosive disorder is prescribed carbamazepine (Tegretol). What type of blood study would be drawn before discharge as a baseline parameter for determining if the client is experiencing adverse effects of the medication?
 1. Fasting blood glucose
 2. Complete blood count (CBC)
 3. Electrolyte tests
 4. Cholesterol studies

Answer: 2. Because carbamazepine has the potential to cause immunosuppression, the nurse should draw blood for a CBC before discharge. Carbamazepine doesn't alter a client's fasting blood glucose. Neither electrolyte tests nor cholesterol studies would be needed because carbamazepine doesn't alter electrolytes (unless the client experiences an overdose) or affect cholesterol or triglyceride levels.

➥ *NCLEX keys*
Client needs category: Safe and effective care environment
Client needs subcategory: Management of care
Cognitive level: Analysis

2. A nurse is caring for a client diagnosed with dissociative amnesia. The client recently experienced a divorce. How should the nurse help the client deal with traumatic memories?

1. Discourage the client from verbalizing feelings because they will be too traumatic.
2. Force the client to confront her memories about the divorce in a direct, confrontational manner.
3. Tell the client that everything will be all right.
4. Encourage the client to verbalize feelings of distress.

Answer: 4. Encouraging the client to verbalize feelings of distress helps her deal with her anxieties before they escalate. Discouraging the client from verbalizing her feelings may cause anxiety to escalate. Forcing the client to confront her memories will increase her anxiety. Telling the client that everything will be all right offers false reassurance.

➡ NCLEX keys
Client needs category: Psychosocial integrity
Client needs subcategory: None
Cognitive level: Application

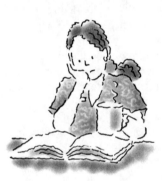

3. A nurse is caring for a client who frequently complains of vague, inconsistent symptoms. Which nursing intervention would be the most appropriate?
1. Screen the client for recent life changes and symptoms of depression, while focusing on physical symptoms.
2. Attempt to minimize physical symptoms, while screening the client for psychological disorders.
3. Exhaust all diagnostic options in ruling out disease before focusing on psychological issues.
4. Refer the client to a psychiatrist.

Answer: 1. It's important not to minimize physical symptoms so that the nurse can demonstrate empathy and establish rapport. The nurse should simultaneously investigate recent life changes and the risk of depression. Although tests and imaging studies may be done in certain cases, review of previous medical records and a physical examination should first be performed to determine the likelihood of physical findings. Referral may be indicated, but not enough information is available.

➡ NCLEX keys
Client needs category: Psychosocial integrity
Client needs subcategory: None
Cognitive level: Analysis

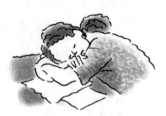

4. A nurse is caring for a client who reports feeling "estranged and separated from himself." How should the nurse describe such symptoms?
1. Intoxication
2. Antimotivational syndrome
3. Existentialism
4. Depersonalization

Answer: 4. Depersonalization is characterized by feelings of separateness from oneself. Intoxication is described as feelings of calm, omnipotence, or euphoria. When a relative lack of motivation occurs within an individual, antimotivational syndrome is present. Existentialism is the philosophy that a person finds meaning in life through experiences.

➡ NCLEX keys
Client needs category: Psychosocial integrity
Client needs subcategory: None
Cognitive level: Comprehension

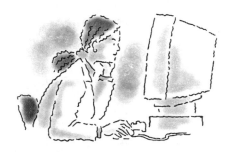

5. A nurse is caring for a client named Susan who has been diagnosed with dissociative identity disorder. Usually, the client arrives to therapy sessions dressed in a tasteful business suit. One day, the client comes to the clinic dressed in a gold lamé mini-dress and insists that her name is Ruby. How should the nurse respond?
1. Ask the client why she's wearing that ridiculous outfit.
2. Refuse to call the client anything but Susan.
3. Ignore the client's behavior.
4. Help the client explore the characteristics of this newly emerged personality.

Answer: 4. The nurse should help the client explore the characteristics of this newly emerged personality to work toward integration. Asking the client about her outfit would further decrease the client's self-esteem. Not calling the client by the name she requests would jeopardize the trusting nurse-client relationship. Ignoring the behavior doesn't help the client work toward integration.

➡ NCLEX keys
Client needs category: Psychosocial integrity
Client needs subcategory: None
Cognitive level: Application

6. A nurse is caring for a client who has a dissociative identity disorder. Which statement about this client is true?
1. The client's sense of selfhood, which sustains an integrated personality structure, is diminished.

2. The client's sense of selfhood continuously sustains an integrated personality structure.
3. The physician has requested that the client dissociate from her usual medical caregivers and be referred to a psychiatrist.
4. The client is experiencing a gender identity crisis.

Answer: 1. Identity is described as a person's sense of selfhood that sustains an integrated personality structure. In a client with a dissociative identity disorder, this sense is altered. The other choices aren't logical.

➡ NCLEX keys
Client needs category: Psychosocial integrity
Client needs subcategory: None
Cognitive level: Comprehension

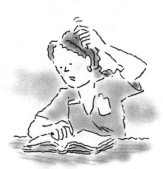

7. A nurse is caring for a client who seems to lack spontaneity, have difficulty distinguishing himself from others, and have difficulty distinguishing between internal and external stimuli. The client describes a vague feeling of estrangement. Which statement would describe this client?
1. He's depressed and should be placed on antidepressants.
2. He may have a depersonalization disorder.
3. He may benefit from electroconvulsive therapy (ECT).
4. He should be placed on suicide precautions.

Answer: 2. The client has characteristics of a depersonalization disorder. He may also suffer from depression, but antidepressants aren't indicated given the available information. ECT wouldn't be appropriate. At this point, the client's behavior doesn't seem suicidal; therefore, such precautions aren't needed.

➡ *NCLEX keys*
Client needs category: Psychosocial integrity
Client needs subcategory: None
Cognitive level: Analysis

8. A nurse is caring for a client who has a depersonalization disorder. Which clear and explicit outcomes should the nurse work toward?
1. Emphasizing strengths, rather than the pathologic condition
2. Focusing on past accomplishments, rather than the current condition
3. Increasing confidence and active participation in planning and implementation of the treatment
4. Eliciting empathetic responses from the client

Answer: 3. Increasing confidence and active participation in planning and implementation of the treatment are measurable outcomes. The active involvement expected of this client will allow for concise documentation. The other options are vague and inappropriate.

➡ *NCLEX keys*
Client needs category: Psychosocial integrity
Client needs subcategory: None
Cognitive level: Application

9. A nurse is caring for a client who has a dissociative disorder. What should the nurse do to assist the client in goal achievement?
1. Provide opportunities for the client to experience success.
2. Praise the client frequently, whether warranted or not.
3. Evaluate components of the client's self-concept.
4. Discuss with the client three categories of behavior commonly associated with an altered self-concept.

Answer: 1. Providing opportunities for the client to experience success would assist him in achieving goals. Praise, if offered in unwarranted situations, will inevitably cause the client to question the caregiver's sincerity.

The other two choices are merely academic exercises and won't assist the client in achieving goals.

➡ *NCLEX keys*
Client needs category: Psychosocial integrity
Client needs subcategory: None
Cognitive level: Application

10. A nurse is caring for a client who has a dissociative disorder and is experiencing amnesia. What could have triggered the amnesia?
1. Severe psychosocial stress
2. Short-acting sedation
3. Conscious sedation
4. Syndrome of inappropriate antidiuretic hormone (SIADH)

Answer: 1. Amnesia in the client with a dissociative disorder can be triggered by severe psychosocial stress. Certain pharmacologic agents given for sedation actually have an amnesic affect, but this doesn't qualify as a dissociative disorder. SIADH isn't associated with amnesia.

➡ *NCLEX keys*
Client needs category: Psychosocial integrity
Client needs subcategory: None
Cognitive level: Analysis

I'm ready to dissociate from this chapter. On to the next one!

Brush up on key concepts

Sexual disorders described in the *Diagnostic and Statistical Manual of Mental Disorders,* Fourth Edition, Text Revision (*DSM-IV-TR*) include **gender identity disorder, paraphilias,** and **sexual dysfunctions.** Gender identity disorder is characterized by an intense and ongoing cross-gender identification. Paraphilias are characterized by an intense, recurring sexual urge centered on inanimate objects or on human suffering and humiliation. Sexual dysfunctions are characterized by a deficiency or loss of desire for sexual activity or by a disturbance in the sexual response cycle.

At any time, you can review the major points of each disorder by consulting the *Cheat sheet* on page 114.

Polish up on client care

This section discusses care for clients with gender identity disorders, paraphilias, and sexual dysfunctions.

Gender identity disorder

Clients with gender identity disorders want to become or be like the opposite sex and are extremely uncomfortable with their assigned gender roles. This disorder can occur in childhood, adolescence, or adulthood.

CONTRIBUTING FACTORS
• Concurrent paraphilias, especially transvestic fetishism
• Feelings of sexual inadequacy and being in the body of the wrong gender

• Generalized anxiety disorder
• Personality disorders

ASSESSMENT FINDINGS
• Anxiety
• Attempts to mask sex organs
• Requests for surgery to remove primary and secondary sex characteristics
• Cross-dressing
• Depression
• Disturbance in body image
• Dreams of cross-gender identification
• Fear of abandonment by family and friends
• Finding one's own genitals "disgusting"
• Ineffective coping strategies
• Peer ostracism
• Persistent distress about sexual orientation
• Preoccupation with appearance
• Self-hatred
• Self-medication such as hormonal therapy
• Strong attraction to stereotypical activities of the opposite sex
• Suicide attempts
• Impairment of social and occupational function

DIAGNOSTIC TEST RESULTS
• Karyotyping for sex chromosomes (not usually indicated) may reveal an abnormality.
• Psychological testing may reveal cross-gender identification or behavior patterns.
• Sex hormones assay (not usually indicated) may reveal an abnormality.

NURSING DIAGNOSES
• Disturbed body image
• Chronic low self-esteem
• Disturbed personal identity
• Ineffective coping
• Risk for suicide

TREATMENT
• Group and individual psychotherapy
• Hormonal therapy

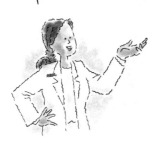

Cheat sheet

Sexual disorders refresher

GENDER IDENTITY DISORDER

Key signs and symptoms
- Dreams of cross-gender identification
- Finding one's own genitals "disgusting"
- Persistent distress about sexual orientation
- Preoccupation with appearance
- Self-hatred

Key test results
- Psychological testing may reveal cross-gender identification or behavior patterns.

Key treatments
- Group and individual psychotherapy
- Hormonal therapy
- Sex-reassignment surgery

Key interventions
- Be careful to demonstrate a nonjudgmental attitude at all times. Don't say anything that would make the client feel ashamed.
- Help the client to identify positive aspects of himself.

PARAPHILIAS

Key signs and symptoms
- Development of a hobby or change in occupation that makes the paraphilia more accessible
- Recurrent paraphilic fantasies
- Social isolation
- Troubled social or sexual relationships

Key treatments
- Individual therapy

Key interventions
- Be careful to demonstrate a nonjudgmental attitude at all times. Don't say anything that would make the client feel ashamed.
- If the client is a threat to others, institute safety precautions per facility protocol.
- Initiate a discussion about how emotional needs for self-esteem, respect, love, and intimacy influence sexual expression.

- Encourage the client to identify feelings, such as pleasure, reduced anxiety, increased control, or shame associated with sexual behavior and fantasies.

SEXUAL DYSFUNCTIONS

Key signs and symptoms
- Anxiety
- Decreased sexual desire (sexual desire disorder)
- Delayed or absent orgasm (orgasmic disorder)
- Depression
- Inability to maintain an erection (sexual arousal disorder)
- Pain with sexual intercourse (sexual pain disorder)
- Premature ejaculation (orgasmic disorder)

Key test results
- Diagnostic tests are used to rule out a physiologic cause for the dysfunction.

Key treatments
- Individual therapy
- Hormone replacement
- Phosphodiesterase inhibitors: sildenafil (Viagra), tadalafil (Cialis), vardenafil (Levitra)

Key interventions
- Encourage the client to discuss feelings and perceptions about his sexual dysfunction.
- Teach the client and his partner alternative ways of expressing sexual intimacy and affection.
- Encourage the client to seek evaluation and therapy from a qualified professional.

Use the Cheat sheet for a quick review of sexual disorders.

- Sex-reassignment surgery

INTERVENTIONS AND RATIONALES
- Be careful to demonstrate a nonjudgmental attitude at all times. Don't say anything that would make the client feel ashamed. *It's the client's needs and feelings, not your opinions, that matter.*
- Provide emotional support and empathy as the client discusses fears and concerns *to help him deal with anxiety.*
- Help the client to identify positive aspects of himself *to alleviate feelings of shame and distress.*
- Encourage the client to participate in support groups *so the client can gain empathy from others and find a safe environment to discuss concerns.*

Teaching topics
- Explanation of the disorder and treatment plan
- Medication use and possible adverse effects
- Available support groups and follow-up care

Paraphilias

A paraphilia is defined as a recurrent, intense sexual urge or fantasy, generally involving nonhuman subjects, children, nonconsenting partners, or the degradation, suffering, and humiliation of the client or partners. The client may report that the fantasy is always present but there are periods when the frequency of the fantasy and intensity of the urge vary. The disorder tends to be chronic and lifelong but, in adults, both the fantasy and behavior commonly diminish with advancing age. Inappropriate sexual behavior may increase in response to psychological stressors, in relation to other mental disorders, or when opportunity to engage in the paraphilia becomes more available.

Common paraphilias include:
- exhibitionism (exposing genitals and occasionally masturbating in public)
- fetishism (use of an object to become sexually aroused)
- frotteurism (rubbing one's genital on another nonconsenting person to become aroused)
- pedophilia (sexual activity with a child)
- sexual masochism (being humiliated or feeling pain to become aroused)
- sexual sadism (causing physical or emotional pain to another to become aroused)
- transvestic fetishism (cross-dressing)
- voyeurism (watching others who are nude or engaging in sex to become aroused).

CONTRIBUTING FACTORS
- Childhood incest
- Concurrent mental disorders
- Emotional trauma
- Gender (more likely in males)
- Personality disorders
- Central nervous system tumors
- Closed head injury
- Neuroendocrine disorders
- Psychosocial stressors
- Lack of knowledge about sex
- Sexual trauma

ASSESSMENT FINDINGS
- Anxiety
- Depression
- Development of a hobby or change in occupation that makes the paraphilia more accessible
- Disturbance in body image
- Guilt or shame
- Ineffective coping
- Multiple paraphilias at the same time
- Obsessive-compulsive tendencies
- Purchase of books, films, or magazines related to the paraphilia
- Recurrent paraphilic fantasies
- Sexual dysfunction
- Social isolation
- Troubled social or sexual relationships

DIAGNOSTIC TEST RESULTS
- Penile plethysmography testing may measure sexual arousal in response to visual imagery; however, the results of this procedure can be unreliable.

NURSING DIAGNOSES
- Ineffective sexuality patterns
- Chronic low self-esteem
- Risk for other-directed violence
- Anxiety
- Impaired social interaction

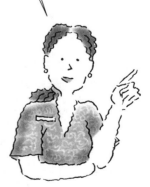

Inappropriate sexual behavior may increase in response to stress.

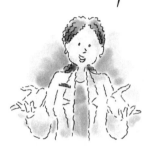

Institute safety precautions if the client with paraphilia is a threat to others.

TREATMENT
• Behavior therapy
• Cognitive therapy
• Individual therapy

INTERVENTIONS AND RATIONALES
• Be careful to demonstrate a nonjudgmental attitude at all times. Don't say anything that would make the client feel ashamed. *It's the client's needs and feelings, not your opinions, that matter.*
• If the client is a threat to others, institute safety precautions per facility protocol *to protect the client and others.*
• Initiate a discussion about how emotional needs for self-esteem, respect, love, and intimacy influence sexual expression *to help the client understand the disorder.*
• Encourage the client to identify feelings, such as pleasure, reduced anxiety, increased control, or shame associated with sexual behavior and fantasies, *to provide insight for developing appropriate interventions.*
• Help the client distinguish practices that are distressing because they don't conform to social norms or personal values from those that may place him or others in serious emotional, medical, or legal jeopardy *to reinforce the need to stop behaviors that could harm the client or others.*

Teaching topics
• Explanation of the disorder and treatment plan
• Contacting Sexaholics Anonymous

Sexual dysfunctions

Sexual dysfunctions are characterized by a disturbance during one or more phases of the sexual response cycle. The most common dysfunctions are:
• orgasmic disorders — The *DSM-IV-TR* lists female orgasmic disorder, male orgasmic disorder, and premature ejaculation. Male and female orgasmic disorders are characterized by a persistent or recurrent delay in or absence of orgasm following a normal sexual excitement phase. Premature ejaculation is marked by persistent and recurrent onset of orgasm and ejaculation with minimal sexual stimulation.
• sexual arousal disorders — These include female sexual arousal disorder and male erectile disorder. With female sexual arousal disorder, the client has a persistent or recurrent inability to attain or maintain adequate lubrication, swelling, and response of sexual excitement until the completion of sexual activity. In male erectile disorder, the client has a persistent or recurrent inability to attain or maintain an adequate erection until completion of sexual activity.
• sexual desire disorders — This category includes hypoactive sexual desire disorder and sexual aversion disorder. The key feature of hypoactive sexual desire disorder is a deficiency or absence of sexual fantasies and the desire for sexual activity. The client usually doesn't initiate sexual activity and may only engage in it reluctantly when it's initiated by the partner. With sexual aversion disorder, the client has an aversion to and active avoidance of genital sexual contact with a sexual partner.
• sexual dysfunction due to a medical condition — Sexual dysfunction may occur as a result of a physiologic problem.
• sexual pain disorders — This category includes dyspareunia and vaginismus. The essential feature of dyspareunia is genital pain associated with sexual intercourse. Most commonly experienced during intercourse, dyspareunia may also occur before or after intercourse. The disorder can occur in males and females. Vaginismus is recurrent or persistent involuntary contraction of the perineal muscles surrounding the outer third of the vagina when vaginal penetration is attempted. In some clients, even the anticipation of vaginal insertion may result in muscle spasm. The contractions may be mild to severe.
• substance-induced sexual dysfunction — This term is used to describe sexual dysfunction resulting from direct physiologic effects of a substance, such as from drug abuse, medication use, or toxin exposure.

CONTRIBUTING FACTORS
• Anger or hostility
• Depression
• Disability

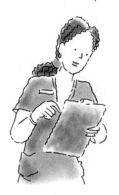

Sexual dysfunction usually accompanies other medical situations, such as surgery, pregnancy, or pharmacologic treatment.

- Drugs or alcohol
- Endocrine disorders
- Genital surgery
- Genital trauma
- Infections
- Lifestyle disruptions
- Medications
- Paraphilia
- Pregnancy
- Religious or cultural taboos that reinforce guilty feelings about sex
- Stress

ASSESSMENT FINDINGS

- Anxiety
- Decreased sexual desire (sexual desire disorder)
- Delayed or absent orgasm (orgasmic disorder)
- Depression
- Disturbance in body image
- Frustration and feelings of being unattractive
- Inability to maintain an erection (sexual arousal disorder)
- Ineffective coping
- Pain with sexual intercourse (sexual pain disorder)
- Poor self-concept
- Premature ejaculation (orgasmic disorder)
- Social isolation

DIAGNOSTIC TEST RESULTS

- Diagnostic tests are used to rule out a physiologic cause for the dysfunction.

NURSING DIAGNOSES

- Impaired social interaction
- Chronic low self-esteem
- Sexual dysfunction

TREATMENT

- Changing medications to decrease symptoms (as appropriate)
- Individual therapy
- Marital or couples therapy
- Penile implant or vacuum pump (for erectile dysfunction)
- Sex therapy
- Treatment of underlying medical condition

- Vaginal dilators
- Vascular surgery for erectile dysfunction

Drug therapy

- Hormone replacement
- Phosphodiesterase inhibitors: sildenafil (Viagra), tadalafil (Cialis), vardenafil (Levitra)
- Alprostadil (Caverject) intracavernously to induce erection

INTERVENTIONS AND RATIONALES

- Establish a therapeutic relationship with the client *to provide a safe and comfortable atmosphere for discussing sexual concerns.*
- Encourage the client to discuss feelings and perceptions about his sexual dysfunction *to help validate his perceptions and reduce emotional distress.*
- Teach the client and his partner alternative ways of expressing sexual intimacy and affection. *Alternative expressions of intimacy may raise the client's self-esteem.*
- Encourage the client to seek evaluation and therapy from a qualified professional *to enable the client to obtain proper diagnosis and treatment.*

Teaching topics

- Explanation of the disorder and treatment plan
- Medication use and possible adverse effects
- Understanding sexual response
- Using alternative sexual positions to promote comfort
- Performing relaxation exercises
- Performing Kegel exercises to improve urethral and vaginal tone
- Contacting self-help groups

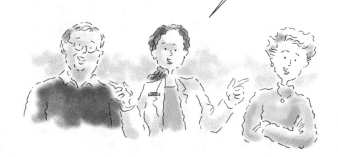

Teach the client and his partner alternative ways of expressing sexual intimacy and affection.

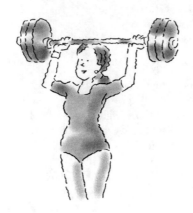

Pump up on practice questions

1. A nurse is caring for a client who's experiencing hypoactive sexual desire. How should the nurse classify this condition?
1. Sexual arousal disorder
2. Sexual pain disorder
3. Sexual desire disorder
4. Orgasmic disorder

Answer: 3. Sexual desire disorders include sexual aversion and hypoactive sexual desire disorder. Sexual arousal disorders include male erectile and female arousal disorders. Examples of sexual pain disorders include dyspareunia and vaginismus. Orgasmic disorders, such as premature ejaculation, affect males and females.

➡ *NCLEX keys*
Client needs category: Psychosocial integrity
Client needs subcategory: None
Cognitive level: Application

2. A nurse is caring for a client who was accused of voyeurism by his neighbors. Which term most appropriately describes such behavior?
1. Paraphilia
2. Depersonalization disorder
3. Dissociative fugue
4. Gender identity disorder

Answer: 1. Paraphilia is a general diagnosis that encompasses such disorders as exhibitionism, fetishism, pedophilia, and voyeurism. Depersonalization disorder is characterized by a feeling of detachment or estrangement from one's self. Dissociative fugue is characterized by sudden, unexpected travel away from home, accompanied by an inability to recall one's past. Gender identity disorder is a separate diagnostic category and isn't related to paraphilias.

➡ *NCLEX keys*
Client needs category: Psychosocial integrity
Client needs subcategory: None
Cognitive level: Application

3. A nurse is caring for a female client who's about to begin thrombolytic therapy to treat an acute myocardial infarction (MI). When the physician questions the client about her last menstrual period, she becomes embarrassed and asks him to leave the room. She then tells the nurse that she underwent sex-reassignment surgery. What should be the nurse's most appropriate response?
1. "I understand your reluctance to tell the physician, but it may have an impact on your treatment."
2. "Based on client confidentiality, I won't tell the physician if you wish."
3. "Your sex change and your hormones have nothing to do with your heart attack."
4. "Tell me about your sexual preference. Are you attracted to men or women?"

Answer: 1. During the history and physical examination of any female client being screened for thrombolytic therapy, the physician must know about the last menstrual period before the MI. Although not an absolute contraindication to thrombolytics, the possibility of pregnancy or menstruation must be documented. According to the ethics of client confidentiality, information may be shared in a professional manner with those who require it for the client's care. Hormones are an important factor in the pathogenesis of MI. Estrogen is cardioprotective, while replacement hormones after sex-reassignment surgery can impact how prone a person is to an MI. The client's sexual preference is of no consequence in this situation.

➡ *NCLEX keys*
Client needs category: Physiological integrity
Client needs subcategory: Reduction of risk potential
Cognitive level: Application

4. A client arrives at her physician's office crying. Her husband of 17 years has asked her for a divorce. She admits that recently she has avoided having sexual intercourse with him. Which response by the nurse would be most appropriate when talking with this client?
1. "Please stop crying so that we can discuss your feelings about the divorce."
2. "Once you have intercourse with him, you'll be able to get your relationship back on track."
3. "I can see how upset you are. Let's sit in the office so that we can talk about how you're feeling."
4. "Find a good lawyer who'll look out for your interests, and then you'll feel better."

Answer: 3. This response validates the client's distress and provides her the opportunity to talk about her feelings. Because a client in crisis has difficulty making decisions, the nurse must be directive as well as supportive. Telling the client to stop crying doesn't provide the client with adequate support. Suggesting that the client have intercourse or hire a lawyer doesn't acknowledge the client's distress. Moreover, the client in crisis can't think beyond the immediate moment, so discussing long-range plans isn't helpful.

➡ NCLEX keys
Client needs category: Psychosocial integrity
Client needs subcategory: None
Cognitive level: Application

5. A client explains to the nurse that she has felt distant from her spouse for a long period. Which question would be appropriate for the nurse to ask this client to assess female sexual functioning?
1. "Have you been spending time with friends?"
2. "What problems are you having with sleep?"
3 "Are you experiencing any signs of depression?"
4. "When did your family allow you to be independent?"

Answer: 3. A client who feels distant from her spouse may be experiencing hypoactive sexual desire disorder, and it may be related to negativity or cognitive distortions. It's important for the nurse to explore the client's feelings of depression and factors that may contribute to decreased sexual desire. Asking about time with friends, sleep problems, and independence doesn't address potential factors that contribute to hypoactive sexual desire disorder.

➡ NCLEX keys
Client needs category: Psychosocial integrity
Client needs subcategory: Psychosocial adaptation
Cognitive level: Application

6. A male client tells the nurse that he's experiencing problems with sexual arousal, and he asks her if he'll get anything out of attending the educational session on sexual disorders. Which response by the nurse would provide useful information to the client?
1. "I'm not sure if the class is appropriate for you; please ask your doctor what he thinks."
2. "I'll be talking about how certain medications can enhance sexual functioning."
3. "If you have a substance abuse problem, the class won't be helpful."
4. "I think that everyone can benefit from an educational class on sexual functioning."

Answer: 2. A male client with a sexual arousal disorder is typically experiencing an erectile disorder. In the educational session the nurse will speak about such medications as sildenafil (Viagra), tadalafil (Cialis), and vardenafil (Levitra), which are used to enhance male sexual functioning. The other responses don't directly answer the client's question about problems with sexual functioning.

➡ NCLEX keys
Client needs category: Psychosocial integrity
Client needs subcategory: Psychosocial adaptation
Cognitive level: Application

7. A client is diagnosed with erectile disorder. Which drug may be beneficial in treating a client with this disorder?
1. Methyldopa (Aldomet)
2. Alprostadil (Caverject)

3.   Benazepril (Lotensin)
4.   Clonidine (Catapres)

Answer: 2. Alprostadil is indicated for erectile disorder. It can be administered intracavern-ously before sexual intercourse. Methyldopa, benazepril, and clonidine are antihypertensive agents that can cause erectile disorder.

➡ *NCLEX keys*

Client needs category: Psychosocial integrity
Client needs subcategory: None
Cognitive level: Analysis

8.   A nurse is caring for a male client await-ing sex-reassignment surgery. When inter-acting with this client, it's important that the nurse:
   1.   discourage the client from under-going the procedure.
   2.   demonstrate a nonjudgmental atti-tude.
   3.   discuss with the client the option of undergoing hypnosis as an alternative to the surgery.
   4.   tell the client that his life will be less complicated and more peaceful after the surgery is complete.

Answer: 2. When caring for a client with gender identity disorder, the nurse should demonstrate a nonjudgmental attitude toward the client. It's the client's needs and feelings that matter most, not the nurse's opinions. The nurse shouldn't discourage the client's decision to go ahead with the procedure. Hypnosis isn't a treatment for gender identity disorder, and it isn't appropriate for the nurse to suggest hyp-nosis to the client. Telling the client his life will be less complicated and more peaceful after surgery offers false reassurance.

➡ *NCLEX keys*

Client needs category: Psychosocial integrity
Client needs subcategory: None
Cognitive level: Analysis

9.   A nurse explains exhibitionism, a sexual disorder, to a mother whose 24-year-old son displays the disorder. Which statement by the woman indicates her understanding of the disorder?
   1.   "The genetic factors make the dis-order out of his control."

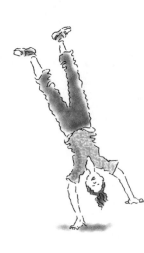

   2.   "There's no real treatment except for aversion therapy."
   3.   "Getting caught is the only thing that will stop this behavior."
   4.   "The pleasure that he got from the behavior reinforced it."

Answer: 4. A client who displays exhibi-tionism will continue to display this behavior when negative consequences don't occur and the pleasure he obtains continues to be reinforced. There are no genetic factors asso-ciated with exhibitionism. Aversion therapy isn't appropriate treatment for exhibitionism. Getting caught doesn't necessarily stop the behavior of this sexual disorder.

➡ *NCLEX keys*

Client needs category: Psychosocial integrity
Client needs subcategory: None
Cognitive level: Application

10.   A 14-year old male who prefers to dress in female clothing is brought to the psychi-atric crisis room by his mother. The client's mother states, "He is always dressing in female clothing. There must be something wrong with him." Which of the following responses from the nurse is most appro-priate?
   1.   "Your son will be evaluated shortly."
   2.   "I will explain to your son that his behavior isn't appropriate."
   3.   "I see you're upset. Would you like to talk?"
   4.   "You're being judgmental. There's nothing wrong with a boy wearing female clothing."

Answer: 3. Acknowledging the mother's feel-ings and offering her an opportunity to ver-balize her concerns provides a forum for open communication. Telling the boy's mother that he will be evaluated shortly doesn't address the mother's concerns. Telling the client that his behavior is inappropriate isn't therapeutic. The nurse shouldn't offer an opinion regarding whether the client's behavior is acceptable.

➡ *NCLEX keys*

Client needs category: Psychosocial integrity
Client needs subcategory: None
Cognitive level: Application

12 Eating disorders

Brush up on key concepts

Eating disorders are characterized by severe disturbances in eating behaviors. The two most common disorders, anorexia nervosa and bulimia nervosa, put the client at risk for severe cardiovascular and GI complications and can ultimately result in death.

Clients with these disorders exhibit severe disturbances in body image and self-perception. Their behavior may include self-starvation, binge eating, and purging. The causes of eating disorders aren't fully understood. They're more prevalent in females (90%) and can be chronic with periods of remission.

At any time, you can review the major points of each disorder by consulting the *Cheat sheet* on page 122.

Polish up on client care

Here's a review of anorexia nervosa and bulimia nervosa, the two most common eating disorders.

Anorexia nervosa

In anorexia nervosa, the client deliberately starves herself or engages in binge eating and purging. A client with anorexia nervosa wants to become as thin as possible and refuses to maintain an appropriate weight. A key clinical finding is a refusal to sustain weight at or above minimum requirements for the client's age and height and an intense fear of gaining weight or becoming fat. If left untreated, anorexia nervosa can be fatal.

CONTRIBUTING FACTORS
- Age (most prominent in adolescents)
- Distorted body image
- Gender (primarily affects females)
- Genetic predisposition
- Low self-esteem
- Neurochemical changes
- Poor family relations
- Poor self-esteem
- Preoccupation with weight and dieting
- Sexual abuse

ASSESSMENT FINDINGS
- Amenorrhea, fatigue, loss of libido, infertility
- Body image disturbance
- Cognitive distortions, such as overgeneralization, dichotomous thinking, or ideas of reference
- Compulsive behavior
- Decreased blood volume, evidenced by lowered blood pressure and orthostatic hypotension
- Dependency on others for self-worth
- Electrolyte imbalance, evidenced by muscle weakness, seizures, or arrhythmias
- Emaciated appearance
- GI complications, such as constipation or laxative dependence
- Guilt associated with eating
- Impaired decision making
- Need to achieve and please others
- Obsessive rituals concerning food
- Overly compliant attitude
- Perfectionist attitude
- Refusal to eat

DIAGNOSTIC TEST RESULTS
- Eating Attitude Test suggests an eating disorder.
- Electrocardiogram reveals non-specific ST interval, prolonged PR interval, and T-wave changes.

Eating disorders refresher

ANOREXIA NERVOSA

Key signs and symptoms
- Decreased blood volume, evidenced by lowered blood pressure and orthostatic hypotension
- Electrolyte imbalance, evidenced by muscle weakness, seizures, or arrhythmias
- Emaciated appearance
- Need to achieve and please others
- Obsessive rituals concerning food
- Refusal to eat

Key test results
- Eating Attitude Test suggests an eating disorder.
- Electrocardiogram reveals nonspecific ST interval, prolonged PR interval, and T-wave changes.
- Laboratory tests show elevated blood urea nitrogen level and electrolyte imbalances.
- Female clients exhibit low estrogen levels.
- Male clients exhibit low serum testosterone levels.

Key treatments
- Individual and group therapy
- Nutritional counseling
- Antianxiety agents: lorazepam (Ativan), alprazolam (Xanax)
- Antidepressants: amitriptyline (Elavil), imipramine (Tofranil)
- Selective serotonin reuptake inhibitors: paroxetine (Paxil), fluoxetine (Prozac), sertraline (Zoloft), citalopram (Celexa)

Key interventions
- Contract with the client for amount to be eaten.
- Provide one-on-one support before, during, and after meals.
- Prevent the client from using the bathroom for 90 minutes after eating.
- Help the client identify coping mechanisms for dealing with anxiety.
- Weigh the client once or twice per week at the same time of day using the same scale.

- Help the client and her family understand the anorectic cycle.
- Monitor for suicidal ideation, maladaptive substance use, and medical complications.

BULIMIA NERVOSA

Key signs and symptoms
- Alternating episodes of binge eating and purging
- Constant preoccupation with food
- Disruptions in interpersonal relationships
- Eroded tooth enamel
- Extreme need for acceptance and approval
- Irregular menses
- Russell sign (bruised knuckles due to induced vomiting)
- Sporadic, excessive exercise

Key test results
- Beck Depression Inventory may reveal depression.
- Eating Attitude Test suggests an eating disorder.
- Metabolic acidosis may occur from diarrhea caused by enemas and excessive laxative use.
- Metabolic alkalosis may occur from frequent vomiting.

Key interventions
- Explain the purpose of a nutritional contract.
- Avoid power struggles around food.
- Prevent the client from using the bathroom for 90 minutes after eating.
- Provide one-on-one support before, during, and after meals.
- Weigh the client once or twice per week at the same time of day using the same scale.
- Help the client and her family identify the cause of the disorder.
- Point out cognitive distortions.

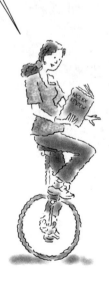

I can use the Cheat sheet to study while I get my exercise.

Management moments

Communication counts

Communication strategies play a key role when caring for the client with anorexia nervosa. Many clients with this disorder communicate on a superficial level and have difficulty forming interpersonal relationships. Therefore, you should focus on developing a therapeutic relationship. Use an accepting, nonjudgmental approach, and encourage the client to discuss her feelings, which may include sadness, depression, and loneliness. Teach the client effective communication techniques that focus on assertiveness skills.

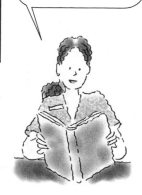

The largest obstacle to treating anorexia is that clients don't want to be treated. Yet quick intervention is essential. Anorexia nervosa can be fatal.

- Laboratory tests show elevated blood urea nitrogen and electrolyte imbalances.
- Female clients exhibit low estrogen levels.
- Leukopenia and mild anemia are apparent.
- Male clients exhibit low serum testosterone levels.
- Thyroid study findings are low.

NURSING DIAGNOSES
- Imbalanced nutrition: Less than body requirements
- Disturbed body image
- Chronic low self-esteem
- Anxiety
- Ineffective coping
- Decreased cardiac output

TREATMENT
- Behavioral modification
- Individual and group therapy
- Nutritional counseling
- Family therapy

Drug therapy
- Antianxiety agents: lorazepam (Ativan), alprazolam (Xanax)
- Antidepressants: amitriptyline (Elavil), imipramine (Tofranil)
- Selective serotonin reuptake inhibitors (SSRIs): paroxetine (Paxil), fluoxetine (Prozac), sertraline (Zoloft), citalopram (Celexa)

INTERVENTIONS AND RATIONALES
- Obtain a complete physical assessment *to identify complications of anorexia nervosa.*
- Contract with the client for amount to be eaten *to avoid conflict between staff members and the client.*

- Provide one-on-one support before, during, and after meals *to foster a strong nurse-client relationship and to ensure that the client is eating.*
- Prevent the client from using the bathroom for 90 minutes after eating *to break the purging cycle.*
- Encourage verbal expression of feelings *to foster open communications about body image.* (See *Communication counts.*)
- Help the client identify coping mechanisms for dealing with anxiety *to promote health-coping techniques.*
- Weigh the client once or twice per week at the same time of day using the same scale *to accurately monitor weight gain.* Be aware of objects in pockets or heavy clothing the client may be wearing in an attempt *to increase her weight.*
- Help the client and her family understand the anorectic cycle *to prevent future anorectic behavior.*
- Discuss the client's perception of her appearance. Explain that she has a right to think of herself as beautiful regardless of how she compares with others *to build self-esteem.*
- Discuss the client's progress with her *to increase awareness of achievements and promote continued effort.*
- Monitor for suicidal ideation, maladaptive subtance use, and medical complications *to better understand the client history.*

Teaching topics
- Explanation of the disorder and treatment plan
- Medication use and possible adverse effects
- Need for gradual weight gain
- Nutritional support measures

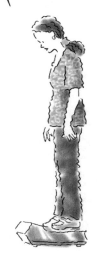

Weigh the client once or twice each week but not more; weighing too often reinforces the focus on weight.

- Treatment options
- Support services and community resources

Bulimia nervosa

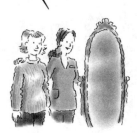

Tell the client that she has a right to think of herself as beautiful regardless of how she compares with others.

Bulimia nervosa is characterized by episodic binge eating, followed by purging in the form of vomiting. The client may also use laxatives, enemas, diuretics, or syrup of ipecac. The client's weight may remain normal or close to normal. The severity of the disorder depends on the frequency of the binge and purge cycle as well as physical complications. The client commonly views food as a source of comfort. The condition can be chronic or intermittent.

CONTRIBUTING FACTORS
- Distorted body image
- History of sexual abuse
- Low self-esteem
- Neurochemical changes
- Poor family relations

ASSESSMENT FINDINGS
- Alternating episodes of binge eating and purging
- Anxiety
- Avoidance of conflict
- Cognitive distortions such as with anorexia nervosa
- Constant preoccupation with food
- Eroded tooth enamel
- Disruptions in interpersonal relationships
- Dissatisfaction with body image
- Extreme need for acceptance and approval
- Feelings of helplessness
- Focus on changing a specific body part
- Frequent lies and excuses to explain behavior
- Guilt and self-disgust
- Irregular menses
- Perfectionist attitude
- Parotid and salivary gland swelling
- Pharyngitis
- Physiologic problems as in anorexia nervosa (amenorrhea, fatigue, loss of libido, infertility, electrolyte imbalance, GI complications)
- Possible use of amphetamines or other drugs to control hunger
- Problems caused by frequent vomiting
- Repression of anger and frustration

- Russell sign (bruised knuckles due to induced vomiting)
- Sporadic, excessive exercise

DIAGNOSTIC TEST RESULTS
- Beck Depression Inventory may reveal depression.
- Eating Attitude Test suggests an eating disorder.
- Metabolic acidosis may occur from diarrhea caused by enemas and excessive laxative use.
- Metabolic alkalosis (the most common metabolic complication) may occur from frequent vomiting.

NURSING DIAGNOSES
- Imbalanced nutrition: Less than body requirements
- Anxiety
- Powerlessness
- Fatigue
- Disturbed body image

TREATMENT
- Cognitive therapy to identify triggers for binge eating and purging
- Family therapy

Drug therapy
- SSRIs: paroxetine (Paxil), fluoxetine (Prozac)
- Topiramate (Topamax) to reduce binge eating and preoccupation with food
Note: Drug therapy is most effective when combined with cognitive therapy.

INTERVENTIONS AND RATIONALES
- Perform a complete physical assessment *to identify complications associated with bulimia nervosa.*
- Explain the purpose of a nutritional contract *to encourage a dietary change without initiating arguments or struggles.*
- Avoid power struggles around food *to keep the focus on establishing and maintaining a positive self-image and self-esteem.*
- Prevent the client from using the bathroom for 90 minutes after eating *to help the client avoid purging behavior.*
- Provide one-on-one support before, during, and after meals *to monitor and assist the client with eating.*

• Encourage the client to express her feelings *to facilitate conversation and promote understanding.*

• Weigh the client once or twice per week at the same time of day using the same scale *to monitor weight.*

• Help the client and her family identify the cause of the disorder *to help her gain understanding and work toward wellness.*

• Point out cognitive distortions *to help identify sources of the problem.*

• Discuss the client's perception of her appearance. Explain that she has a right to think of herself as beautiful regardless of how she compares with others *to build self-esteem.*

• Discuss the client's progress with her *to increase awareness of achievements and promote continued effort.*

Teaching topics

• Explanation of the disorder and treatment plan

• Medication use and possible adverse effects

• Need to gain weight gradually

• Treatment options

• Support services and community resources

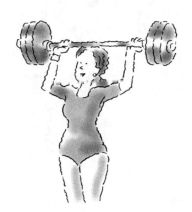

Pump up on practice questions

1. During the health history, a 16-year-old female client is looking for her prescription medication in her purse. The nurse notices a bottle of ipecac among the contents. Which concern should this observation cause the nurse?

1. Does the client frequently self-induce vomiting?

2. Will the client sell this drug to a minor at school?

3. Is the client aware that it's illegal to have this drug?

4. How should the nurse notify the client's parents about the client's possession of this drug?

Answer: 1. The only reason a client would have a bottle of ipecac is to self-induce vomiting. This information strongly indicates the possibility that the client has an eating disorder. Ipecac isn't an illegal drug and it would be unlikely that the client would sell it at school. The nurse isn't mandated to report possession of this drug to the client's parents.

➡ **NCLEX keys**

Client needs category: Physiological integrity
Client needs subcategory: Reduction of risk potential
Cognitive level: Application

2. A nurse is monitoring a client diagnosed with anorexia nervosa. In addition to monitoring the client's eating, the nurse should do which of the following after meals?

1. Encourage the client to go for a walk to get some exercise.

2. Prevent the client from using the bathroom for 90 minutes after eating.

3. Tell the client to lie down for 2 hours after eating.

4. Instruct the client to get plenty of exercise.

Answer: 2. After observing the client while she eats, the nurse should prevent the client from using the bathroom for at least 90 minutes to break the purging cycle. Exercise should be restricted until the client has shown adequate weight gain, and then it should be encouraged in moderation. It isn't necessary for the client to lie down for 90 minutes after eating.

➡ **NCLEX keys**

Client needs category: Physiological integrity
Client needs subcategory: Reduction of risk potential
Cognitive level: Application

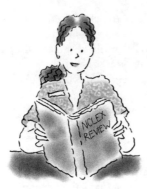

3. A nurse has taken the health history of a client who admits to binge eating. Which health concern should the nurse assess further during the next meeting with the client?

1. Adolescent turmoil
2. Emotional hunger
3. Disorganized behavior
4. Extreme restlessness

Answer: 2. A client who engages in binge eating will commonly eat when already feeling full and as a way to cope with emotions that aren't being handled effectively. A history of adolescent turmoil isn't necessarily associated with binge eating. Disorganized behavior and extreme restlessness are associated with bipolar disorder, not binge eating.

➟ NCLEX keys
Client needs category: Psychosocial integrity
Client needs subcategory: None
Cognitive level: Analysis

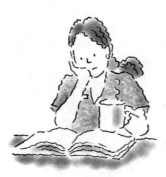

4. A nurse overhears a female client with bulimia nervosa talk in a disparaging way about herself to another client before the beginning of the group therapy session. Which intervention should the nurse initiate during group therapy?

1. Help the client realize and admit that she has socialization problems.
2. Discuss with the client ways to acknowledge and accept her angry feelings.
3. Encourage the client to recognize and change misperceptions about herself.
4. Teach the client to identify and tolerate frustrations about her daily life.

Answer: 3. A client who has distorted perceptions about herself would benefit from recognizing and changing these distorted perceptions. The nurse needs to address the issue of negative verbalizations about the self, rather than focus on socialization issues, anger management, or tolerance of frustrations.

➟ NCLEX keys
Client needs category: Psychosocial integrity
Client needs subcategory: None
Cognitive level: Analysis

5. A nurse is taking a history from a woman diagnosed with bulimia nervosa and suspects that the client may also have a substance abuse disorder. Which illicit drug should the nurse ask the client if she has used?

1. Amphetamines
2. Sedatives
3. Hallucinogens
4. Cannabis

Answer: 1. Clients with bulimia nervosa will commonly use amphetamines as an additional way to control weight. Sedatives, hallucinogens, and cannabis aren't typically used by bulimic clients to control weight.

➟ NCLEX keys
Client needs category: Psychosocial integrity
Client needs subcategory: None
Cognitive level: Application

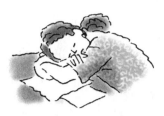

6. A client with bulimia nervosa tells the nurse that she wants to stop her binge eating. Which intervention should the nurse use to meet the client's request for help?

1. Discuss the binge-purge cycle and identify where the cycle could be interrupted.
2. Address the defense mechanism of projection and talk about underlying conflicts.
3. Provide anger management counseling and later involve the client's family in the treatment.
4. Focus on dysfunctional family and peer relationships and teach positive self-talk.

Answer: 1. Educating a client with bulimia nervosa about the binge-purge cycle can assist her to change her eating behavior and regain control over her eating. The defense mechanism commonly seen in a client with an eating disorder is denial, not projection. Anger management and learning positive self-talk wouldn't be the interventions of choice for assisting someone to stop binge eating behavior.

➡ *NCLEX keys*
Client needs category: Physiological integrity
Client needs subcategory: Reduction of risk potential
Cognitive level: Application

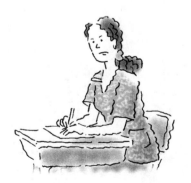

7. A nurse is caring for a client who has bulimia. Which treatment option is most effective?

1. Antidepressants
2. Cognitive-behavioral therapy
3. Antidepressants and cognitive-behavioral therapy
4. Total parenteral nutrition (TPN) and antidepressants

Answer: 3. The combined approach of antidepressants and cognitive-behavioral therapy has been effective, even when clients don't present with depression. TPN isn't indicated.

➡ *NCLEX keys*
Client needs category: Physiological integrity
Client needs subcategory: Pharmacological and parenteral therapies
Cognitive level: Application

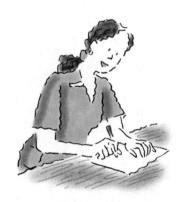

8. A nurse is caring for several clients who have eating disorders. Based on appearance, how would the nurse distinguish bulimic clients from anorectic clients?

1. By their teeth
2. By body size and weight
3. By looking for Mallory-Weiss tears
4. The clients are indistinguishable upon physical examination

Answer: 2. Behaviors of the anorectic client and the bulimic client are commonly similar, especially because both implement rituals to lose weight; however, the bulimic client tends to eat much more, due to binge episodes, and therefore can be near-normal weight. Not all persons with the purge disorder have loss of enamel on teeth, especially if the disorder has developed recently. Mallory-Weiss tears are small tears in the esophageal mucosa caused by forceful vomiting, but they aren't always present in bulimic clients.

➡ **NCLEX keys**
Client needs category: Physiological integrity
Client needs subcategory: Physiological adaptation
Cognitive level: Application

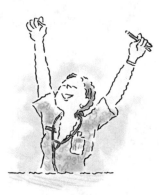

9. A client newly diagnosed with bulimia nervosa is working with the nurse to prepare for a family meeting. Which educational topic should the nurse discuss with the client's family during the meeting?
1. The family emphasis on individualism
2. The myth of the perfect family
3. The need to stop pharmacological intervention
4. The correlation of learning disabilities with disordered eating

Answer: 2. A client with a diagnosis of bulimia nervosa commonly comes from a family in which there's strong parental criticism. The family also places a high value on the idea of being perfect in all aspects of someone's life; the nurse needs to begin dismantling the myth of the perfect family. The emphasis on individualism wouldn't contribute to an eating disorder. Pharmacological intervention is frequently a necessary part of treatment and isn't discontinued in the early phase of treatment. There's no correlation between learning disabilities and eating disorders.

➡ **NCLEX keys**
Client needs category: Physiological integrity
Client needs subcategory: Reduction of risk potential
Cognitive level: Analysis

10. A nurse is caring for a client who has an eating disorder. Which nursing interventions would be appropriate for this client?
1. Weigh the client once or twice per week, and contract for amount of food to be eaten.
2. Weigh the client daily, and allow the client to use the bathroom ½ hour after eating.
3. Provide one-on-one support before meals.
4. Contract amount of food to be eaten, and weigh the client twice daily.

Answer: 1. Weighing the client more often than once or twice per week reinforces the client's excessive emphasis on weight. The client shouldn't be allowed to use the bathroom any sooner than 90 minutes after eating without supervision. One-on-one support for the client must be undertaken before, during, and after meals — not just before meals.

➡ **NCLEX keys**
Client needs category: Physiological integrity
Client needs subcategory: Physiological adaptation
Cognitive level: Application

It's been a long, strange trip through the mind, so give your brain a rest. Then move on to the next section.

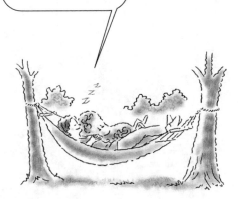

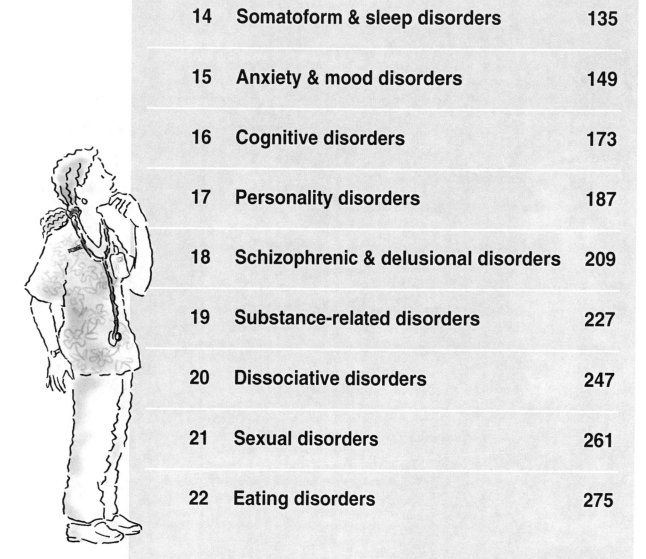

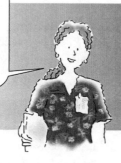

Before you take the tests relating to psychiatric care, take this test relating to tests (and treatments, too) in psychiatric care.

Chapter 13
Essentials of psychiatric nursing

1. A 50-year-old client is scheduled for electroconvulsive therapy (ECT). ECT is most commonly prescribed for which condition?
1. Major depression
2. Antisocial personality disorder
3. Chronic schizophrenia
4. Somatoform disorder

2. A patient with bipolar disorder becomes verbally aggressive in a group therapy session. Which response by the nurse would be best?
1. "You're behaving in an unacceptable manner, and you need to control yourself."
2. "If you continue to talk like that, no one will want to be around you."
3. "You're frightening everyone in the group. Leave the room immediately."
4. "Other people are disturbed by your profanity. I'll walk with you down the hall to help release some of that energy."

3. A newly admitted client is extremely hostile toward a staff member he has just met, without apparent reason. According to Freudian theory, the nurse should suspect that the client is exhibiting which phenomena?
1. Intellectualization
2. Transference
3. Triangulation
4. Splitting

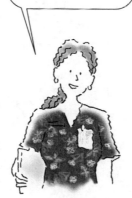

All of these options might be acceptable, but which is *best*?

1. 1. ECT is most commonly used for the treatment of major depression in clients who haven't responded to antidepressants or who have medical problems that contraindicate the use of antidepressants. ECT isn't commonly used for treatment of personality disorders. ECT doesn't appear to be of value to individuals with chronic schizophrenia and isn't the treatment of choice for clients with somatoform disorders.
CN: Psychosocial integrity; CNS: None; CL: Application

2. 4. This response informs the client that, although the behavior is unacceptable, the client is still worthy of help. The other responses are nontherapeutic and blaming.
CN: Safe, effective care environment; CNS: Management of care; CL: Application

3. 2. Transference is the unconscious assignment of negative or positive feelings evoked by a significant person in the client's past to another person. Intellectualization is a defense mechanism in which the client avoids dealing with emotions by focusing on facts. Triangulation refers to conflicts involving three family members. Splitting is a defense mechanism commonly seen in clients with personality disorders in which the world is perceived as all good or all bad.
CN: Psychosocial integrity; CNS: None; CL: Analysis

4. Which intervention would be typical of a nurse using a cognitive-behavioral approach to a client experiencing low self-esteem?
  1. Use of unconditional positive regard
  2. Analysis of free associations
  3. Classical conditioning
  4. Examination of negative thought patterns

4. 4. Popular cognitive-behavioral approaches examine the validity of habitual patterns of thinking and belief systems that influence feelings and behaviors. "Unconditional positive regard" is a phrase from Carl Rogers's client-centered therapy and describes a supportive, nonjudgmental, neutral approach by a therapist. Analysis of free associations is characteristic of Freudian psychoanalysis. Classical conditioning is characteristic of a pure behavioral intervention.
CN: Psychosocial integrity; CNS: None; CL: Application

5. During group therapy, a client listening to another client's description of an abusive incident that occurred during childhood says, "I didn't think anyone else felt like I did as a child." The nurse recognizes this statement as a reflection of which curative factor of group therapy, as identified by Yalom?
  1. Altruism
  2. Universality
  3. Catharsis
  4. Existential factors

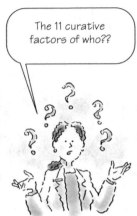

5. 2. One of the 11 curative factors of group therapy identified by Yalom is universality, which assists group participants in recognizing common experiences and responses. This action helps reduce anxiety and allows other group members to provide support and understanding. Altruism, catharsis, and existential factors are other curative factors Yalom described, but they don't describe this particular incident. Altruism refers to finding meaning through helping others; catharsis is an open expression of previously suppressed feelings; and existential factors describe the recognition that one has control over the quality of one's life.
CN: Psychosocial integrity; CNS: None; CL: Application

6. Which statement best describes the key advantage of using groups in psychotherapy?
  1. Decreases the focus on the individual
  2. Fosters the physician–client relationship
  3. Confronts individuals with their shortcomings
  4. Fosters a new learning environment

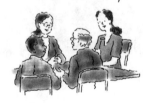

6. 4. In a group, the individual has the opportunity to learn that others have the same problems and needs. The group can also provide an arena where new methods of relating to others can be tried. Decreasing focus on the individual isn't a key advantage (and sometimes isn't an advantage at all). Groups don't, by themselves, foster the physician–client relationship, and they aren't always used to confront individuals.
CN: Psychosocial integrity; CNS: None; CL: Analysis

7. A client who has recently lost his wife and children in a car collision is being treated at the outpatient psychiatric clinic. Which therapy should be most effective with this client?
  1. Electroconvulsive therapy (ECT)
  2. Group therapy
  3. Hypnotherapy
  4. Individual therapy

7. 2. The client history strongly suggests posttraumatic stress disorder. Group therapy has been especially effective with this diagnosis. ECT, hypnotherapy, and individual therapy may be useful to this client, but these therapies aren't as strongly advocated as group therapy.
CN: Psychosocial integrity; CNS: None; CL: Analysis

CN: Client needs category   CNS: Client needs subcategory   CL: Cognitive level

8. During a group therapy session, a teenage girl says that she's fat and ugly and that everybody makes fun of her. This statement reflects which common adolescent fear or anxiety?
1. Fear of the unknown
2. Fear of loss of respect, love, and emerging self-esteem
3. Anxiety related to guilt
4. Anxiety about body image and changes in physical appearance

9. After telling a nurse to "pray for me," a client gives away personal possessions and shows a sudden calmness. The nurse recognizes that this behavior may signal which condition?
1. Major depression
2. Panic attack
3. Suicidal ideation
4. Severe anxiety

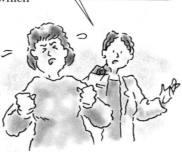

In psychiatric care, the nurse needs to recognize verbal as well as physical clues.

10. A client recently lost his spouse. Which of the following behaviors indicates that the client is going through a normal stage of grieving?
1. The client starts using chemicals.
2. The client becomes an overachiever.
3. The client shows signs of hyperactivity.
4. The client shows a loss of warmth when interacting with others.

11. Two 16-year-old clients are being treated in an adolescent unit. During a recreational activity, they begin to physically fight. How should the nurse intervene?
1. Remove the teenagers to separate areas and set limits.
2. Remind the teenagers of the unit rules.
3. Obtain an order to place the teenagers in seclusion.
4. Obtain an order to place the teenagers in restrains.

8. 4. Anxiety about body image and changes in physical appearance is a common fear of adolescents. Fear of the unknown is associated with toddlerhood. Fear of loss of respect, love, and emerging self-esteem is associated with the school-age developmental phase. Anxiety related to guilt is also associated with the school-age developmental phase.
CN: Psychosocial integrity; CNS: None; CL: Application

9. 3. Verbal clues to suicidal ideation include such statements as "Pray for me," and "I won't be here when you get back." Nonverbal clues include giving away personal possessions, a sudden calmness, and risk-taking behaviors. The nurse should recognize the combination of these signs as indicating suicidal ideation —not depression, panic, or anxiety. Clients with major depression generally don't exhibit suicidal behavior until their outlook on their problems begins to improve (an improvement in behavior should raise suspicion, especially if accompanied by sudden calmness).
CN: Psychosocial integrity; CNS: None; CL: Application

10. 4. Hostile reactions, such as loss of warmth when interacting with others, occur during normal grieving. Chemical use, overachieving, and hyperactivity commonly correlate with complicated grieving.
CN: Psychosocial integrity; CNS: None; CL: Application

11. 1. Setting limits and removing the clients from the situation is the best way to handle aggression. Reminders of appropriate behavior aren't likely to be effective at this time and seclusion and restraints are reserved for more serious situations.
CN: Psychosocial integrity; CNS: None; CL: Application

12. A client is prescribed sertraline (Zoloft), a selective serotonin reuptake inhibitor. Which information about this drug's adverse effects should the nurse include when creating a medication teaching plan? Select all that apply:

1. Agitation
2. Agranulocytosis
3. Sleep disturbance
4. Intermittent tachycardia
5. Dry mouth
6. Seizures

13. A physician prescribes lithium for a client diagnosed with bipolar disorder. The nurse needs to provide appropriate education for the client on this drug. Which topics should the nurse cover? Select all that apply:

1. The potential for addiction
2. Signs and symptoms of drug toxicity
3. The potential for tardive dyskinesia
4. A low-tyramine diet
5. The need to consistently monitor blood levels
6. The expected time frame for noticing improvements in mood

14. A physician starts a client on the antipsychotic medication haloperidol (Haldol). The nurse is aware that this medication has extrapyramidal adverse effects. Which measures should the nurse take during haloperidol administration? Select all that apply:

1. Review subcutaneous injection technique.
2. Closely monitor vital signs, especially temperature.
3. Provide the client with the opportunity to pace.
4. Monitor blood glucose levels.
5. Provide the client with hard candy.
6. Monitor for signs and symptoms of urticaria.

12. 1, 3, 5. Common adverse effects of sertraline include agitation, sleep disturbance, and dry mouth. Agranulocytosis, intermittent tachycardia, and seizures are adverse effects of clozapine (Clozaril).

CN: Physiological integrity; CNS: Pharmacological and parenteral therapies; CL: Application

13. 2, 5, 6. Client education should cover the signs and symptoms of drug toxicity as well as the need to report them to the physician. The client should be instructed to monitor his lithium levels on a regular basis to avoid toxicity. The nurse should explain that 7 to 21 days may pass before the client notes a change in his mood. Lithium doesn't have addictive properties. Tardive dyskinesia isn't associated with lithium. Tyramine is a potential concern for clients taking monoamine-oxidase inhibitors.

CN: Physiological integrity; CNS: Pharmacological and parenteral therapies; CL: Application

14. 2, 3, 5. Neuroleptic malignant syndrome is a life-threatening adverse effect of antipsychotic medications such as haloperidol. It's associated with a rapid increase in temperature. The most common extrapyramidal adverse effect, akathisia, is a form of psychomotor restlessness that can typically be relieved by pacing. Haloperidol and the anticholinergic medications that are provided to alleviate its extrapyramidal effects can result in a dry mouth. Providing the client with hard candy to suck on can help with this problem. Haloperidol isn't given subcutaneously and doesn't affect blood glucose levels. Urticaria isn't usually associated with haloperidol administration.

CN: Physiological integrity; CNS: Pharmacological and parenteral therapies; CL: Analysis

Here's to you! You've just zipped through another important NCLEX topic.

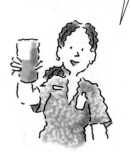

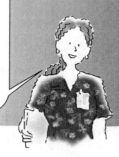

Can't remember much about a particular somatoform disorder? Type this address into your Web browser: **www.emedicine.com.** Then search for the disorder.

Chapter 14
Somatoform & sleep disorders

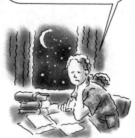

I hope I stay awake long enough to finish these questions.

1. The nurse is teaching a student nurse about somatoform disorders. Which of the following statements by the nurse would be the most accurate in describing somatoform disorders?
  1. They usually seek medical attention.
  2. They have organic pathologic disorders.
  3. They regularly attend psychotherapy sessions without encouragement.
  4. They're eager to discover the true reasons for their physical symptoms.

2. A nurse is caring for a client with a somatoform disorder. In providing education to the family, the nurse discusses that these disorders:
  1. are limited to one organ system.
  2. occur with a recent physical illness.
  3. are physical conditions with organic pathologic causes.
  4. occur in the absence of organic findings.

3. Which rationale best explains the physical symptoms experienced by a client with a somatoform disorder?
  1. The client complains of physical symptoms that can be explained by a known physiologic cause.
  2. The client complains of physical symptoms to gain attention.
  3. The client experiences physical symptoms in response to anxiety.
  4. The client complains of physical symptoms to cope with delusional thinking.

1. 1. A client with a somatization disorder usually seeks medical attention. These clients have a history of multiple physiologic complaints without associated demonstrable organic pathologic causes. The expected behavior for this type of disorder is to seek treatment from several medical physicians for somatic complaints, not psychiatric evaluation.
CN: Health promotion and maintenance; CNS: None; CL: Application

2. 4. The essential feature of somatoform disorders is a physical or somatic complaint without any demonstrable organic findings to account for the complaint. Somatic complaints aren't limited to one organ system. There are no known physiologic mechanisms to explain the findings. The diagnostic criteria for somatoform disorders state that the client has a history of many physical complaints beginning before age 30 that occur over several years.
CN: Psychosocial integrity; CNS: None; CL: Application

3. 3. In a client with a somatoform disorder, physical symptoms are manifestations of psychological distress, such as anxiety and depression, that have no apparent physiologic cause. The physical symptoms enable the client to avoid unpleasant emotions, not seek individual attention intentionally. The attention received, if any, is a secondary gain that stems from the primary gain of anxiety relief. Somatic delusions are characteristic of schizophrenia.
CN: Psychosocial integrity; CNS: None; CL: Analysis

CN: Client needs category   CNS: Client needs subcategory   CL: Cognitive level

4. A nurse is caring for a client who's demonstrating an ego defense mechanism. Which finding supports the nurse's observations?

1. Repression of anger
2. Suppression of grief
3. Denial of depression
4. Preoccupation with pain

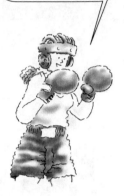

Remember, you're looking for a defense mechanism.

4. 1. One psychodynamic theory states that somatization is the transformation of aggressive and hostile wishes toward others into physical complaints. Repressed anger originating from past disappointments and unfilled needs for nurturing and caring are expressed by soliciting other people's concern and rejecting them as ineffective. Denial, suppression, and preoccupation aren't the defense mechanisms underlying the dynamics of somatization disorders.

CN: Psychosocial integrity; CNS: None; CL: Application

5. An 86-year-old client in an extended care facility is anxious most of the time and frequently complains of a number of vague symptoms that interfere with his ability to eat. These symptoms indicate which disorder?

1. Conversion disorder
2. Hypochondriasis
3. Severe anxiety
4. Sublimation

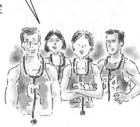

Accurate nursing diagnoses make sure all staff are working toward the same goal!

5. 2. Complaints of vague physical symptoms that have no apparent medical causes are characteristic of clients with hypochondriasis. In many cases, the GI system is affected. Conversion disorders are characterized by one or more neurologic symptoms. The client's symptoms don't suggest severe anxiety. A client experiencing sublimation channels maladaptive feelings or impulses into socially acceptable behavior.

CN: Psychosocial integrity; CNS: None; CL: Analysis

6. Which nursing diagnosis is <u>most appropriate</u> for the disorder known as hypochondriasis?

1. *Risk for injury*
2. *Grieving*
3. *Risk for situational low self-esteem*
4. *Deficient diversional activity*

6. 3. Hypochondriasis is a disorder manifested by fear, risk for situational low self-esteem, and feelings of worthlessness. *Risk for injury, Grieving,* and *Deficient diversional activity* have no correlation to the disorder.

CN: Safe, effective care environment; CNS: Management of care; CL: Application

7. A college student frequently visited the health center during the past year with multiple vague complaints of GI symptoms before course examinations. Although physical causes have been eliminated, the student continues to express her belief that she has a serious illness. These symptoms are typical of which disorder?

1. Conversion disorder
2. Depersonalization
3. Hypochondriasis
4. Somatization disorder

7. 3. Hypochondriasis in this case is shown by the client's belief that she has a serious illness, although pathologic causes have been eliminated. The disturbance usually lasts at least 6 months, and the GI system is commonly affected. Exacerbations are usually associated with identifiable life stressors such as, in this case, course examinations. Conversion disorders are characterized by one or more neurologic symptoms. Depersonalization refers to persistent, recurrent episodes of feeling detached from one's self or body. Somatoform disorders generally have a chronic course with few remissions.

CN: Psychosocial integrity; CNS: None; CL: Analysis

8. A nursing goal for a client diagnosed with hypochondriasis should focus on which area?
1. Determining the cause of the sleep disturbance
2. Relieving the fear of serious illness
3. Recovering the lost or altered function
4. Giving positive reinforcement for accomplishments related to physical appearance

9. Which nursing intervention is appropriate for a client diagnosed with hypochondriasis?
1. Teach the client adaptive coping strategies.
2. Help the client eliminate the stress in her life.
3. Confront the client with the statement, "It's all in your head."
4. Encourage the client to focus on identification of physical symptoms.

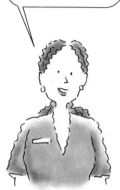

Accurate nursing diagnoses make sure all staff are working toward the same goal!

10. After repeated office visits, physical examinations, and diagnostic tests for assorted complaints, a client is referred to a psychiatrist. The client later tells a friend, "I can't imagine why my doctor wants me to see a psychiatrist." Which statement is the <u>most likely</u> explanation for the client's statement?
1. The client probably believes psychiatrists are only for "crazy" people.
2. The client probably doesn't understand the correlation of symptoms and stress.
3. The client probably believes his physician has made an error in diagnosis.
4. The client probably believes his physician wants to get rid of him as a client.

11. Which therapeutic strategy is used to reduce anxiety in a client diagnosed with hypochondriasis?
1. Suicide precautions
2. Relaxation exercises
3. Electroconvulsive therapy (ECT)
4. Aversion therapy

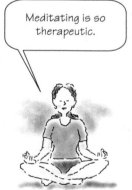

Meditating is so therapeutic.

8. 2. The nursing goal for hypochondriasis is relief of fear. For insomnia, the goal is focused on determining the cause of the sleep disturbance. The nursing goal for a conversion disorder focuses on the recovery of the lost or altered function. An appropriate goal for body dysmorphic disorder focuses on positive reinforcement for accomplishments related to physical appearance.
CN: Psychosocial integrity; CNS: None; CL: Application

9. 1. Because of weak ego strength, a client with hypochondriasis is unable to use coping mechanisms effectively. The nursing focus is to teach adaptive coping mechanisms. It isn't realistic to eliminate all stress. A client should never be confronted with the statement, "It's all in your head," because this wouldn't facilitate a long-term therapeutic relationship, which is necessary to offer reassurance that no physical disease is present. Calling attention to physical symptoms is counterproductive to treatment.
CN: Psychosocial integrity; CNS: None; CL: Application

10. 3. The preoccupation in hypochondriasis is related to bodily functions or physical sensations. Repeated physical examinations, diagnostic tests, and reassurance from the physician don't allay the concerns about bodily disease. There's a belief that a health care professional has poor insight if he sees the concern about having a serious illness as excessive or unreasonable. The other responses aren't valid.
CN: Psychosocial integrity; CNS: None; CL: Analysis

11. 2. Relaxation exercises help to decrease anxiety in a client with hypochondriasis. In a hypochondriasis disorder, no threat of suicide exists. ECT and aversion therapy aren't therapeutic strategies for hypochondriasis.
CN: Psychosocial integrity; CNS: None; CL: Application

12. A client is given triazolam (Halcion) for a sleep disorder. The nurse is reinforcing some teaching precautions concerning the medication. The nurse determines that the client understands the precautions when the client states:
1. "I take the medication with citrus juice."
2. "I shouldn't confuse this medication with Haldol."
3. "It's okay to take a short drive after taking the medication."
4. It's okay to smoke while I take this medication."

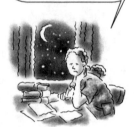

Who needs help to sleep?

13. Which measure should be included when teaching a client strategies to help sleep?
1. Keep the room warm.
2. Eat a large meal before bedtime.
3. Schedule bedtime when you feel tired.
4. Avoid caffeine, excessive fluid intake, alcohol, and stimulating drugs before bedtime.

14. A nurse is interviewing a client newly admitted to the unit. While stating a list of medications, the client falls asleep. The nurse understands that the client is most likely exhibiting which sleep disorder?
1. Hypersomnia
2. Insomnia
3. Narcolepsy
4. Parasomnia

15. Treatments for sleep disorders include which method?
1. Behavior therapy
2. Biofeedback
3. Group therapy
4. Insight-oriented psychotherapy

12. 2. Haldol is an antipsychotic that has a spelling similar to Halcion and is used for clients with psychoses, Tourette's syndrome, severe behavioral problems in children, and emergency sedation of severely agitated psychotic clients. Halcion is one of a group of sedative-hypnotic medications that can be used only for a limited time because of the risk of dependence. Grapefruit and grapefruit juices can alter the absorption of Halcion. The client should avoid driving and other tasks that require alertness or motor skills because the medication may cause drowsiness. Smoking reduces drug effectiveness.
CN: Physiological integrity; CNS: Pharmacological and parenteral therapies; CL: Analysis

13. 4. Caffeine, excessive fluid intake, alcohol, and stimulating drugs act as stimulants; avoiding them should promote sleep. Maintaining a cool temperature in the room will better facilitate sleeping. Excessive fullness or hunger may interfere with sleep. Setting a regular bedtime and wake-up time facilitates physiologic patterns.
CN: Health promotion and maintenance; CNS: None; CL: Application

14. 3. Narcolepsy is also known as sleep attacks. Hypersomnia, or somnolence, refers to excessive sleepiness or seeking excessive amounts of sleep. Insomnia is a sleep disorder in which an individual has difficulty initiating or maintaining sleep. Parasomnia refers to unusual or undesired behavior that occurs during sleep, such as nightmares and sleepwalking.
CN: Physiological integrity; CNS: Physiological adaptation; CL: Analysis

15. 2. Biofeedback, relaxation therapy, and psychopharmacology are appropriate treatments for sleep disorders. Behavior therapy, group therapy, and insight-oriented psychotherapy are treatments related to somatoform disorders.
CN: Physiological integrity; CNS: Basic care and comfort; CL: Application

CN: Client needs category   CNS: Client needs subcategory   CL: Cognitive level

16. Which nursing intervention would be the most appropriate for a depressed client with a nursing diagnosis of *Disturbed sleep pattern related to external factors*?
1. Consult the physician about prescribing a bedtime sleep medication.
2. Allow the client to sit at the nurses' station for comfort.
3. Allow the client to watch television until he's sleepy.
4. Encourage the client to take a warm bath before retiring.

17. Which condition characterizes rapid eye movement (REM) sleep?
1. Disorientation and disorganized thinking
2. Jerky limb movements and position changes
3. Pulse rate slowed by 5 to 10 beats/minute
4. Highly active brain and physiologic activity levels

18. A client with sleep terror disorder might have autonomic signs of intense anxiety. Which autonomic sign or symptom should the nurse monitor?
1. Tachycardia
2. Pupil constriction
3. Cool, clammy skin
4. Decreased muscle tone

19. Which consideration is important in planning care for a client experiencing sleep deprivation?
1. Sleep is influenced by biological rhythms.
2. The natural body clock follows a 24-hour cycle.
3. Long sleepers have more rapid eye movement periods.
4. Prolonged periods of sleep deprivation can lead to ego disorganization, hallucinations, and delusions.

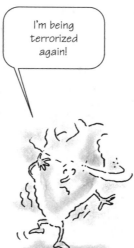

I'm being terrorized again!

16. 4. Sleep-inducing activities, such as a warm bath, help promote relaxation and sleep. Although consulting a physician about prescribing a bedtime sleep medication is possible, it wouldn't be the best nursing intervention for this client. Encouraging the client to watch television or sit at the nurses' station wouldn't necessarily promote sleep. In fact, these activities may provide too much stimulation, further preventing sleep.
CN: Physiological integrity; CNS: Basic care and comfort; CL: Application

17. 4. Highly active brain and physiologic activity levels characterize REM stage. Stages 3 and 4 of non-REM sleep are characterized by disorientation and disorganization. During REM sleep, body movement ceases except for the eyes. The pulse rate slows by 5 or 10 beats/minute during non-REM sleep, not REM sleep.
CN: Physiological integrity; CNS: Physiological adaptation; CL: Analysis

18. 1. Autonomic arousal includes tachycardia, which should be closely monitored by the nurse to prevent the occurrence of further complications such as arrhythmia. Sweating, increased muscle tone, and pupillary dilation are responses that may also occur but aren't considered life-threatening.
CN: Physiological integrity; CNS: Physiological adaptation; CL: Application

19. 4. Sleep deprivation can lead to hallucinations and delusions. Uninterrupted sleep is an important nursing consideration in planning care. All other data are expected and shouldn't cause sleep deprivation.
CN: Physiological integrity; CNS: Physiological adaptation; CL: Application

20. A nurse is instructing a 38-year-old male client undergoing treatment for anxiety and insomnia. The practitioner has prescribed lorazepam (Ativan) 1 mg by mouth three times per day. The nurse determines that the teaching regarding the client's medication has been effective when the client gives which of the following responses?
1. "I'll avoid caffeine."
2. "I'll avoid aged cheese."
3. "I'll avoid sunlight."
4. "I'll maintain adequate salt intake."

21. A client diagnosed with a sleep disorder awakens abruptly with a piercing scream. Which disorder best explains this behavior?
1. Hypersomnia
2. Nightmare disorder
3. Sleep terror disorder
4. Sleepwalking

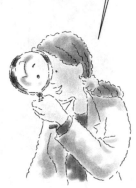

In question 20, you're looking for what could exacerbate the client's symptoms

22. Which nursing diagnosis is appropriate for a client with a sleep disorder?
1. *Fear*
2. *Risk for injury*
3. *Risk for situational low self-esteem*
4. *Disturbed sensory perception (auditory)*

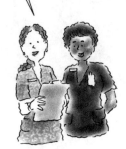

Nursing diagnoses are the professional language of nursing.

23. A 35-year-old female client is diagnosed with conversion disorder with paralysis of the legs. What's the best nursing intervention for the nurse to use?
1. Discuss with the client ways to live with the paralysis.
2. Focus interactions on results of medical tests.
3. Encourage the client to move her legs as much as possible.
4. Avoid focusing on the client's physical limitations.

20. 1. Lorazepam is a benzodiazepine used to treat various forms of anxiety and insomnia. Caffeine is contraindicated because it's a stimulant and increases anxiety. A client on a monoamine oxidase inhibitor should avoid aged cheeses. Clients taking certain antipsychotic medications should avoid sunlight. Salt intake has no effect on lorazepam.
CN: Physiological integrity CNS: Pharmacological and parenteral therapies; CL: Analysis

21. 3. Sleep terror disorder refers to an abrupt arousal from sleep with a piercing scream or cry. Hypersomnia is excessive sleepiness or seeking excessive amounts of sleep. Nightmares are frightening dreams that lead to awakenings from sleep and are severe enough to interfere with social or occupational functioning. Sleepwalking refers to motor activity initiated during sleep in which the individual may leave the bed and walk around.
CN: Psychosocial integrity; CNS: None; CL: Analysis

22. 2. A client with a sleep disorder may be at *Risk for injury* due to drowsiness and decreased concentration. *Fear* may be applicable to hypochondriasis. *Risk for situational low self-esteem* may be related to an alteration in self-concept or self-esteem. No evidence of a *Disturbed sensory perception (auditory)* problem exists.
CN: Safe, effective care environment; CNS: Management of care; CL: Analysis

23. 4. The paralysis is used as an unhealthy way of expressing unmet psychological needs. The nurse should avoid speaking about the vparalysis to shift the client's attention to the mental aspect of the disorder. The other options focus too much on the paralysis, which doesn't allow for recognition of the underlying psychological motivations.
CN: Psychological integrity; CNS: None; CL: Application

24. Which statement is correct about conversion disorders?
1. The symptoms can be controlled.
2. The psychological conflict is repressed.
3. The client is aware of the psychological conflict.
4. The client shouldn't be made aware of the conflicts underlying the symptoms.

25. A client is admitted for abrupt onset of paralysis in his left arm. Although no physiologic cause has been found, the symptoms are exacerbated when he speaks of losing custody of his children in a recent divorce. These assessment findings are characteristic of which of the following disorders?
1. Body dysmorphic disorder
2. Conversion disorder
3. Delusional disorder
4. Malingering

26. A client has been hospitalized with a diagnosis of conversion-disorder blindness. Which statement best explains this manifestation?
1. The client is suppressing her true feelings.
2. The client's anxiety has been relieved through her physical symptoms.
3. The client is acting indifferent because she doesn't want to show her actual fear.
4. The client's needs are being met, so she doesn't need to be anxious.

27. A client with hypochondriasis complains of pain in his right side that he hasn't had before. Which response is the most appropriate?
1. "It's time for group therapy now."
2. "Tell me about this new pain you're having. You'll miss group therapy today."
3. "I'll report this pain to your physician. In the meantime, group therapy starts in 5 minutes. You must leave now to be on time."
4. "I'll call your physician and see whether he'll order a new pain medication. Why don't you get some rest for now?"

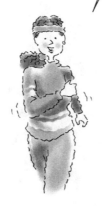

You've run through 24 questions. You're almost there.

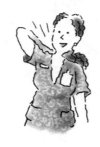

You deserve a pat on the back for answering these questions.

24. 2. In conversion disorder, physical symptoms are manifestations of a repressed psychological conflict. The client isn't able to control or produce symptoms and is unaware of the psychological conflict. Understanding the principles and conflicts behind the symptoms can prove helpful during a client's therapy.
CN: Psychosocial integrity; CNS: None; CL: Analysis

25. 2. Conversion disorders are characterized by one or more neurologic symptoms associated with psychological conflict. Body dysmorphic disorder is an imagined belief that there's a defect in the appearance of all or part of the body. The client doesn't have a delusion; this is the sole manifestation of a delusional disorder. Malingering is the intentional production of symptoms to avoid obligations or obtain rewards.
CN: Psychosocial integrity; CNS: None; CL: Analysis

26. 2. Conversion accomplishes anxiety reduction through the production of a physical symptom symbolically linked to an underlying conflict. The client isn't aware of the internal conflict. Hospitalization doesn't remove the source of the conflict.
CN: Psychosocial integrity; CNS: None; CL: Analysis

27. 3. The amount of time focused on discussing physical symptoms should be decreased. Lack of positive reinforcement may help stop the maladaptive behavior. However, avoiding the statement altogether demeans the client and doesn't address the underlying problem. Asking the client to further explain the pain emphasizes physical symptoms and prevents the client from attending group therapy. All physical complaints need to be evaluated for physiologic causes by the physician.
CN: Psychosocial integrity; CNS: None; CL: Application

28. Which intervention would help a client with conversion-disorder blindness to eat?
1. Direct the client to independently locate items on the tray and feed himself.
2. See to the needs of the other clients in the dining room; then feed this client last.
3. Establish a "buddy" system with other clients who can feed the client at each meal.
4. Expect the client to feed himself after explaining the location of food on the tray.

29. A client diagnosed with conversion disorder who's experiencing left-sided paralysis tells the nurse that he has received a lot of attention in the hospital and that it's unfortunate that others outside the hospital don't find him interesting. Which nursing diagnosis is appropriate for this client?
1. *Interrupted family processes*
2. *Ineffective health maintenance*
3. *Ineffective coping*
4. *Social isolation*

30. To help a client with conversion disorder increase self-esteem, which nursing intervention is appropriate?
1. Set large goals so the client can see positive gains.
2. Focus attention on the client as a person rather than on the symptom.
3. Discuss the client's childhood to link present behaviors with past traumas.
4. Encourage the client to use avoidant-interactional patterns rather than assertive patterns.

31. A nurse is caring for a client with a conversion disorder. What sign or symptom should she expect to observe or have the client report?
1. Delusions
2. Feelings of depression or euphoria
3. A feeling of dread accompanied by somatic signs
4. One or more neurologic symptoms associated with psychological conflict or need

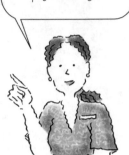

A client with a disorder of psychologic origin may need the same interventions as one with a disorder of physical origin.

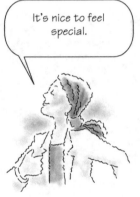

It's nice to feel special.

28. 4. The client is expected to maintain some level of independence by feeding himself, while at the same time the nurse provides some direction and is supportive in a matter-of-fact way. Feeding the client leads to dependence.
CN: Psychosocial integrity; CNS: None; CL: Application

29. 3. The client can't express his internal conflicts in appropriate ways. There are no defining characteristics to support the other nursing diagnoses.
CN: Psychosocial integrity; CNS: None; CL: Application

30. 2. Focusing on the client directs attention away from the symptom. This approach eventually reduces the client's need to gain attention through physical symptoms. Small goals ensure success and reinforce self-esteem. Discussion of childhood has no correlation with self-esteem. Avoiding interactional situations doesn't foster self-esteem.
CN: Psychosocial integrity; CNS: None; CL: Application

31. 4. Symptoms of conversion disorders are neurologic in nature (paralysis, blindness). Delusional disorders are characterized by delusions. Mood disorders are characterized by abnormal feelings of depression or euphoria. Anxiety is characterized by a feeling of dread.
CN: Health promotion and maintenance; CNS: None; CL: Application

CN: Client needs category   CNS: Client needs subcategory   CL: Cognitive level

32. Which nursing diagnosis is appropriate for a client with conversion disorder who has little energy to expend on activities or interactions with friends?
1. *Powerlessness*
2. *Hopelessness*
3. *Impaired social interaction*
4. *Compromised family coping*

33. A client diagnosed with conversion disorder has a nursing diagnosis of *Interrupted family processes related to the client's disability.* Which goal is appropriate for this client?
1. The client will resume former roles and tasks.
2. The client will take over roles of other family members.
3. The client will rely on family members to meet all client needs.
4. The client will focus energy on problems occurring in the family.

34. A new client admitted to a psychiatric unit is diagnosed with conversion disorder. The client shows a lack of concern for his sudden paralysis, although his athletic abilities have always been a source of pride to him. The nurse understands that the client is demonstrating:
1. acute dystonia.
2. *la belle indifference.*
3. malingering.
4. secondary gain.

35. Which nursing intervention is the <u>most appropriate</u> for a client who had pseudoseizures and is diagnosed with conversion disorder?
1. Explain that the pseudoseizures are imaginary.
2. Promote dependence so that unfilled dependency needs are met.
3. Encourage the client to discuss his feelings about the pseudoseizures.
4. Promote independence, and withdraw attention from the pseudoseizures.

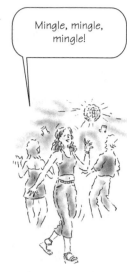

Mingle, mingle, mingle!

32. 3. When clients focus their mental and physical energy on somatic symptoms, they have little energy to expend on social or diversional activities. Such a client needs nursing assistance to become involved in social interactions. Although the other diagnoses are common for a client with conversion disorder, the information given in the question doesn't support them.
CN: Psychosocial integrity; CNS: None; CL: Application

33. 1. The client who uses somatization has typically adopted a sick role in the family, characterized by dependence. Increasing independence and resumption of former roles are necessary to change this pattern. The client shouldn't be expected to take on the roles or responsibilities of other family members. Focusing energy on problems occuring in the family doesn't address the nursing diagnosis and related factors.
CN: Psychosocial integrity; CNS: None; CL: Application

34. 2. *La belle indifference* is a lack of concern about the present illness. Acute dystonia refers to muscle spasms. Malingering is voluntary production of symptoms. Secondary gain refers to the benefits of illness.
CN: Psychosocial integrity; CNS: None; CL: Application

35. 4. Successful performance of independent activities enhances self-esteem. Telling the client that the symptoms are imaginary may jeopardize the nurse-client relationship. Positive reinforcement encourages the use of maladaptive responses. Focus shouldn't be on the disability because it may provide positive gains for the client.
CN: Psychosocial integrity; CNS: None; CL: Application

36. Which therapeutic approach would enable a client to cope effectively with life stress without using conversion?
1. Focus on the symptoms.
2. Ask for clarification of the symptoms.
3. Listen to the client's symptoms in a matter-of-fact manner.
4. Point out that the client's symptoms are an escape from dealing with conflict.

37. Which statement made by a client with a pain disorder shows the nurse that the goal of stress management was attained?
1. "My arm hurts."
2. "I enjoy being dependent on others."
3. "I don't really understand why I'm here."
4. "My muscles feel relaxed after that progressive relaxation exercise."

38. Which nursing diagnosis is appropriate for a client with hypochondriasis disorder?
1. *Disturbed sensory perception (visual)*
2. *Hopelessness*
3. *Imbalanced nutrition: Less than body requirements*
4. *Risk for other-directed violence*

39. A nurse is teaching the family of a client diagnosed with a somatoform pain disorder. Which of the following statements by the nurse most accurately describes this disorder?
1. A preoccupation with pain in the absence of physical disease
2. A physical or somatic complaint without any demonstrable organic findings
3. A morbid fear or belief that one has a serious disease where none exists
4. One or more neurologic symptoms associated with psychological conflict or need

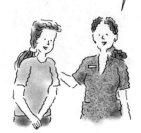

Focus on what the client is saying.

36. 3. Listening in a matter-of-fact manner doesn't focus on the client's symptoms. All other interventions focus on the client's symptoms, which draw attention to the physical symptoms, not the underlying cause.
CN: Health promotion and maintenance; CNS: None; CL: Application

37. 4. The client is experiencing positive results from the relaxation exercise. All other responses alert the nurse that the client needs further interventions.
CN: Physiological integrity; CNS: Basic care and comfort; CL: Analysis

38. 3. A client with hypochondriasis has a preoccupying fear of having a serious disease and is at risk for not getting adequate nutrition. Delusions are not a symptom of hypochondriasis. Although hopelessness may be present, it is not the primary focus. Clients with hypochondriasis are not prone to violence toward themselves or others.
CN: Safe, effective care environment; CNS: Management of care; CL: Application

39. 1. Somatoform pain disorder is a preoccupation with pain in the absence of physical disease. A physical or somatic complaint refers to somatoform disorders in general. A morbid fear of serious illness is hypochondriasis. Neurologic symptoms are associated with conversion disorders.
CN: Psychosocial integrity; CNS: None; CL: Application

40. By which process does a client conceal the true motivations for his thoughts, actions, or feelings?
1. Displacement
2. Rationalization
3. Regression
4. Substitution

What a relief!

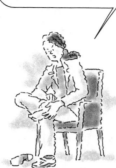

41. Which nursing goal is appropriate for a client with a pain disorder?
1. The client will express less fear.
2. The client will increase independence.
3. The client will express relief from pain.
4. The client will adapt coping strategies to deal with stress.

42. Which conditions or situations are most likely to result in difficulty sleeping? Select all that apply:
1. Shift work
2. Sleep apnea
3. Reduction of external stimuli
4. Caffeine intake in the evening
5. Consistent bedtime routine
6. Excessive worry or anxiety

43. Based on a nursing diagnosis of *Ineffective coping* for a client with somatoform pain disorder, which nursing goal is most realistic?
1. The client will be free from injury.
2. The client will recognize sensory impairment.
3. The client will discuss beliefs about spiritual issues.
4. The client will verbalize the absence or significant reduction of physical symptoms.

40. 2. Rationalization is a process by which an individual deals with emotional conflict or internal or external stressors by concealing the true motivations for his thoughts, actions, and feelings through the elaboration of reassuring or self-serving, but incorrect, explanations. This process isn't a defense mechanism related to pain disorders. Displacement, substitution, and regression are defense mechanisms that would be expected from a client with a pain disorder.
CN: Psychosocial integrity; CNS: None; CL: Application

41. 3. Relief of pain should be a priority for clients experiencing pain. Expression of less fear applies to a client with hypochondriasis. A focus on independence is appropriate for a client diagnosed with conversion disorder. The development of coping strategies would be beneficial for a client with a somatization disorder.
CN: Physiological integrity; CNS: Physiological adaptation; CL: Application

42. 1, 2, 4, 6. Shift work can disrupt the circadian rhythm. Sleep apnea can cause a reduction in oxygen to the brain, which can reduce the quality of rest. Caffeine is a stimulant and, if taken too close to bedtime, can interfere with falling asleep. Excessive worry or anxiety causes an increase in adrenaline, which enhances alertness and reduces sleepiness. A consistent bedtime routine and reduction of external stimuli promote good sleep.
CN: Health promotion and maintenance; CNS: None; CL: Analysis

43. 4. Expression of feelings enables the client to ventilate emotions, which decreases anxiety and draws attention away from the physical symptoms. The client isn't experiencing a safety issue. There's no apparent correlation with any sensory-perceptual alterations. Spiritual issues are related to spiritual distress, and no evidence exists to support that the client is having spiritual distress.
CN: Physiological integrity; CNS: Basic care and comfort; CL: Analysis

44. Which statement made by a client best meets the diagnostic criteria for pain disorder?
1. "I can't move my right leg."
2. "I'm having severe stomach and leg pain."
3. "I'm so afraid I might have human immunodeficiency virus."
4. "I'm having chest pain and pain radiating down my left arm that began more than 1 hour ago."

Remember, diagnostic criteria for psychologic problems come from the latest edition of the Diagnostic and Statistical Manual of Mental Disorders, currently known as DSM-IV-TR.

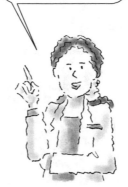

44. 2. The diagnostic criteria for pain disorders state that pain in one or more anatomic sites is the predominant focus of the clinical presentation and is of sufficient severity to warrant clinical attention. A client with a conversion disorder can experience a motor neurologic symptom such as paralysis. Hypochondriasis is a morbid fear or belief that one has a serious disease where none exists. Unremitting chest pain with radiation of pain down the left arm is symptomatic of a myocardial infarction.
CN: Psychosocial integrity; CNS: None; CL: Application

45. Which nursing diagnosis is appropriate for a client with somatoform pain disorder?
1. *Interrupted family processes*
2. *Disturbed body image*
3. *Ineffective denial*
4. *Ineffective coping*

45. 4. A somatoform pain disorder is closely associated with the client's inability to handle stress and conflict. Although *Interrupted family processes* and *Ineffective denial* may be present, they aren't the primary focus. *Disturbed body image* isn't directly correlated with this disorder.
CN: Safe, effective care environment; CNS: Management of care; CL: Application

46. Which statement made by a nurse will help a client diagnosed with somatoform pain disorder become independent in self-care?
1. "I'll call you for all the group activities."
2. "I'll help you on a daily basis with your care."
3. "The staff will help you with your basic needs for today."
4. "We'll wait until you have no more pain before you participate in activities."

46. 3. Limited time in assisting a client will help the client develop independence. All other options would promote dependence on the staff.
CN: Safe, effective care environment; CNS: Management of care; CL: Application

What is the initial intervention?

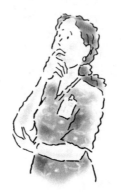

47. Which <u>initial</u> therapeutic intervention is the most appropriate for a client diagnosed with ineffective coping related to a pain disorder?
1. Make an accurate assessment.
2. Promote expression of feelings.
3. Promote insight into the disorder.
4. Help the client develop alternative coping strategies.

47. 1. It's essential to accurately assess the client first before any interventions. Promoting expression of feelings and insight and helping the client develop coping strategies are appropriate interventions that can be implemented after the initial assessment.
CN: Psychosocial integrity; CNS: None; CL: Application

48. A client with a somatoform pain disorder may obtain secondary gain. Which statement refers to a secondary gain?
1. It brings some stability to the family.
2. It decreases the preoccupation with the physical illness.
3. It enables the client to avoid some unpleasant activity.
4. It promotes emotional support or attention for the client.

48. 4. Secondary gain refers to the benefits of the illness that allow the client to receive emotional support or attention. A dysfunctional family may disregard the real issue, although some conflict is relieved. Somatoform pain disorder is a preoccupation with pain in the absence of physical disease. Primary gain enables the client to avoid some unpleasant activity.
CN: Psychosocial integrity; CNS: None; CL: Analysis

CN: Client needs category   CNS: Client needs subcategory   CL: Cognitive level

49. Which nursing intervention is appropriate for a client diagnosed with a somatoform pain disorder?

1. Reinforce the client's behavior when it isn't focused on pain.
2. Allow the client to verbalize anxieties related to body image.
3. Allow the client to verbalize relief of fear related to the illness.
4. Assist the client in recovery of the lost or altered function of a body part.

50. A client has primary insomnia and requires pharmaceutical assistance to sleep. The physician orders secobarbital sodium (Seconal) 75 mg by mouth at bedtime. The nurse has secobarbital sodium 25-mg tablets on hand. How many tablets should the nurse administer to the client? Record your answer using a whole number.

_____ tablets

51. A home health nurse is caring for a client diagnosed with a conversion disorder manifested by paralysis in the left arm. An organic cause for the deficit has been ruled out. Which nursing intervention is the most appropriate for this client?

1. Perform all physical tasks for the client to foster dependence.
2. Allot an hour each day to discuss the paralysis and its cause.
3. Identify primary or secondary gains that the physical symptom provides.
4. Allow the client to withdraw from all physical activities.

52. A client with somatoform disorder states that her frequent headaches result from a brain tumor. However, a tumor hasn't shown up on diagnostic tests. The nurse identifies the client's form of somatization as which disorder?

1. Conversion disorder
2. Pain disorder
3. Hypochondriasis
4. Body dysmorphic disorder

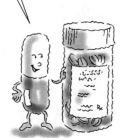

Remember to use the correct formula when calculating the appropriate drug dose.

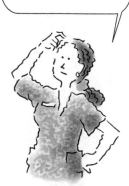

Have you sorted out the various forms of somatization? Don't try to rush. You can do it!

49. 1. Help the client get attention and see himself as valuable without using pain. Verbalization of anxieties related to body image may be beneficial in a client with body dysmorphic disorder. Fear of illness is related to hypochondriasis. The recovery of a lost or altered function of a part is related to conversion disorders.
CN: Psychosocial integrity; CNS: None; CL: Application

50. 3. Each tablet contains 25 mg of the medication. The correct formula to calculate this drug dose is:

Dose of each tablet × X = Prescribed dose
25 mg × X (# of tablets) = 75 mg
25X = 75
X = 75/25
X = 3

CN: Physiological integrity; CNS: Pharmacological and parenteral therapies; CL: Analysis

51. 3. Primary or secondary gains should be identified because they're etiological factors that can be used in problem resolution. The nurse should encourage the client to be as independent as possible and should intervene only when the client requires assistance. The nurse shouldn't focus on the disability. The nurse should encourage the client to perform physical activities to the greatest extent possible.
CN: Psychosocial integrity; CNS: None; CL: Application

52. 3. In hypochondriasis, a physical symptom is interpreted as severe or life-threatening and causes exaggerated worry. In conversion disorder, the client loses a motor or sensory function but lacks appropriate concern about the loss. In pain disorder, pain is the dominant feature. In body dysmorphic disorder, the client is preoccupied with a perceived defect in appearance.
CN: Psychosocial integrity; CNS: None; CL: Application

53. A college student frequently visited the health center before course examinations. Physical causes for these visits have been eliminated. Based on the following progress note entry in the client's chart, the nurse suspects which disorder?

Progress notes	
9/9/10	19-year-old client states I'm having
2130	abdominal discomfort. It happens on
	and off, especially the last week while
	I'm trying to study for mid-term
	exams. I know that there's something
	really wrong. Client denies that these
	symptoms are related to eating. Normal
	bowel sounds auscultated. Abdomen soft
	and nontender to palpation. Vital signs:
	Temp, 98.2°F; BP, 114/72 mm Hg; heart
	rate, 76 beats/minute; respiratory rate,
	20 breaths/minute. Client denies
	nausea, vomiting, diarrhea or loss of
	appetite. ———— Natalie Jones, RN

1. Conversion disorder
2. Depersonalization
3. Hypochondriasis
4. Somatoform disorder

54. A 26-year-old client is diagnosed with somatoform disorder. When discussing the care plan with the client's wife, the nurse should give which instruction?
1. "Tell your husband that his symptoms are all in his head to force him to deal with reality."
2. "Tell your husband that his symptoms are an attempt to get attention and that you'll be more attentive."
3. "Accept the reality of the symptoms as your husband presents them, and don't dispute them."
4. "Realize that your husband is creating the symptoms on purpose."

55. A client with a diagnosis of somatoform disorder has been admitted to the psychiatric unit and has difficulty breathing, numbness, and loss of movement in his left arm. He seems unusually calm and unconcerned about his loss. The nurse recognizes these symptoms as which disorder?
1. Conversion disorder
2. Hypochondriasis
3. Body dysmorphic disorder
4. Pain disorder

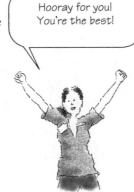

Hooray for you! You're the best!

53. 3. Hypochondriasis in this case is shown by the client's belief that she has a serious illness, although pathologic causes have been eliminated. The disturbance usually lasts at least 6 months, and the GI system is commonly affected. Exacerbations are usually associated with identifiable life stressors that, in this case, can be related to the client's examinations. Conversion disorders are characterized by one or more neurologic symptoms. Depersonalization refers to persistent, recurrent, episodes of feeling detached from one's self or body. Somatoform disorders generally have a chronic course with few remissions.
CN: Psychosocial integrity; CNS: None; CL: Analysis

54. 3. For a client with somatoform disorder, caregivers should accept the symptoms and avoid disputing them. The symptoms aren't contrived or all in the client's head. They're neither an attempt to get attention nor created "on purpose."
CN: Psychosocial integrity; CNS: None; CL: Application

55. 1. Conversion disorder is characterized by loss of motor, sensory, or visceral functioning accompanied by the client's indifference to the loss. In hypochondriasis, the client interprets a physical symptom as severe or life-threatening and worries over it excessively. Body dysmorphic disorder is a preoccupation with a perceived defect in appearance. In pain disorder, pain is the dominant physical symptom.
CN: Psychosocial integrity; CNS: None; CL: Application

CN: Client needs category   CNS: Client needs subcategory   CL: Cognitive level

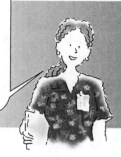

Chapter 15
Anxiety & mood disorders

1. Which statement is <u>typical</u> of a client who experiences periodic panic attacks while sleeping?
1. "Yesterday, I sat up in bed and just felt so scared."
2. "I have difficulty sleeping because I'm so anxious."
3. "Sometimes I have the most wild and vivid dreams."
4. "When I drink beer, I fall asleep without any problems."

2. A client with generalized anxiety disorder states, "I'm afraid I'm going to die from cancer. My mother had cancer." Which of the following responses by the nurse would be the most therapeutic?
1. "We all live in fear of dying from cancer."
2. "Did your father also have cancer?"
3. "I wouldn't worry about it just yet. You seem to be in good health."
4. "Has something happened that is causing you to worry?"

3. A client with a history of panic attacks who says, "I felt so trapped," right after an attack <u>most likely</u> has which fear?
1. Loss of control
2. Loss of identity
3. Loss of memory
4. Loss of maturity

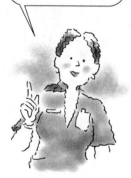

Question 1 is typical of what you'll be asked throughout the test.

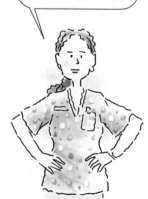

Remember: You're in control, so read the question carefully and choose the most likely response.

1. 1. A person who suffers a panic attack while sleeping experiences an abrupt awakening and feelings of fear. People with severe anxiety commonly have symptoms related to a sleep disorder; they wouldn't typically experience a sleep panic attack. A panic attack while sleeping often causes an inability to remember dreams. Intake of alcohol initially produces a drowsy feeling, but after a short period of time alcohol causes restless, fragmented sleep and strange dreams.
CN: Psychosocial integrity; CNS: None; CL: Analysis

2. 4. By asking the client about what is making them worry, the nurse assists the client in determining the cause of the anxiety. The other responses deflect and minimize the client's concerns.
CN: Psychosocial integrity; CNS: None; CL: Analysis

3. 1. People who fear loss of control during a panic attack commonly make statements about feeling trapped, getting hurt, or having little or no personal control over their situations. People who experience panic attacks don't tend to have loss of identity or memory impairment. People who have panic attacks also don't regress or become immature.
CN: Psychosocial integrity; CNS: None; CL: Application

CN: Client needs category   CNS: Client needs subcategory   CL: Cognitive level

4. A nurse is caring for a client with a panic disorder. On morning rounds, the physician orders alprazolam (Xanax). In reviewing the client's medical history, the nurse calls the physician regarding:
1. intermittent insomnia.
2. acute-angle glaucoma.
3. seizure disorder.
4. tartrazine hypersensitivity.

5. Which nursing intervention is given priority in a care plan for a client having an acute panic attack?
1. Tell the client to take deep breaths.
2. Have the client talk about the anxiety.
3. Encourage the client to verbalize feelings.
4. Ask the client about the cause of the attack.

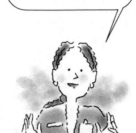

Don't panic! Stay calm and remember to prioritize.

6. Which instruction should a nurse include in a teaching session about panic disorder for clients and their families?
1. Identifying when anxiety is escalating
2. Determining how to stop a panic attack
3. Addressing strategies to reduce physical pain
4. Preventing the client from depending on others

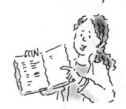

For the NCLEX, you should memorize the definitions of common fears such as agoraphobia.

7. Which question should a nurse ask to determine how <u>agoraphobia</u> affects the life of a client who has panic attacks?
1. How realistic are your goals?
2. Are you able to go shopping?
3. Do you struggle with impulse control?
4. Who else in your family has panic disorder?

4. 2. Acute-angle glaucoma is a medical problem that contraindicates the use of alprazolam. Alprazolam causes drowsiness and sedation, so sleep shouldn't be interrupted. Seizure disorder isn't a contraindication for the use of alprazolam. Tartrazine hypersensitivity is associated with yellow dye used in some convenience foods and isn't a contraindication for the use of alprazolam.
CN: Physiological integrity; CNS: Pharmacological and parenteral therapies; CL: Application

5. 1. During a panic attack, the nurse should remain with the client and direct what's said toward changing the physiologic response, such as taking deep breaths. During an attack, the client is unable to talk about anxious situations and isn't able to address feelings, especially uncomfortable feelings and frustrations. While having a panic attack, the client is also unable to focus on anything other than the symptoms, so the client won't be able to discuss the cause of the attack.
CN: Safe, effective care environment; CNS: Management of care; CL: Analysis

6. 1. By identifying the presence of anxiety, it's possible to take steps to prevent its escalation. A panic attack can't be stopped. The nurse can take steps to assist the client safely through the attack. Later, the nurse can assist the client to alleviate the precipitating stressors. Clients who experience panic disorder don't tend to be in physical pain. The client experiencing a panic disorder may need to periodically depend on other people when having a panic attack.
CN: Psychosocial integrity; CNS: None; CL: Application

7. 2. The client with agoraphobia typically restricts himself to home and can't carry out normal socializing and life-sustaining activities. Clients with panic disorder are able to set realistic goals and tend to be cautious and reclusive rather than impulsive. Although there's a familial tendency toward panic disorder, information about client needs must be obtained to determine how agoraphobia affects the client's life.
CN: Psychosocial integrity; CNS: None; CL: Application

8. Which fact would be helpful to include when teaching a female client who's considering life-style changes as part of a behavior modification program to treat her panic attacks?
1. Cigarettes can trigger panic episodes.
2. Fermented foods can cause panic attacks.
3. Hormonal therapy can induce panic attacks.
4. Tryptophan can predispose a person to panic attacks.

9. Which intervention should a nurse initially implement when caring for a client with panic disorder?
1. Make the client role-play the panic attack.
2. Assist the client to develop an exercise program.
3. Teach the client to identify cognitive distortions.
4. Teach the client to identify sources of anxiety.

10. Which nursing intervention is appropriate to include when planning care for a client with panic disorder?
1. Identify childhood trauma.
2. Monitor nutritional intake.
3. Institute suicide precautions.
4. Monitor episodes of disorientation.

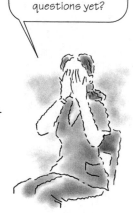

I'm too anxious to look. Have you finished 10 questions yet?

11. A client diagnosed with panic disorder with agoraphobia is talking with the nurse about the progress made in treatment. Which statement indicates a positive client response?
1. "I went to the mall with my friend last Saturday."
2. "I'm hyperventilating only when I have a panic attack."
3. "Today I decided that I can stop taking my medication."
4. "Last night I decided to eat more than a bowl of cereal."

8. 1. Cigarettes contain nicotine, which can be a stimulant, a depressant, or a tranquilizer, and can trigger panic attacks. None of the other options causes panic attacks.
CN: Psychosocial integrity; CNS: None; CL: Application

9. 4. The client must be aware of the connection between sources of anxiety and the symptoms of a panic attack. Role-playing a panic attack isn't useful. Role-playing coping strategies would be useful for the client. Later in treatment, the client can develop an exercise program as part of the overall plan to handle stress. Learning to identify cognitive distortions is a useful strategy to teach the client after he's begun to work on identifying sources of anxiety.
CN: Psychosocial integrity; CNS: None; CL: Analysis

10. 3. Clients with panic disorder are at risk for suicide because they can be impulsive. Childhood trauma is associated with posttraumatic stress disorder, *not* panic disorder. Nutritional problems don't typically accompany panic disorder. Clients aren't typically disoriented; they may have a temporary altered sense of reality, but that lasts only for the duration of the attack.
CN: Psychosocial integrity; CNS: None; CL: Application

11. 1. Clients with panic disorder tend to be socially withdrawn. Going to the mall is a sign of working on avoidance behaviors. Hyperventilation is a key symptom of panic disorder. Teaching breathing control is a major intervention for clients with panic disorder. The client taking medications for panic disorder, such as tricyclic antidepressants and benzodiazepines, must be weaned off these drugs. Most clients with panic disorder with agoraphobia don't have nutritional problems.
CN: Psychosocial integrity; CNS: None; CL: Analysis

12. Which group therapy intervention should be of <u>primary</u> importance to a client with panic disorder?
1. Explore how secondary gains are derived from the disorder.
2. Discuss new ways of thinking and feeling about panic attacks.
3. Work to eliminate manipulative behavior used for meeting needs.
4. Learn the risk factors and other demographics associated with panic disorder.

13. A nurse is caring for a client with social phobia. A symptom that should be addressed in a team meeting is the client's tendency toward:
1. self-harm.
2. poor self-esteem.
3. compulsive behavior.
4. avoidance of social situations.

14. Which statement is typical of a client with social phobia?
1. "Without people around, I just feel so lost."
2. "There's nothing wrong with my behavior."
3. "I like to be the center of attention."
4. "I know I can't accept that award for my brother."

15. Clients with a social phobia would most likely fear which situation?
1. Dental procedures
2. Meeting strangers
3. Being bitten by a dog
4. Having a car collision

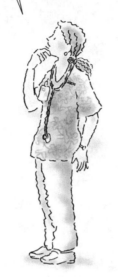

Which intervention is of primary importance?

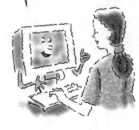

Don't be shy about answering this question.

12. 2. Restructuring an anxiety-producing event allows the client to gain control over the situation. Discussing new ways of thinking and feeling about panic attacks can enable others to learn and benefit from a variety of intervention strategies. There are usually no secondary gains obtained from having a panic disorder. People with panic disorder aren't using the disorder as a way to manipulate others. Learning the risk factors could be accomplished in another format such as a psychoeducational program.
CN: Psychosocial integrity; CNS: None; CL: Analysis

13. 4. Clients with social phobia avoid social situations for fear of being humiliated or embarrassed. They generally don't tend to be at risk for self-harm and usually don't demonstrate compulsive behavior. Not all individuals with social anxiety have low self-esteem.
CN: Psychosocial integrity; CNS: None; CL: Application

14. 4. People who have a social phobia usually undervalue themselves and their talents. They don't like to be in feared social situations or around many people. They tend to stay away from situations in which they may feel humiliated and embarrassed. They fear social gatherings and dislike being the center of attention. They're very critical of themselves and believe that others also will be critical.
CN: Psychosocial integrity; CNS: None; CL: Application

15. 2. Fear of meeting strangers is a common example of social phobia. Fears of having a dental procedure, being bitten by a dog, or having a collision are *not* social phobias.
CN: Psychosocial integrity; CNS: None; CL: Application

CN: Client needs category   CNS: Client needs subcategory   CL: Cognitive level

16. Which factor should the nurse find most helpful in assessing a client for a blood-injection-injury phobia?
1. Episodes of fainting
2. Gregarious personality
3. Difficulty managing anger
4. Dramatic, overreactive personality

17. Which individual counseling approach should be used to assist a client with a phobic disorder?
1. Have the client keep a daily journal.
2. Help the client identify the source of the anxiety.
3. Teach the client effective ways to problem-solve.
4. Develop strategies to prevent the client from using substances.

18. Which behavior modification technique is useful in the treatment of phobias?
1. Aversion therapy
2. Imitation or modeling
3. Positive reinforcement
4. Systematic desensitization

19. Which statement would be useful when teaching the client and family about phobias and the need for a strong support system?
1. The use of a family support system is only temporary.
2. The need to be assertive can be reinforced by the family.
3. The family needs to set limits on inappropriate behaviors.
4. The family plays a role in promoting client independence.

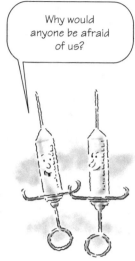

Why would anyone be afraid of us?

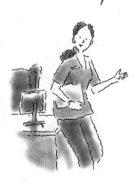

Along with assessment, you also need to familiarize yourself with common treatments.

16. 1. Many people with a history of blood-injection-injury phobia report frequently fainting when exposed to this type of situation. All personality styles can develop phobias, so personality type doesn't provide information for assessing phobias. Information about a client's difficulty managing anger isn't related to a specific phobic disorder. Individuals with blood-injection-injury phobias aren't being dramatic or overreactive.
CN: Psychosocial integrity; CNS: None; CL: Analysis

17. 2. By understanding the source of the anxiety, the client will understand how this anxiety has been displaced as a phobic response. Keeping a journal is an effective method in many situations; however, its use is limited in the treatment of phobias. Problem solving is a more useful technique for clients with obsessive-compulsive disorder than for clients with phobias. People with phobias don't tend to self-medicate like clients with other psychiatric disorders.
CN: Psychosocial integrity; CNS: None; CL: Application

18. 4. Systematic desensitization is a common behavior modification technique successfully used to help treat phobias. Aversion therapy and positive reinforcement are *not* behavior modification techniques used with treatment of phobias. Imitation and modeling are social learning techniques, not behavior modification techniques.
CN: Psychosocial integrity; CNS: None; CL: Application

19. 4. The family plays a vital role in supporting the client in treatment and preventing the client from using the phobia to obtain secondary gains. Family support must be ongoing, not temporary. The family can be more helpful by focusing on effective handling of anxiety, rather than focusing on developing assertiveness skills. People with phobias are already restrictive in their behavior; more restrictions aren't necessary.
CN: Psychosocial integrity; CNS: None; CL: Analysis

20. Which nursing intervention is of primary importance during the administration of paroxetine (Paxil) to a depressed client with a phobic disorder?
1. Monitor renal function.
2. Determine electrocardiogram (ECG) changes.
3. Assess for sleeping difficulties.
4. Observe for extrapyramidal symptoms.

21. A client suspected of having posttraumatic stress disorder should be assessed for which problem?
1. Eating disorder
2. Schizophrenia
3. Suicide
4. "Sundown" syndrome

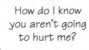
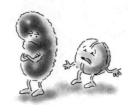

How do I know you aren't going to hurt me?

22. Which action explains why tricyclic antidepressant medication is given to a client who has severe posttraumatic stress disorder?
1. It prevents hyperactivity and purposeless movements.
2. It increases the client's ability to concentrate.
3. It helps prevent experiencing the trauma again.
4. It facilitates the grieving process.

23. Which nursing action should be included in a care plan for a client with posttraumatic stress disorder who states that the experience was "bad luck"?
1. Encourage the client to verbalize the experience.
2. Assist the client in defining the experience as a trauma.
3. Work with the client to take steps to move on with life.
4. Help the client accept positive and negative feelings.

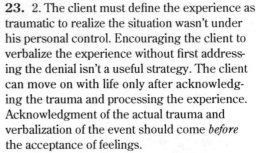

Don't deny it. You're doing great!

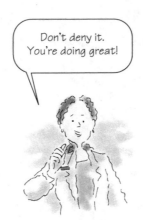

20. 1. Clients with impaired renal function shouldn't take paroxetine. ECG changes aren't adverse effects of paroxetine. Other than a transient period of drowsiness occurring when the client begins to take the drug, sleep difficulties don't tend to be a problem. Extrapyramidal symptoms aren't seen with paroxetine.
CN: Physiological integrity; CNS: Pharmacological and parenteral therapies; CL: Analysis

21. 3. Clients who experience posttraumatic stress disorder are at high risk for suicide and other forms of violent behaviors. Eating disorders are possible but aren't a common complication of posttraumatic stress disorder. Clients with posttraumatic stress disorder don't usually have their extreme anxiety manifest itself as schizophrenia. "Sundown" syndrome is an increase in agitation accompanied by confusion. It's commonly seen in clients with dementia, not clients with posttraumatic stress disorder.
CN: Psychosocial integrity; CNS: None; CL: Application

22. 3. Tricyclic antidepressant medication will decrease the frequency of reenactment of the trauma for the client. It will help memory problems and sleeping difficulties and will decrease numbing. The medication won't prevent hyperactivity and purposeless movements nor increase the client's concentration. No medication will facilitate the grieving process.
CN: Physiological integrity; CNS: Pharmacological and parenteral therapies; CL: Application

23. 2. The client must define the experience as traumatic to realize the situation wasn't under his personal control. Encouraging the client to verbalize the experience without first addressing the denial isn't a useful strategy. The client can move on with life only after acknowledging the trauma and processing the experience. Acknowledgment of the actual trauma and verbalization of the event should come *before* the acceptance of feelings.
CN: Psychosocial integrity; CNS: None; CL: Analysis

24. Which instruction should a nurse include about relationships for the client with posttraumatic stress disorder?
1. Encourage the client to resume former roles as soon as possible.
2. Assess the client's discomfort when talking about feelings to family members.
3. Explain that avoiding emotional attachment protects against anxiety.
4. Warn the client that he'll have a tendency to be overdependent in relationships.

25. Which approach should a nurse use with the family when a posttraumatic stress disorder client states, "My family doesn't believe anything about posttraumatic stress disorder"?
1. Provide the family with information.
2. Teach the family about problem solving.
3. Discuss the family's view of the problem.
4. Assess for the presence of family violence.

Caring for clients commonly means working with their families—a skill you can expect the exam to test.

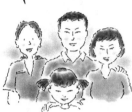

26. While caring for a client with posttraumatic stress disorder, the family notices that loud noises cause a serious anxiety response. Which explanation should help the family understand the client's response?
1. Environmental triggers can cause the client to become hyperaroused and have exaggerated startle reactions.
2. Clients commonly experience extreme fear about normal environmental stimuli.
3. After a trauma, the client can't respond to stimuli in an appropriate manner.
4. The response indicates that another emotional problem needs investigation.

27. Which psychological symptom should a nurse expect to find in a hospitalized client who's the only survivor of a train collision?
1. Denial
2. Indifference
3. Perfectionism
4. Trust

24. 3. The client may tend to avoid interpersonal relationships to protect himself against unrelieved anxiety. Because relationships tend to be avoided, the client won't express feelings to family members at this time and won't resume roles and responsibilities for a while. Clients with posttraumatic stress disorder don't tend to become overdependent in relationships but do tend to withdraw from them.
CN: Psychosocial integrity; CNS: None; CL: Application

25. 1. If the family can understand posttraumatic stress disorder, they can more readily participate in the client's care and be supportive. Learning problem-solving skills doesn't help clarify posttraumatic stress disorder. After being given information about posttraumatic stress disorder, the family can then ask questions and present its views. The family must first have information about posttraumatic stress disorder; then the discussion about violence to self or others can be addressed.
CN: Safe, effective care environment; CNS: Management of care; CL: Application

26. 1. Repeated exposure to environmental triggers can cause the client to experience a hyperarousal state because there's a loss of physiologic control of incoming stimuli. After experiencing a trauma, the client may have strong reactions to stimuli similar to those that occurred during the traumatic event. However, not *all* stimuli will cause an anxiety response. The client's anxiety response is typically seen after a traumatic experience and doesn't indicate the presence of another problem.
CN: Psychosocial integrity; CNS: None; CL: Application

27. 1. Denial can act as a protective response. The client tends to be overwhelmed and disorganized by the trauma, not indifferent to it. Perfectionism is more commonly seen in clients with eating disorders, not in clients with posttraumatic stress disorder. Clients who have had a severe trauma commonly experience an inability to trust others.
CN: Psychosocial integrity; CNS: None; CL: Analysis

28. If a client suffering from posttraumatic stress disorder says, "I've decided to just avoid everything and everyone," the nurse might suspect the client is at greatest risk for which behavior?
1. Becoming homeless
2. Exhausting finances
3. Terminating employment
4. Using substances

29. Which action would be most appropriate when speaking with a client with posttraumatic stress disorder about the trauma?
1. Obtain validation of what the client says from another party.
2. Request that the client write down what's being said.
3. Ask questions to convey an interest in the details.
4. Listen attentively and remain with the client.

30. Which client statement indicates an understanding of survivor guilt?
1. "I think I can see the purpose of my survival."
2. "I can't help but feel that everything is their fault."
3. "I now understand why I'm not able to forgive myself."
4. "I wish I could stop sabotaging my family relationships."

31. Which nursing intervention would best help a client with posttraumatic stress disorder and his family handle interpersonal conflict at home?
1. Have the family teach the client to identify defensive behaviors.
2. Have the family discuss how to change dysfunctional family patterns.
3. Have the family agree not to tell the client what to do about problems.
4. Have the family arrange for the client to participate in social activities.

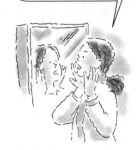

Mirror, mirror, on the wall, what's the greatest risk of all?

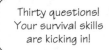

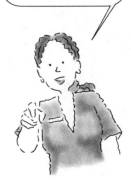

Thirty questions! Your survival skills are kicking in!

28. 4. The use of substances is a way for the client to deny problems and self-medicate distress. There are few homeless people with posttraumatic stress disorder as the cause of their homelessness. Most clients with posttraumatic stress disorder can manage money and maintain employment.
CN: Psychosocial integrity; CNS: None; CL: Application

29. 4. An effective communication strategy for a nurse to use with a posttraumatic stress disorder client is listening attentively and staying with the client. There's no need to obtain validation about what the client says by asking for information from another party, asking the client to write what's being said, or distracting him by asking questions.
CN: Psychosocial integrity; CNS: None; CL: Application

30. 3. Survivor guilt occurs when the person has almost constant thoughts about the other people who perished in the event. The survivor doesn't understand why he survived when a friend or loved one didn't. Blaming self, not others, is a component of survivor guilt. Survivor guilt and impaired interpersonal relationships are two different categories of responses to trauma.
CN: Psychosocial integrity; CNS: None; CL: Analysis

31. 2. Discussion of dysfunctional family patterns allows the family to determine why and how these patterns are maintained. Having family members point out the defensive behaviors of the client may inadvertently produce more defensive behavior. Families can be a source of support and assistance; therefore, inflexible rules aren't useful to either the client or the family. The family shouldn't be encouraged to arrange social activities for the client. Social activities outside of the home don't help the family handle conflict within the home.
CN: Psychosocial integrity; CNS: None; CL: Application

CN: Client needs category   CNS: Client needs subcategory   CL: Cognitive level

32. The family members of a client diagnosed with posttraumatic stress disorder can't understand why the client has this disorder, especially because the client didn't directly experience a personal trauma. Which topic should the nurse discuss with the family?
  1. Advise them to obtain a second psychiatric evaluation.
  2. Ask them what they perceive the client's problem to be.
  3. Explain the effect of learning about another's experience.
  4. Identify the time period the client manifested symptoms.

32. 3. Posttraumatic stress disorder can occur if a person has experienced the traumatic event, witnessed the event happening to another person, or learned that trauma has happened to a family member or close friend. After educating the family about posttraumatic stress disorder, a second evaluation may not be necessary. Encouraging family members to discuss the situation and share their perceptions can be helpful, but it isn't their responsibility or within their abilities to diagnose the health problem. Symptoms of posttraumatic stress disorder usually appear 6 or more months after the event has occurred for at least a 1-month duration. This information isn't as important as an explanation of what constitutes a traumatic event.
CN: Psychosocial integrity; CNS: None; CL: Analysis

33. The effectiveness of monoamine oxidase (MAO) inhibitor drug therapy in a client with posttraumatic stress disorder can be demonstrated by which client self-report?
  1. "I'm sleeping better and don't have nightmares."
  2. "I'm not losing my temper as much."
  3. "I've lost my craving for alcohol."
  4. "I've lost my phobia for water."

33. 1. MAO inhibitors are used to treat sleep problems, nightmares, and intrusive daytime thoughts in individuals with posttraumatic stress disorder. MAO inhibitors aren't used to help control flashbacks or phobias or to decrease the craving for alcohol.
CN: Physiological integrity; CNS: Pharmacological and parenteral therapies; CL: Analysis

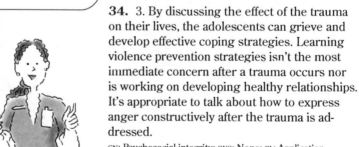

The term *major purpose* indicates that there may be more than one right answer. You need to choose the best answer.

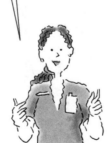

34. Which result is the <u>major purpose</u> of group therapy for adolescents who witnessed the violent death of a peer?
  1. To learn violence prevention strategies
  2. To talk about appropriate expression of anger
  3. To discuss the effect of the trauma on their lives
  4. To develop trusting relationships among their peers

34. 3. By discussing the effect of the trauma on their lives, the adolescents can grieve and develop effective coping strategies. Learning violence prevention strategies isn't the most immediate concern after a trauma occurs nor is working on developing healthy relationships. It's appropriate to talk about how to express anger constructively after the trauma is addressed.
CN: Psychosocial integrity; CNS: None; CL: Application

35. Which symptom of posttraumatic stress disorder would indicate that hypnosis is an appropriate treatment modality?
  1. Addiction
  2. Confabulation
  3. Dissociation
  4. Hallucinations

35. 3. Hypnosis is one of the main therapies for clients who dissociate. Hypnosis isn't a treatment of choice for clients with addictive disorders or hallucinations. Confabulation isn't a symptom of posttraumatic stress disorder.
CN: Psychosocial integrity; CNS: None; CL: Application

36. Which nursing behavior would demonstrate caring to a client with a diagnosis of anxiety disorder?
1. Verbalize concern about the client.
2. Arrange group activities for the client.
3. Have the client sign the treatment plan.
4. Hold psychoeducational groups on medications.

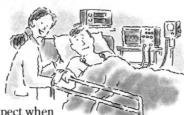

It's important for the client to know you care.

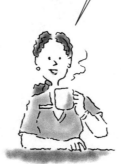

37. Which finding should a nurse expect when talking about school to a child diagnosed with a generalized anxiety disorder?
1. The child has been fighting with peers for the past month.
2. The child can't stop lying to parents and teachers.
3. The child has gained 15 (6.8 kg) pounds in the past month.
4. The child expresses concerns about grades.

38. A client with a generalized anxiety disorder also may have which concurrent diagnosis?
1. Bipolar disorder
2. Gender identity disorder
3. Panic disorder
4. Schizoaffective disorder

What do you know about the relationship between anxiety and caffeine?

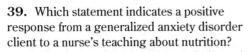

39. Which statement indicates a positive response from a generalized anxiety disorder client to a nurse's teaching about nutrition?
1. "I've stopped drinking so much diet cola."
2. "I've reduced my intake of carbohydrates."
3. "I now eat less at dinner and before bedtime."
4. "I've cut back on my use of dairy products."

36. 1. The nurse who verbally expresses concern about a client's well-being is acting in a caring and supportive manner. Arranging for group activities may be an action where the nurse has no direct client contact and is therefore unable to have interpersonal contact with clients. Having a client sign the treatment plan may not be viewed as a sign of caring. Having a psychoeducational group on medications may be viewed by clients as a teaching experience and not interpersonal contact, because the nurse may have limited interactions with them.
CN: Psychosocial integrity; CNS: None; CL: Application

37. 4. Children with generalized anxiety disorder will worry about how well they're performing in school. Children with generalized anxiety disorder don't tend to be involved in conflict. They're more oriented toward good behavior. Children with generalized anxiety disorder don't tend to lie to others. They would want to do their best and try to please others. A weight gain of 15 pounds isn't a typical characteristic of a child with anxiety disorder.
CN: Psychosocial integrity; CNS: None; CL: Analysis

38. 3. Approximately 75% of clients with generalized anxiety disorder also may have a diagnosis of phobia, panic disorder, or substance abuse. Clients with generalized anxiety disorder don't tend to have a coexisting diagnosis of gender identity disorder, bipolar disorder, or schizoaffective disorder.

CN: Psychosocial integrity; CNS: None; CL: Application

39. 1. Clients with generalized anxiety disorder can decrease anxiety by eliminating caffeine from their diets. It isn't necessary for clients with generalized anxiety to decrease their carbohydrate intake, eat less at dinner or before bedtime (unless there are other compelling health reasons), or cut back on their use of dairy products.
CN: Physiological integrity; CNS: Basic care and comfort; CL: Application

CN: Client needs category   CNS: Client needs subcategory   CL: Cognitive level

40. A client with generalized anxiety disorder is prescribed a benzodiazepine, but the client doesn't want to take the medication. Which explanation by the client for this behavior would be most likely?
1. "I don't think the psychiatrist likes me."
2. "I want to solve my problems on my own."
3. "The voices tell me that I don't have to take the medication."
4. "I think my family gains by keeping me medicated."

41. Which factor should a nurse consider when assisting a client with generalized anxiety disorder in verbalizing feelings?
1. The client may intellectualize the anxiety.
2. The client may regard the problem as genetic.
3. The client may decide that verbalizing feelings isn't beneficial.
4. The client may believe only medications are useful.

42. Which of the following statements would most likely be associated with an adult client who has a long-standing history of generalized anxiety disorder?
1. "I was, and still am, an impulsive person."
2. "I've always been hyperactive, but not in useful ways."
3. "When I was in college, I never thought I would finish."
4. "All my life I've had intrusive dreams and scary nightmares."

43. Which symptom would a client with generalized anxiety disorder most likely display when assessed for muscle tension?
1. Difficulty sleeping
2. Restlessness
3. Strong startle response
4. Tachycardia

40 down, 54 to go!

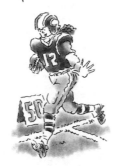

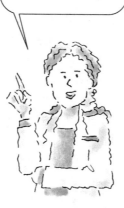

Certain psychological disorders tend to appear at particular ages—that's information to know for the NCLEX.

40. 2. It's common for a client with generalized anxiety disorder to refuse to take medication because he believes that using a medication is a sign of personal weakness and that he can't solve problems by himself. Fear that the psychiatrist dislikes him reflects paranoid thinking that isn't usually seen in a client with generalized anxiety disorder. Auditory hallucinations and paranoia about the motives of friends and family members aren't characteristic of clients with generalized anxiety disorder.
CN: Psychosocial integrity; CNS: None; CL: Analysis

41. 1. Clients who experience generalized anxiety disorder commonly need assistance acknowledging anxiety instead of denying or intellectualizing it. Although scientists believe that there may be a tendency for anxiety to be familial, the problem isn't regarded as genetic. A client who's unwilling to express feelings may not view therapy as helpful. The most effective treatment of generalized anxiety disorder combines psychotherapy and pharmacotherapy.
CN: Psychosocial integrity; CNS: None; CL: Analysis

42. 3. For many people who have a generalized anxiety disorder, the age of onset is during young adulthood. The symptoms of impulsiveness and hyperactivity aren't commonly associated with a diagnosis of generalized anxiety disorder. Intrusive dreams and nightmares are associated with posttraumatic stress disorder rather than generalized anxiety disorder.
CN: Psychosocial integrity; CNS: None; CL: Analysis

43. 2. Restlessness is a symptom associated with muscle tension. Difficulty sleeping and a strong startle response are considered symptoms of vigilance and scanning of the environment, not muscle tension. Tachycardia is classified as a symptom of autonomic hyperactivity, not muscle tension.
CN: Physiological integrity; CNS: Physiological adaptation; CL: Application

44. Which intervention should be given <u>priority</u> for a client with generalized anxiety disorder who's working to develop coping skills?

1. Determine whether the client has fears or obsessive thinking.
2. Monitor the client for overt and covert signs of anxiety.
3. Teach the client how to use effective communications skills.
4. Assist the client to identify coping mechanisms used in the past.

45. Which instruction should help a nurse deal with escalating client anxiety?

1. Explore feelings about current life stressors.
2. Discuss the need to flee from painful situations.
3. Have the client develop a realistic view of self.
4. Provide appropriate phone numbers for hotlines and clinics.

46. Which of the following points would a nurse include in teaching for the family of an adult client with generalized anxiety disorder?

1. Explain how the family can handle the confusion related to memory loss.
2. Teach the family to assist the client with coping strategies as needed.
3. Teach the family how to cope with the client's sudden and unexpected travel behavior.
4. Have the family determine when and for what reasons the client should take medication.

47. A client with a diagnosis of generalized anxiety disorder wants to stop taking his lorazepam (Ativan). Which important fact should the nurse discuss with the client about discontinuing the medication?

1. Stopping the drug may cause depression.
2. Stopping the drug increases cognitive abilities.
3. Stopping the drug decreases sleeping difficulties.
4. Stopping the drug can cause withdrawal symptoms.

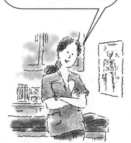

Thorough teaching plans typically include ways to contact support organizations.

You should be familiar with the symptoms that discontinuing key medications may cause.

44. 4. To help a client develop effective coping skills, the nurse must know the client's baseline functioning. Determining whether the client has fears or obsessive thinking, monitoring for signs of anxiety, and teaching about effective communications skills are later priorities, not initial ones.
CN: Safe, effective care environment; CNS: Management of care; CL: Application

45. 4. By having information on hotlines and clinics, the client can pursue help when the anxiety is escalating. Discussion about current life stressors isn't useful when focusing on how best to handle the client's escalating anxiety. Fleeing from painful situations and discussing views of oneself aren't the best strategies; neither allows for problem solving.
CN: Psychosocial integrity; CNS: None; CL: Application

46. 2. The family can be there for support, but they negate the client's ability to function if they take control of the situation and don't allow the client to use his own coping skills. A client who has confusion related to memory loss is commonly struggling with dissociative amnesia, not a generalized anxiety disorder. Sudden and unexpected travel behavior is a problem for families who have members with dissociative identity disorder, not generalized anxiety disorder. The client must handle and use medication as prescribed.
CN: Psychosocial integrity; CNS: None; CL: Application

47. 4. Stopping antianxiety drugs such as benzodiazepines can cause the client to have withdrawal symptoms. Stopping a benzodiazepine doesn't tend to cause depression, increase cognitive abilities, or decrease sleeping difficulties.
CN: Physiological integrity; CNS: Pharmacological and parenteral therapies; CL: Application

CN: Client needs category   CNS: Client needs subcategory   CL: Cognitive level

48. Five days after running out of medication, a client taking clonazepam (Klonopin) says to the nurse, "I know I shouldn't have just stopped the drug like that, but I'm OK." Which response would be best?
1. "Let's monitor you for problems, in case something else happens."
2. "You could go through withdrawal symptoms for up to 2 weeks."
3. "You have handled your anxiety, and you now know how to cope with stress."
4. "If you're fine now, chances are you won't experience withdrawal symptoms."

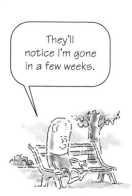

They'll notice I'm gone in a few weeks.

48. 2. Withdrawal syndrome symptoms can appear after 1 or 2 weeks because the benzodiazepine has a long half-life. Looking for another problem unrelated to withdrawal isn't the nurse's best strategy. The act of discontinuing an antianxiety medication doesn't indicate that a client has learned to cope with stress. Every client taking medication needs to be monitored for withdrawal symptoms when the medication is stopped abruptly.
CN: Physiological integrity; CNS: Pharmacological and parenteral therapies; CL: Analysis

49. A client taking alprazolam (Xanax) reports light-headedness and nausea every day while getting out of bed. Which action should the nurse take to objectively validate this client's problem?
1. Take the client's blood pressure.
2. Monitor body temperature.
3. Teach the Valsalva maneuver.
4. Obtain a blood chemical profile.

49. 1. The nurse should take a blood pressure reading to validate orthostatic hypotension. A body temperature reading or chemistry profile won't yield useful information about hypotension. The Valsalva maneuver is performed to lower the heart rate and isn't an appropriate intervention.
CN: Physiological integrity; CNS: Reduction of risk potential; CL: Application

50. A client with generalized anxiety disorder complains of a headache and upset stomach. In assessing this client, the nurse is aware that a client with generalized anxiety disorder may experience which of the following?
1. May have a variety of somatic symptoms.
2. Undergo an alteration in his self-care skills.
3. Is prone to unhealthy binge eating episodes.
4. Will experience secondary gains from mental illness.

50. 1. Clients with anxiety disorders commonly experience somatic symptoms. They don't usually experience problems with self-care. Eating problems aren't a typical part of the diagnostic criteria for anxiety disorders. Not all clients obtain secondary gains from mental illness.
CN: Psychosocial integrity; CNS: None; CL: Application

51. Which communication guideline should a nurse use when talking with a client experiencing mania?
1. Address the client in a light and joking manner.
2. Focus and redirect the conversation as necessary.
3. Allow the client to talk about several different topics.
4. Ask only open-ended questions to facilitate conversation.

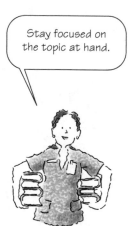

Stay focused on the topic at hand.

51. 2. To decrease stimulation, the nurse should attempt to redirect and focus the client's communication, not allow the client to talk about different topics. By addressing the client in a light and joking manner, the conversation may contribute to the client's feeling out of control. For a manic client, it's best to ask closed questions because open-ended questions may enable the client to talk endlessly, again possibly contributing to the client's feeling out of control.
CN: Psychosocial integrity; CNS: None; CL: Application

52. Which adverse effect should a nurse explain to a client with bipolar disorder and his family when providing preprocedure teaching for electroconvulsive therapy (ECT)?
1. Cholestatic jaundice
2. Hypertensive crisis
3. Mouth ulcers
4. Respiratory distress

53. A client who has just had electroconvulsive therapy (ECT) asks for a drink. Which assessment is a <u>priority</u> when meeting the client's request?
1. Take the client's blood pressure.
2. Monitor the gag reflex.
3. Obtain a body temperature.
4. Determine the level of consciousness.

54. A nurse is caring for a client with hypomania. In performing the assessment, which behavior should she expect?
1. A hypomanic client is on the verge of experiencing depression and crisis.
2. A hypomanic client is indecisive and vacillating, with a diminished ability to think.
3. A hypomanic client is irritable, with an elevated mood and symptoms of mania.
4. A hypomanic client is disorganized and tends to exhibit impaired judgment.

55. A client with bipolar disorder who complains of headache, agitation, and indigestion is most likely experiencing which of the following problems?
1. Depression
2. Cyclothymia
3. Hypomania
4. Mania

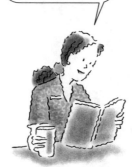

What harm could result from a glass of water?

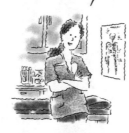

The words *most likely* can help you focus on the answer.

52. 4. Respiratory distress or even arrest may occur as a complication of the anesthesia used with ECT. Cholestatic jaundice, hypertensive crisis, and mouth ulcers don't occur during or as a result of ECT.
CN: Physiological integrity; CNS: Physiological adaptation; CL: Application

53. 2. The nurse must check the client's gag reflex before allowing the client to have a drink after an ECT procedure. Blood pressure and body temperature don't influence whether the client may have a drink after the procedure. The client would obviously be conscious if he's requesting a glass of water.
CN: Physiological integrity; CNS: Physiological adaptation; CL: Analysis

54. 3. When a client is hypomanic, there's evidence of an elevated and irritable mood, along with mild or beginning symptoms of mania. A hypomanic client is experiencing a period of mild elation, not a depression or crisis. Indecision and vacillation with a diminished ability to think are symptoms more likely seen in a major depressive episode than in a hypomanic episode. A client with hypomania tends to be creative and more productive than usual, rather than disorganized with impaired judgment.
CN: Psychosocial integrity; CNS: None; CL: Analysis

55. 4. Headache, agitation, and indigestion are symptoms suggestive of mania in a client with a history of bipolar disorder. These symptoms are *not* suggestive of depression, cyclothymia, or hypomania.
CN: Physiological integrity; CNS: Physiological adaptation; CL: Application

CN: Client needs category   CNS: Client needs subcategory   CL: Cognitive level

56. A client with bipolar disorder has abruptly stopped taking his prescribed medication. Which high-risk behavior would indicate the client has experienced a manic episode?
1. Binge eating
2. Relationship avoidance
3. Sudden relocation
4. Thoughtless spending

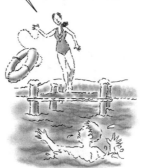

Know the high-risk behaviors associated with each disorder.

57. Which intervention would assist a client with bipolar disorder to maintain adequate nutrition during a manic episode?
1. Determine the client's metabolic rate.
2. Make the client sit down for each meal and snack.
3. Give the client foods to be eaten while he's active.
4. Have the client interact with a dietitian twice a week.

58. A nurse is providing discharge teaching to a client being discharged on lithium. The nurse would emphasize that the client should report which of the following?
1. Black tongue
2. Increased lacrimation
3. Periods of excitability
4. Persistent GI upset

Lithium has adverse effects specifically associated with pregnancy.

59. Which information is important to teach a client with bipolar disorder who's pregnant and taking lithium?
1. Use of lithium usually results in serious congenital problems.
2. Thyroid problems can occur in the first trimester of the pregnancy.
3. Lithium causes severe urine retention and increased risk of toxicity.
4. Women who take lithium are very likely to have a spontaneous abortion.

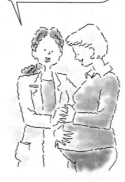

56. 4. Thoughtless or reckless spending is a common symptom of a manic episode. Binge eating isn't a behavior that's characteristic of a client during a manic episode. Relationship avoidance doesn't occur in a client experiencing a manic episode; during episodes of mania, a client may in fact interact with many people and participate in unsafe sexual behavior. Sudden relocation isn't a characteristic of impulsive behavior demonstrated by a client with bipolar disorder.
CN: Psychosocial integrity; CNS: None; CL: Application

57. 3. By giving the client high-caloric foods that can be eaten while he's active, the nurse facilitates the client's nutritional intake. Determining the client's metabolic rate isn't useful information when the client is experiencing mania. During a manic episode, the client can't be still or focused long enough to interact with a dietitian or sit still long enough to eat.
CN: Physiological integrity; CNS: Basic care and comfort; CL: Application

58. 4. Persistent GI upset indicates a mild-to-moderate toxic reaction. Black tongue is an adverse reaction of mirtazapine (Remeron), not lithium. Increased lacrimation and periods of excitability aren't adverse effects of lithium.
CN: Physiological integrity; CNS: Pharmacological and parenteral therapies; CL: Application

59. 1. Use of lithium during pregnancy results in congenital defects, especially cardiac defects. Thyroid problems don't occur in the first trimester of the pregnancy. In lithium toxicity, a condition called nontoxic goiter may occur. An adverse effect of lithium is polyuria, not urine retention. The rate of spontaneous abortion for women taking lithium is no greater than for non-users.
CN: Physiological integrity; CNS: Pharmacological and parenteral therapies; CL: Application

60. A nurse is teaching a client with bipolar disorder about the drug carbamazepine (Tegretol). The teaching has been effective when the client states which of the following?
1. "My hair will fall out if I take this drug."
2. "I will drink plenty of water so I don't develop kidney problems."
3. "I need to have my blood counts checked periodically."
4. "I can't take any other drugs with this one."

61. A nurse is leading a team conference. Suggestions are given for a client with bipolar disorder. Which one should the nurse enter on the care plan?
1. Obtain medication for sleep.
2. Work on solving a problem.
3. Exercise before bedtime.
4. Develop a sleep ritual.

62. Which topic should the nurse discuss with the family of a client with bipolar disorder if the family is distressed about the client's episodes of manic behavior?
1. Ways to protect oneself from client's behavior
2. How to proceed with an involuntary commitment
3. How to confront the client about the reckless behavior
4. When to safely increase medication during manic periods

63. Which statement regarding lithium blood levels represents the <u>most accurate</u> client teaching for a bipolar client?
1. Lithium levels are obtained to determine liver and renal damage.
2. Lithium levels demonstrate whether the client is taking a therapeutic dose range of the drug.
3. Lithium levels indicate whether the drug has passed through the blood-brain barrier.
4. Lithium levels are unnecessary if the client takes the drug as ordered.

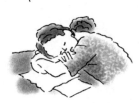

My immediate sleep goal is a 10-minute nap.

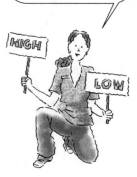

Monitoring blood levels helps ensure that adequate doses of lithium are being administered.

60. 3. The most dangerous adverse effect of carbamazepine is bone marrow depression. Other medications may be taken with carbamazepine. Hair loss doesn't occur in clients taking carbamazepine. Clients who take lithium, not carbamazepine, must be closely monitored for nephrogenic diabetes insipidus. The interactions of all drugs being taken must be monitored because some drugs can either increase or decrease the blood level of carbamazepine.
CN: Physiological integrity; CNS: Pharmacological and parenteral therapies; CL: Analysis

61. 4. A sleep ritual or nighttime routine helps the client to relax and prepare for sleep. Obtaining sleep medication is a temporary solution. Working on problem solving may excite the client rather than tire him. Exercise before retiring is inappropriate.
CN: Physiological integrity; CNS: Reduction of risk potential; CL: Application

62. 1. Family members need to assess their needs and develop ways to protect themselves. Clients who have symptoms of impulsive or reckless behavior might not be candidates for hospitalization. Confronting the client during a manic episode may escalate the behavior. The family must never increase the dosage of prescribed medication without first consulting the primary health care provider.
CN: Safe, effective care environment; CNS: Safety and infection control; CL: Application

63. 2. Lithium levels determine whether an effective dose of lithium is being given to maintain a therapeutic level of the drug. The drug is contraindicated for clients with renal, cardiac, or liver disease. Lithium levels aren't drawn for the purpose of determining whether the drug passes through the blood-brain barrier. Taking the drug as ordered doesn't eliminate the need for blood work.
CN: Physiological integrity; CNS: Pharmacological and parenteral therapies; CL: Application

CN: Client needs category   CNS: Client needs subcategory   CL: Cognitive level

64. What information is important to include in the <u>nutritional counseling</u> of a family with a member who has bipolar disorder?
1. If sufficient roughage isn't eaten while taking lithium, bowel problems will occur.
2. If the intake of carbohydrates increases, the lithium level will increase.
3. If the intake of calories is reduced, the lithium level will increase.
4. If the intake of sodium increases, the lithium level will decrease.

65. Which statement made by a client with bipolar disorder indicates that the nurse's teaching on coping strategies was effective?
1. "I can decide what to do to prevent family conflict."
2. "I can handle problems without asking for any help."
3. "I can stay away from my friends when I feel distressed."
4. "I can ignore things that go wrong instead of getting upset."

66. A client with depression is admitted to the inpatient unit because of attempted suicide. Which of the following nursing goals should be given the <u>highest priority</u>?
1. The client will seek out the nurse when feeling self-destructive.
2. The client will identify and discuss actual and perceived losses.
3. The client will learn strategies to promote relaxation and self-care.
4. The client will establish healthy and mutually caring relationships.

67. A nurse is caring for a client who reports that he thinks about suicide every day. In conferring with the treatment team, which recommendation by the nurse would be the <u>most</u> appropriate for this client?
1. A no-suicide contract
2. Weekly outpatient therapy
3. A second psychiatric opinion
4. Intensive inpatient treatment

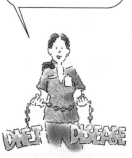

It's important to know how medications interact with foods.

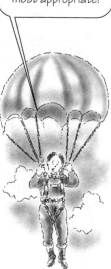

You shouldn't have to ask what short-term goal is most appropriate!

64. 4. Any time the level of sodium increases, such as with a change in dietary intake, the level of lithium will decrease. The intake of roughage and carbohydrates in the diet isn't related to the metabolism of lithium. Reducing the number of calories the client eats doesn't affect the lithium level in the body.
CN: Physiological integrity; CNS: Reduction of risk potential; CL: Analysis

65. 1. The client should be focusing on his strengths and abilities to prevent family conflict. Not being able to ask for help is problematic and not a good coping strategy. Avoiding problems also isn't a good coping strategy. It's better to identify and handle problems as they arise. Ignoring situations that cause discomfort won't facilitate solutions or allow the client to demonstrate effective coping skills.
CN: Psychosocial integrity; CNS: None; CL: Analysis

66. 1. By seeking out the nurse when feeling self-destructive, the client can feel safe and begin to see that there are coping skills to assist in dealing with self-destructive tendencies. Discussion of losses also is important when dealing with feelings of depression, but the priority intervention is still to promote immediate client safety. Although relationship building and learning strategies to promote relaxation and self-care are important goals, safety is the priority intervention.
CN: Safe, effective care environment; CNS: Management of care; CL: Analysis

67. 4. For a client thinking about suicide on a daily basis, inpatient care would be the best intervention. Although a no-suicide contract is an important strategy, this client needs additional care. The client needs a more intensive level of care than weekly outpatient therapy. Immediate intervention is paramount, not a second psychiatric opinion.
CN: Safe, effective care environment; CNS: Management of care; CL: Application

68. Which <u>short-term goal</u> should a nurse focus on for a client who makes statements about not deserving things?
1. Identify distorted thoughts.
2. Describe self-care patterns.
3. Discuss family relationships.
4. Explore communication skills.

69. Which intervention should be of primary importance to a nurse working with a client to modify the client's negative expectations?
1. Encourage the client to discuss spiritual matters.
2. Assist the client to learn how to problem-solve.
3. Help the client explore issues related to loss.
4. Have the client identify positive aspects of self.

70. Which intervention strategy is <u>most</u> appropriate to use with a client with depression who may be suicidal?
1. Speak to family members to ascertain whether the client is suicidal.
2. Talk to the client to determine whether the client is an attention seeker.
3. Arrange for the client to be placed on immediate suicidal precautions.
4. Ask a direct question such as, "Do you ever think about killing yourself?"

71. Which instruction should a nurse include when teaching the family of a client with <u>major depression</u>?
1. Address how depression is a lifelong illness.
2. Explain that depression is an illness and can be treated.
3. Describe how depression masks a person's true feelings.
4. Teach how depression causes frequent disorganized thinking.

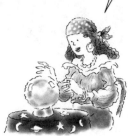

You're doing great in the short term, and your long-term goal is in sight.

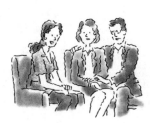

Depression affects the entire family.

68. 1. It's important to identify distorted thinking because self-deprecating thoughts lead to depression. Self-care patterns don't necessarily reflect distorted thinking. Family relationships might not influence distorted thinking patterns. A form of communication called negative self-talk would be explored only after distorted thinking patterns were identified.
CN: Psychosocial integrity; CNS: None; CL: Application

69. 4. An important intervention used to counter negative expectations is to focus on the positive and have the client explore positive aspects of himself. Discussion of spiritual matters doesn't address the need to change negative expectations. Learning how to problem-solve won't modify the client's negative expectations. If the client dwells on the negative and focuses on loss, it will be natural to have negative expectations.
CN: Psychosocial integrity; CNS: None; CL: Application

70. 4. The best approach to determining whether a client is suicidal is to ask about thoughts of suicide in a direct and caring manner. Assessing for attention-seeking behaviors doesn't deal directly with the problem. The client should be assessed directly, not through family members. Assessment must be performed before determining whether suicide precautions are necessary.
CN: Psychosocial integrity; CNS: None; CL: Application

71. 2. The nurse must help the family understand depression, its impact on the family, and recommended treatments. Depression doesn't need to be a lifelong illness. It's important to help families understand that depression can be successfully treated and that, in some situations, depression can reoccur during the life cycle. The feelings expressed by the client are genuine; they reflect cognitive distortions and disillusionment. Disorganized thinking is more commonly associated with schizophrenia rather than with depression.
CN: Psychosocial integrity; CNS: None; CL: Application

CN: Client needs category   CNS: Client needs subcategory   CL: Cognitive level

72. A client with major depression asks why he is taking mirtazapine (Remeron) instead of imipramine hydrochloride (Tofranil). Which explanation is most accurate?
1. The newer serotonin reuptake inhibitor drugs are better-tested drugs.
2. The serotonin reuptake inhibitors have few adverse effects.
3. The serotonin reuptake inhibitors require a low dose of antidepressant drug.
4. The serotonin reuptake inhibitors are as good as other antidepressant drugs.

72. 2. The serotonin reuptake inhibitors are drugs with few adverse effects and are unlikely to be toxic in an overdose. All drugs must be tested through a government-specified protocol. Comparison of two different types of antidepressant medications isn't useful. The final statement doesn't give the client helpful information.
CN: Physiological integrity; CNS: Pharmacological and parenteral therapies; CL: Analysis

73. A nurse is caring for a client with depression. Which of the following interventions will best meet the client's goal of enhancing self-esteem?
1. Playing cards
2. Praying daily
3. Taking medication
4. Writing poetry

73. 4. Writing poetry or engaging in some other creative outlet will enhance self-esteem. Playing cards and praying don't necessarily promote self-esteem. Taking medication will decrease symptoms of depression after a blood level is established, but it won't, by itself, promote self-esteem.
CN: Psychosocial integrity; CNS: None; CL: Application

74. An adolescent who is depressed and is reported by his parents as having difficulty in school is brought to the community mental health center to be evaluated. Which other health problem should the nurse suspect?
1. Anxiety disorder
2. Behavioral difficulties
3. Cognitive impairment
4. Labile moods

74. 2. Adolescents tend to demonstrate severe irritability and behavioral problems rather than simply a depressed mood. Anxiety disorder is more commonly associated with small children rather than with adolescents. Cognitive impairment is typically associated with delirium or dementia. Labile mood is more characteristic of a client with cognitive impairment or bipolar disorder.
CN: Psychosocial integrity; CNS: None; CL: Analysis

75. Which nursing intervention is most effective in lowering a client's risk of suicide?
1. Using a caring approach
2. Developing a strong relationship with the client
3. Establishing a suicide contract to ensure his safety
4. Encouraging avoidance of over-stimulating activities

You've completed 75 questions. The rest should be smooth sailing.

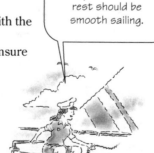

75. 3. Establishing a suicide contract with the client demonstrates that the nurse's concern for his safety is a priority and that his life is of value. When a client agrees to a suicide contract, it decreases his risk of a successful attempt. Caring alone ignores the underlying mechanism of the client's wish to commit suicide. Merely developing a strong relationship with the client isn't addressing the potential the client has for harming himself. Encouraging the client to stay away from activities could cause isolation, which would be detrimental to the client's well-being.
CN: Psychosocial integrity; CNS: None; CL: Application

76. Which nursing diagnosis would the nurse expect to find on the care plan of a client with a phobia about elevators?
1. *Social isolation related to a lack of social skills*
2. *Disturbed sleep pattern related to a fear of elevators*
3. *Ineffective coping related to poor coping skills*
4. *Anxiety related to fear of elevators*

77. Which behavior modification technique is useful in the treatment of phobias?
1. Aversion therapy
2. Imitation or modeling
3. Positive reinforcement
4. Systematic desensitization

78. Which statement would be useful when teaching a client and her family about phobias and the need for a strong support system?
1. The use of a family support system is only temporary.
2. The need to be assertive can be reinforced by the family.
3. The family must set limit on inappropriate behaviors.
4. The family plays a role in promoting client independence.

79. A client with an anxiety disorder is taking alprazolam (Xanax). The nurse should instruct the client to avoid:
1. shellfish.
2. alcohol.
3. coffee.
4. cheese.

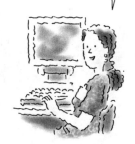

No need to fear this question-focus on which technique would be useful.

76. 3. Poor coping skills can cause ineffective coping. Such a client isn't relegated to social isolation, and lack of social skills has nothing to do with phobia. Fear of elevators is a manifestation, not the cause of altered thoughts and anxiety.
CN: Psychosocial integrity; CNS: None; CL: Analysis

77. 4. Systematic desensitization is a common behavior modification technique that has been successfully used to help treat phobia. Aversion therapy and positive reinforcement aren't behavior modification techniques used with the treatment of phobias. The techniques of imitation or modeling are social learning techniques, not behavior modification techniques.
CN: Psychosocial integrity; CNS: None; CL: Application

78. 4. The family plays a vital role in supporting a client in treatment and in preventing the client from using the phobia to obtain secondary gains. Family support must be ongoing, not temporary. The family can be more helpful by focusing on effective handling of anxiety, rather than focusing energy on developing assertiveness skills. People with phobias are already restrictive in their behavior; more restrictions aren't necessary.
CN: Psychosocial integrity; CNS: None; CL: Analysis

79. 2. Alcohol should be avoided because of additive depressive effects. Ingestion of shellfish, coffee, and cheese isn't problematic.
CN: Physiological integrity; CNS: Pharmacological and parenteral therapies; CL: Application

80. A female client describes her unpredictable episodes of acute anxiety as "just awful." She says that she feels like she's about to die and can hardly breathe. The nurse recognizes that the symptoms described by the client are associated with which condition?
1. Agoraphobia
2. Dissociative disorder
3. Posttraumatic stress disorder (PTSD)
4. Panic disorder

81. A client taking antidepressants for major depression for about 3 weeks is expressing that he's feeling better. Which complication should he now be assessed for?
1. Manic depression
2. Potential for violence
3. Substance abuse
4. Suicidal ideation

82. A 40-year-old female client has been brought to the hospital by her husband because she has refused to get out of bed for 2 days. She won't eat, she's been neglecting household responsibilities, and she's tired all the time. Her diagnosis on admission is major depression. Which question is most appropriate for the admitting nurse to ask <u>at this point</u>?
1. "What has been troubling you?"
2. "Why do you dislike yourself?"
3. "How do you feel about your life?"
4. "What can we do to help?"

83. A client with bipolar disorder has been receiving lithium (Eskalith) for 2 weeks. He also has been taking chemotherapeutic drugs that cause him to feel nauseated and anorexic, making it difficult to distinguish early signs of lithium toxicity. Which sign would indicate lithium toxicity at serum drug levels below 1.5 mEq/L?
1. Hyperpyrexia
2. Marked analgesics and lethargy
3. Hypotonic reflexes with muscle weakness
4. Oliguria

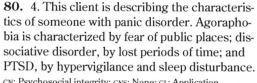
Don't panic if the answer isn't immediately clear—read through the question carefully and eliminate the obvious incorrect options first.

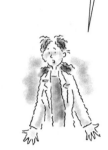

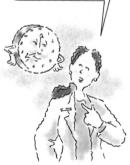
Timing is critical here. Read the question again if you have any doubts about what's being asked.

80. 4. This client is describing the characteristics of someone with panic disorder. Agoraphobia is characterized by fear of public places; dissociative disorder, by lost periods of time; and PTSD, by hypervigilance and sleep disturbance.
CN: Psychosocial integrity; CNS: None; CL: Application

81. 4. After a client has been on antidepressants and is feeling better, he commonly then has the energy to harm himself. Manic depression isn't treated with antidepressants. Nothing in the client's history suggests a potential for violence. There are no signs or symptoms suggesting substance abuse.
CN: Safe, effective care environment; CNS: Safety and infection control; CL: Analysis

82. 3. The nurse must develop nursing interventions based on the client's perceived problems and feelings. Asking the client to draw a conclusion may be difficult for her at this time. *Why* questions can place the client in a defensive position. Requiring the client to find possible solutions is beyond the scope of her pre-sent abilities.
CN: Psychosocial integrity; CNS: None; CL: Analysis

83. 3. Lithium alters sodium transport in nerve and muscle cells, slowing the speed of impulse transmission, so look for hypotonic reflexes and muscle weakness. Lithium has no known effect on body temperature or on the transmission of pain impulses. The drug doesn't cause lethargy. Oliguria and other signs of renal failure occur late in severe lithium toxicity.
CN: Physiologic integrity; CNS: Pharmacological and parenteral therapies; CL: Application

84. A client came to the psychiatric unit 2 days ago. He has a history of bipolar disorder, is in the manic phase, and stopped taking lithium (Eskalith) 2 weeks ago. Which finding should the nurse be likely to see?
 1. Flight of ideas
 2. Echolalia
 3. Clang associations
 4. Neologism

85. An acutely manic client kisses a nurse on the lips and asks her to marry him. The nurse is taken by surprise. Which response would be best?
 1. Seclude the client for his inappropriate behavior.
 2. Ask the client what he's trying to prove by his behavior.
 3. Ask the client to fold some laundry.
 4. Tell the client his behavior is offensive.

86. Which discharge instruction is most important for a client taking lithium (Eskalith)?
 1. Limit fluids to 1,500 ml daily.
 2. Maintain a high fluid intake.
 3. Take advantage of the warm weather by exercising outside whenever possible.
 4. When feeling a cold coming, it's OK to take over-the-counter (OTC) remedies.

87. A client in an outpatient psychiatric facility is diagnosed with dysthymic disorder. Which statement would the nurse include in the teaching for this client?
 1. It involves a mood range from moderate depression to hypomania.
 2. It involves a single manic episode.
 3. It's a form of depression that occurs in the fall and winter.
 4. It's a mood disorder similar to major depression but of mild to moderate severity.

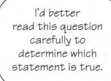

I'd better read this question carefully to determine which statement is true.

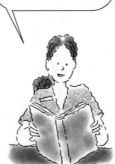

84. 1. Flight of ideas is a speech pattern characterized by rapid transition from topic to topic, typically without finishing one idea. It's common in mania. Echolalia (repetition of words heard), clang associations (use of rhyming), and neologism (inverted words) aren't seen in mania states.
CN: Psychosocial integrity; CNS: None; CL: Application

85. 3. Having the client help with laundry rechannels his energy in a positive activity. The client needs direction and structure, not seclusion. Asking the client what he's trying to prove ignores his impaired judgment and poor impulse control. Telling the client that his behavior is offensive doesn't assist him in controlling his behavior.
CN: Psychosocial integrity; CNS: None; CL: Application

86. 2. Clients taking lithium need to maintain a high fluid intake. Exercising outside may not be safe; photosensitivity occurs with lithium use, and activity in warm weather could increase sodium loss, predisposing the client to lithium toxicity. The client shouldn't take OTC drugs without the physician's approval.
CN: Physiological integrity; CNS: Pharmacological and parenteral therapies; CL: Application

87. 4. Dysthymic disorder is a mood disorder similar to major depression, but it remains mild to moderate in severity. Cyclothymic disorder is a mood disorder characterized by a mood range from moderate depression to hypomania. Bipolar I disorder is characterized by a single manic episode with no past major depressive episodes. Seasonal affective disorder is a form of depression occurring in the fall and winter.
CN: Psychosocial integrity; CNS: None; CL: Application

88. A depressed client taking a prescribed tricyclic antidepressant tells a nurse he's sleepy all the time and doesn't feel like doing anything. Which nursing action is appropriate?

1. Tell the client to stop taking the drug until he sees his physician.
2. Advise the client to continue taking the drug to see whether these effects wear off.
3. Ask the physician whether the medication can be given in one dose at bedtime.
4. Advise the client to get another opinion.

89. A depressed client is taking trazodone (Desyrel), an atypical antidepressant. On discharge, the nurse will instruct the client to take the medication:

1. in the morning.
2. at bedtime.
3. at any time during the day.
4. when he has an urge for a cigarette.

90. Which instruction should a nurse provide when teaching a client about tricyclic antidepressants?

1. "This drug causes photosensitivity."
2. "Avoid milk and dairy products."
3. "Notify your physician if your mood doesn't improve within 7 days."
4. "Mood improvement takes up to 28 days."

91. Which intervention by the nurse would be the most appropriate when caring for a client newly diagnosed with insulin-dependent diabetes mellitus who also has blood-injection-injury phobia?

1. Teach the client to avoid fainting by tensing the muscles of the legs and abdomen.
2. Quickly expose the client to feared situations.
3. Have the client avoid as much medical care as possible.
4. Focus on treating the symptoms with an antianxiety medication.

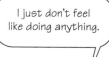

I just don't feel like doing anything.

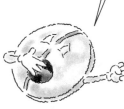

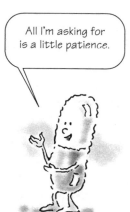

All I'm asking for is a little patience.

88. 3. Many tricyclic antidepressants can be given safely in one dose; when an antidepressant is taken at bedtime, the adverse effect of drowsiness can help the client sleep. It's inappropriate for the nurse to tell the client to stop taking the drug, to continue taking it until the undesired effects wear off, or to seek a second opinion.

CN: Physiological integrity; CNS: Pharmacological and parenteral therapies; CL: Application

89. 2. Trazodone has a strong sedative effect and is commonly prescribed as a sleep aid to be taken at bedtime. Wellbutrin is used for smoking cessation.

CN: Physiological integrity; CNS: Pharmacological and parenteral therapies; CL: Application

90. 4. The client's mood may not improve until the 3rd or 4th week of tricyclic antidepressant therapy. The client needs to be reassured that the drug works slowly. The drug doesn't cause photosensitivity or interact with milk and dairy products.

CN: Physiological integrity; CNS: Pharmacological and parenteral therapies; CL: Application

91. 1. The client may be able to avoid fainting and relieve hypotension by tensing the larger muscle groups. Desensitization by slowly, not quickly, exposing the client to blood injection is indicated to reduce fear. Clients with blood-injection-injury phobia may avoid all medical care, which is dangerous to their health. Antianxiety medications may help on a short-term basis only.

CN: Psychosocial integrity; CNS: None; CL: Application

92. A client with the nursing diagnosis of *Fear related to being embarrassed in the presence of others* exhibits symptoms of social phobia. What should the goals be for this client? Select all that apply:
1. Manage his fear in group situations.
2. Develop a plan to avoid situations that may cause stress.
3. Verbalize feelings that occur in stressful situations.
4. Develop a plan for responding to stressful situations.
5. Deny feelings that may contribute to irrational fears.
6. Use suppression to deal with underlying fears.

92. 1, 3, 4. Improving stress-management skills, verbalizing feelings, and anticipating and planning for stressful situations are adaptive responses to stress. Avoidance, denial, and suppression are maladaptive defense mechanisms.
CN: Psychosocial integrity; CNS: None; CL: Application

93. The nurse recognizes improvement in a client with the nursing diagnosis of *Ineffective role performance related to the need to perform rituals*. Which behavior indicates improvement? Select all that apply:
1. The client refrains from performing rituals during stress.
2. The client verbalizes that he uses "thought stopping" when obsessive thoughts occur.
3. The client verbalizes the relationship between stress and ritualistic behaviors.
4. The client avoids stressful situations.
5. The client rationalizes ritualistic behavior.
6. The client performs ritualistic behaviors in private.

93. 1, 2, 3. Refraining from rituals demonstrates that the client manages stress appropriately. Using "thought stopping" demonstrates the client's ability to employ appropriate interventions for obsessive thoughts. Verbalizing the relationship between stress and behaviors indicates that the client understands the disease process. Avoiding, rationalizing, and hiding behaviors demonstrate maladaptive methods for managing stress and anxiety.
CN: Psychosocial integrity; CNS: None; CL: Analysis

94. After interviewing a client diagnosed with recurrent depression, the nurse determines the client's potential to commit suicide. Which factors should the nurse consider as contributors to the client's potential for suicide? Select all that apply:
1. Psychomotor retardation
2. Impulsive behaviors
3. Overwhelming feelings of guilt
4. Chronic, debilitating illness
5. Decreased physical activity
6. Repression of anger

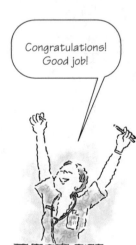

Congratulations! Good job!

94. 2, 3, 4, 6. Impulsive behavior, overwhelming guilt, chronic illness, and anger repression are factors that contribute to suicide potential. Psychomotor retardation and decreased activity are symptoms of depression but don't typically lead to suicide because the client doesn't have the energy to harm himself.
CN: Psychosocial integrity; CNS: None; CL: Analysis

CN: Client needs category   CNS: Client needs subcategory   CL: Cognitive level

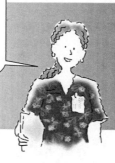

This chapter covers a host of cognitive disorders. Are your own cognitive powers ready? OK, let's go!

Chapter 16
Cognitive disorders

1. A nurse is assessing a client with dementia. Which disorder is the client most likely to have?
1. Alcohol withdrawal
2. Alzheimer's disease
3. Obsessive-compulsive disorder
4. Postpartum depression

1. 2. Dementia occurs in Alzheimer's disease and is generally progressive and deteriorating. The symptoms related to alcohol withdrawal result from alcohol intoxication. Effects of alcohol on the central nervous system include loss of memory, concentration, insight, and motor control. Obsessive-compulsive disorders are recurrent ideas, impulses, thoughts, or patterns of behavior that produce anxiety if resisted. Postpartum depression doesn't lead to dementia.
CN: Physiological integrity; CNS: Physiological adaptation; CL: Application

2. A physician diagnoses a client with dementia of the Alzheimer's type. Which statement about possible causes of this disorder is most accurate?
1. Alzheimer's disease is most commonly caused by cerebral abscess.
2. Chronic alcohol abuse plays a significant role in Alzheimer's disease.
3. Multiple small brain infarctions typically lead to Alzheimer's disease.
4. The cause of Alzheimer's disease is currently unknown.

2. 4. Several hypotheses suggest genetic factors, trauma, accumulation of aluminum, alterations in the immune system, or alterations in acetylcholine as contributing to the development of Alzheimer's disease, but the exact cause of Alzheimer's disease is unknown.
CN: Health promotion and maintenance; CNS: None; CL: Application

The key to the answer is the word reversible.

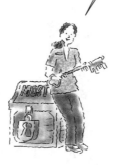

3. Of the following conditions that can cause symptoms similar to Alzheimer's disease, which is <u>reversible</u>?
1. Multiple sclerosis
2. Electrolyte imbalance
3. Multiple small brain infarctions
4. Human immunodeficiency virus infection

3. 2. Electrolyte imbalance is a correctable metabolic abnormality. The other conditions are irreversible.
CN: Physiological integrity; CNS: Physiological adaptation; CL: Application

4. In the <u>early</u> stages of Alzheimer's disease, which symptom is expected?
1. Dilated pupils
2. Rambling speech
3. Elevated blood pressure
4. Significant recent memory impairment

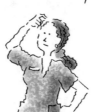

The answer is on the tip of my tongue, but I just can't remember.

4. 4. Significant recent memory impairment, indicated by the inability to verbalize remembrances after several minutes to an hour, can be assessed in the early stages of Alzheimer's disease. Dilated pupils, rambling speech, and increased blood pressure are expected symptoms of delirium.
CN: Physiological integrity; CNS: Physiological adaptation; CL: Application

5. A nurse is caring for a client with delirium. Which nursing intervention has the <u>highest</u> priority?
1. Providing a safe environment
2. Offering recreational activities
3. Providing a structured environment
4. Instituting measures to promote sleep

5. 1. The nurse's highest priority when caring for a client with delirium is to ensure client safety. Offering recreational activities, providing a structured environment, and promoting sleep are all appropriate interventions after safety measures are in place.
CN: Safe, effective care environment; CNS: Management of care; CL: Analysis

6. Which assessment finding shows impairment in abstract thinking and reasoning?
1. The client can't repeat a sentence.
2. The client has problems calculating simple problems.
3. The client doesn't know the name of the president of the United States.
4. The client can't find similarities and differences between related words or objects.

6. 4. Abstract thinking is assessed by noting similarities and differences between related words or objects. Not being able to repeat a sentence or do a simple calculation shows a client's inability to concentrate and focus on thoughts. Not knowing the president of the United States is a deficiency in general knowledge.
CN: Physiological integrity; CNS: Physiological adaptation; CL: Analysis

7. In addition to disturbances in cognition and orientation, a client with Alzheimer's disease may also show changes in which area?
1. Appetite
2. Energy levels
3. Hearing
4. Personality

7. 4. Personality change is common in dementia. There shouldn't be a remarkable change in appetite, energy level, or hearing.
CN: Physiological integrity; CNS: Physiological adaptation; CL: Application

A gentle, calm approach is comforting and nonthreatening.

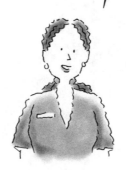

8. Which interventions should help a client diagnosed with Alzheimer's disease perform activities of daily living?
1. Have the client perform all basic care without help.
2. Tell the client morning care must be done by 9 a.m.
3. Give the client a written list of activities he's expected to do.
4. Encourage the client, and give ample time to complete basic tasks.

8. 4. Clients with Alzheimer's disease respond to the effect of those around them. A gentle, calm approach is comforting and nonthreatening, and a tense, hurried approach may agitate the client. The client has problems performing independently. The inherent expectations of deadlines and activity lists may lead to frustration.
CN: Physiological integrity; CNS: Basic care and comfort; CL: Application

CN: Client needs category   CNS: Client needs subcategory   CL: Cognitive level

9. Which of the following medications for Alzheimer's disease will improve cognition and functional autonomy?

1. Bupropion (Wellbutrin)
2. Haloperidol (Haldol)
3. Donepezil (Aricept)
4. Triazolam (Halcion)

10. A nurse places an object in the hand of a client with Alzheimer's disease and asks the client to identify the object. Which term represents the client's inability to name the object?

1. Agnosia
2. Aphasia
3. Apraxia
4. Perseveration

11. Which nursing intervention will help a client with progressive memory deficit function in his environment?

1. Help the client do simple tasks by giving step-by-step directions.
2. Avoid frustrating the client by performing basic care routines for the client.
3. Stimulate the client's intellectual functioning by bringing new topics to the client's attention.
4. Promote the use of the client's sense of humor by telling jokes or riddles and discussing cartoons.

12. Which intervention is an important part of providing care to a client diagnosed with Alzheimer's disease?

1. Avoid physical contact.
2. Confine the client to his room.
3. Provide a high level of sensory stimulation.
4. Monitor the client carefully.

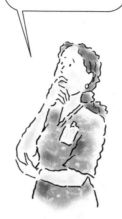

What is the term for the inability to recognize familiar objects?

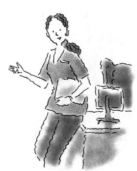

Look for the answer that makes the most safety sense.

9. 3. Donepezil is used to improve cognition and functional autonomy in mild to moderate dementia of the Alzheimer's type. Bupropion is used for depression. Haloperidol is used for agitation, aggression, hallucinations, thought disturbances, and wandering. Triazolam is used for sleep disturbances.

CN: Physiological integrity; CNS: Pharmacological and parenteral therapies; CL: Application

10. 1. Agnosia is the inability to recognize familiar objects. Aphasia is characterized by an impaired ability to speak. Apraxia refers to the client's inability to use objects properly. All three impairments usually occur in stage 3 of Alzheimer's disease. Perseveration is continued repetition of a meaningless word or phrase that occurs in stage 2 of Alzheimer's disease.

CN: Health promotion and maintenance; CNS: None; CL: Application

11. 1. Clients with cognitive impairment should do all the tasks they can. By receiving simple directions in a step-by-step fashion, the client can better process information and perform tasks. Stimulation of intellect can be accomplished by discussing familiar topics with them; changes in topics may add to their confusion. Clients with cognitive impairment may not be able to understand the joke or riddle, and cartoons may add to their confusion.

CN: Psychosocial integrity; CNS: None; CL: Application

12. 4. Whenever client safety is at risk, careful observation and supervision are of ultimate importance in avoiding injury. Physical contact is implemented during basic care. Confining the client may cause agitation and combativeness. A high level of sensory stimulation may be too stimulating and distracting.

CN: Safe, effective care environment; CNS: Management of care; CL: Application

13. Which nursing intervention is the <u>most important</u> in caring for a client diagnosed with Alzheimer's disease?
1. Make sure the environment is safe to prevent injury.
2. Make sure the client receives food she likes to prevent hunger.
3. Make sure the client meets other clients to prevent social isolation.
4. Make sure the client takes care of her daily physical care to prevent dependence.

14. Which medication is used to decrease the agitation, violence, and bizarre thoughts associated with dementia?
1. Diazepam (Valium)
2. Ergoloid (Hydergine)
3. Haloperidol (Haldol)
4. Tacrine (Cognex)

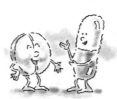

I reduce agitation, violence, and bizarre thoughts. How about you?

15. A client diagnosed with Alzheimer's disease tells the nurse that today she has a luncheon date with her daughter, *who is not visiting that day*. Which response by the nurse would be <u>most appropriate</u> for this situation?
1. "Where are you planning on having your lunch?"
2. "You're confused and don't know what you're saying."
3. "I think you need some more medication, and I'll bring it to you."
4. "Today is Monday, March 8, and we'll be eating lunch in the dining room."

16. Which feature is characteristic of cognitive disorders?
1. Catatonia
2. Depression
3. Feeling of dread
4. Deficit in memory

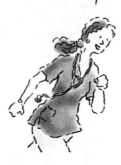

You're already at question 15 and doing great. Keep going!

13. 1. Providing client safety is the number one priority when caring for any client but particularly when a client is already compromised and at greater risk for injury. The other options may be part of caring for a client with Alzheimer's disease but they are not the priority.
CN: Safe, effective care environment; CNS: Safety and infection control; CL: Application

14. 3. Haloperidol is an antipsychotic that decreases the symptoms of agitation, violence, and bizarre thoughts. Diazepam is used for anxiety and muscle relaxation. Ergoloid is an adrenergic blocker used to block vascular headaches. Tacrine is used for improvement of cognition.
CN: Physiological integrity; CNS: Reduction of risk potential; CL: Application

15. 4. The best nursing response is to reorient the client to the date and environment. Humoring the client isn't therapeutic. Medication won't provide immediate relief for memory impairment. Confrontation can provoke an outburst.
CN: Psychosocial integrity; CNS: None; CL: Application

16. 4. Cognitive disorders represent a significant change in cognition or memory from a previous level of functioning. Catatonia is a type of schizophrenia characterized by periods of physical rigidity, negativism, excitement, and stupor. Depression is a feeling of sadness and apathy and is part of major depressive and other mood disorders. A feeling of dread is characteristic of an anxiety disorder.
CN: Physiological integrity; CNS: Physiological adaptation; CL: Application

CN: Client needs category   CNS: Client needs subcategory   CL: Cognitive level

17. A nurse is assessing an elderly client who is admitted with progressive deterioration in cognition. The client most likely has which degenerative disorder?
   1. Delirium
   2. Dementia
   3. Neurosis
   4. Psychosis

18. A nurse is teaching the family of a client with dementia. Which of the following responses by the nurse would be the most accurate definition of dementia?
   1. Personal neglect in self-care
   2. Poor judgment, especially in social situations
   3. Memory loss occurring as a natural consequence of aging
   4. Loss of intellectual abilities sufficient to impair the ability to perform basic care

19. Asking a client with a suspected dementia disorder to recall what she ate for breakfast would assess which area?
   1. Food preferences
   2. Recent memory
   3. Remote memory
   4. Speech

20. Which factor is the most important to determine when collecting data for a definitive diagnosis of a dementia disorder?
   1. Prognosis
   2. Genetic information
   3. Degree of impairment
   4. Implications for treatment

21. What is considered the primary causative factor for vascular dementia?
   1. Head trauma
   2. Genetic factors
   3. Acetylcholine alteration
   4. Interruption of blood flow to the brain

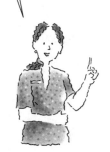

Only one of these disorders is degenerative.

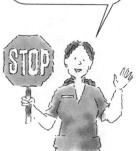

This question is asking specifically about vascular dementia.

17. 2. Dementia is progressive and often associated with aging or underlying metabolic or organic deterioration. Delirium is characterized by abrupt, spontaneous cognitive dysfunction with an underlying organic mental disorder. Neurosis and psychosis are psychological diagnoses.
CN: Physiological integrity; CNS: Physiological adaptation; CL: Application

18. 4. The ability to perform self-care is an important measure of the progression of dementia. Memory loss reflects underlying physical, metabolic, and pathologic processes. Personal neglect and poor judgment typically occur in dementia but aren't considered defining characteristics.
CN: Physiological integrity; CNS: Physiological adaptation; CL: Application

19. 2. Persons with dementia have difficulty in recent memory or learning, which may be a key to early detection. Assessing food preferences may be helpful in determining what the client likes to eat, but this assessment has no direct correlation in assessing dementia. Speech difficulties, such as rambling, irrelevance, and incoherence, may be related to delirium.
CN: Health promotion and maintenance; CNS: None; CL: Application

20. 4. The progression of biological impairment in the central nervous system is a function of the underlying pathologic states, so it's important to collect data and treat the underlying cause. Prognosis isn't the most important factor when making a diagnosis. Genetic information isn't relevant. The degree of impairment is necessary information for developing a care plan.
CN: Health promotion and maintenance; CNS: None; CL: Analysis

21. 4. The cause of vascular dementia is directly related to an interruption of blood flow to the brain. Head trauma, genetic factors, and acetylcholine alteration are causative factors related to dementia of the Alzheimer's type.
CN: Physiological integrity; CNS: Physiological adaptation; CL: Application

22. The family of a client recently admitted with vascular dementia asks the nurse about the cause of the client's condition. Which of the following would be the most accurate response by the nurse?
   1. "It is caused by high blood pressure."
   2. "It is caused by low oxygen levels."
   3. "It is caused by an infection."
   4. "It is caused by toxins."

23. Which assessment finding is expected for a client with vascular dementia?
   1. Hypersomnolence
   2. Insomnia
   3. Restlessness
   4. Small-stepped gait

24. The spouse of a client diagnosed with vascular dementia asks the nurse how this disorder differs from Alzheimer's disease. Which response from the nurse is most appropriate?
   1. "Vascular dementia has a more abrupt onset."
   2. "Vascular dementia develops slowly."
   3. "Personality change is common in vascular dementia."
   4. "The inability to perform motor activities occurs in vascular dementia."

25. A progression of symptoms that occurs in steps rather than a gradual deterioration indicates which type of dementia?
   1. Alzheimer's dementia
   2. Parkinson's dementia
   3. Substance-induced dementia
   4. Vascular dementia

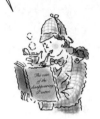

Let's see! What is the cause?

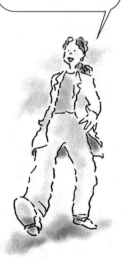

You've taken the first steps towards understanding the many types of dementia.

22. 1. Vascular dementia is a result of small strokes that can either destroy or damage cerebral tissue. Strokes may be caused by high blood pressure, high cholesterol levels, heart disease, or diabetes. Hypoxia, infection, and toxins aren't causes of dementia.
CN: Physiological integrity; CNS: Physiological adaptation; CL: Application

23. 4. Focal neurologic signs commonly seen with vascular dementia include weakness of the limbs, small-stepped gait, and difficulty with speech. Insomnia, hypersomnolence, and restlessness are symptoms related to delirium.
CN: Physiological integrity; CNS: Physiological adaptation; CL: Application

24. 1. Vascular dementia differs from Alzheimer's disease in that it has a more abrupt onset and runs a highly variable course. Personality change is common in Alzheimer's disease. The inability to carry out motor activities is common in Alzheimer's disease.
CN: Health promotion and maintenance; CNS: None; CL: Application

25. 4. Vascular dementia differs from Alzheimer's disease in that vascular dementia has a more abrupt onset and progresses in steps. At times the dementia seems to clear up, and the individual shows fairly lucid thinking. Dementia of the Alzheimer's type has a slow onset with a progressive and deteriorating course. Dementia of Parkinson's sometimes resembles the dementia of Alzheimer's disease. Substance-induced dementia is related to the persisting effects of use of a substance.
CN: Physiological integrity; CNS: Physiological adaptation; CL: Analysis

CN: Client needs category   CNS: Client needs subcategory   CL: Cognitive level

26. Which pathophysiological change in the brain causes the symptoms of Alzheimer's disease?
1. Glucose inadequacy
2. Atrophy of the frontal lobe
3. Degeneration of the cholinergic system
4. Intracranial bleeding in the limbic system

27. An elderly client has experienced memory and attention deficits that developed over a 3-day period. These symptoms are characteristic of which disorder?
1. Alzheimer's disease
2. Amnesia syndrome
3. Delirium
4. Dementia

28. Which age-group is at high risk for developing a state of delirium?
1. Adolescent
2. Elderly
3. Middle-aged
4. School-aged

29. Which nursing diagnosis is best for an elderly client experiencing visual and auditory hallucinations?
1. *Interrupted family processes*
2. *Ineffective role performance*
3. *Impaired verbal communication*
4. *Disturbed sensory perception (visual, auditory)*

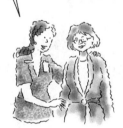

Which one of these changes is a cause of Alzheimer's symptoms?

Age is an important factor when assessing a client.

26. 3. Research related to Alzheimer's disease indicates that the enzyme needed to produce acetylcholine is dramatically reduced. The other pathophysiological changes don't cause the symptoms of Alzheimer's disease.
CN: Physiological integrity; CNS: Physiological adaptation; CL: Analysis

27. 3. Delirium is characterized by an abrupt onset of fluctuating levels of awareness, clouded consciousness, perceptual disturbances, and disturbed memory and orientation. Alzheimer's disease is a progressive dementia. Amnesia refers to recent short-term and long-term memory loss. Dementia is characterized by general impairment in intellectual functioning and occurs in a progressive, irreversible course.
CN: Physiological integrity; CNS: Physiological adaptation; CL: Application

28. 2. The elderly population, because of normal physiological changes, is highly susceptible to delirium. All the other options are incorrect.
CN: Health promotion and maintenance; CNS: None; CL: Application

29. 4. The client is experiencing visual and auditory hallucinations related to a sensory alteration. The other options don't address the hallucinations the client is experiencing.
CN: Health promotion and maintenance; CNS: None; CL: Application

30. Which intervention is the <u>most appropriate</u> for clients with cognitive disorders?
1. Promote socialization.
2. Maintain optimal physical health.
3. Provide frequent changes in personnel.
4. Provide an overstimulating environment.

31. A newly admitted client diagnosed with delirium has a history of hypertension and anxiety. The client had been taking digoxin, furosemide (Lasix), and diazepam (Valium) for anxiety. This client's impairment may be related to which condition?
1. Infection
2. Metabolic acidosis
3. Drug intoxication
4. Hepatic encephalopathy

32. Which environment is the most appropriate for a client experiencing sensory-perceptual alterations?
1. A softly lit room around the clock
2. A brightly lit room around the clock
3. Sitting by the nurses' desk while out of bed
4. A quiet, well-lit room without glare during the day and a darkened room for sleeping

33. As a nurse enters a client's room, the client says, "They're crawling on my sheets! Get them off my bed!" Which assessment is the most accurate?
1. The client is experiencing aphasia.
2. The client is experiencing dysarthria.
3. The client is experiencing a flight of ideas.
4. The client is experiencing visual hallucinations.

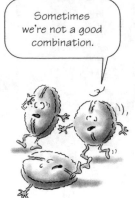

Sometimes we're not a good combination.

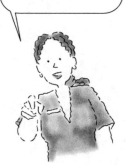

Your clients depend on you for meeting their environmental needs as well as their physical ones.

30. 2. A client's cognitive impairment may hinder self-care abilities. More socialization, frequent changes in staff members, and an overstimulating environment would only increase anxiety and confusion.
CN: Health promotion and maintenance; CNS: None; CL: Application

31. 3. This client was taking several medications that have a propensity for producing delirium; digoxin (a cardiac glycoside), furosemide (a thiazide diuretic), and diazepam (a benzodiazepine). Sufficient supporting data don't exist to suspect the other options as causes.
CN: Physiological integrity; CNS: Physiological adaptation; CL: Analysis

32. 4. A quiet, shadow-free environment produces the fewest sensory-perceptual distortions for a client with cognitive impairment associated with delirium.
CN: Psychosocial integrity; CNS: None; CL: Application

33. 4. The presence of a sensory stimulus correlates with the definition of a hallucination, which is a false sensory perception. Aphasia refers to a communications problem. Dysarthria is difficulty in speech production. Flight of ideas is rapid shifting from one topic to another.
CN: Psychosocial integrity; CNS: None; CL: Application

CN: Client needs category   CNS: Client needs subcategory   CL: Cognitive level

34. A delirious client is shouting for someone to get the bugs off her. Which response is the most appropriate?

1. "Don't worry, I'll stay here and brush away the bugs for you."
2. "Try to relax. The crawling sensation will go away sooner if you can relax."
3. "There are no bugs on your legs. It's just your imagination playing tricks on you."
4. "I know you're frightened. I don't see bugs crawling on your legs, but I'll stay here with you."

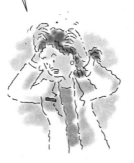

This question is really starting to bug me.

34. 4. Never argue about hallucinations with a client. Instead, promote an environment of trust and safety by acknowledging the client's perceptions.

CN: Physiological integrity; CNS: Basic care and comfort; CL: Application

35. Which description of a client's experience and behavior can be assessed as an illusion?

1. The client tries to hit the nurse when vital signs must be taken.
2. The client says, "I keep hearing a voice telling me to run away."
3. The client becomes anxious whenever the nurse leaves the bedside.
4. The client looks at the shadows on a wall and tells the nurse she sees frightening faces on the wall.

35. 4. An illusion is an inaccurate perception or false response to a sensory stimulus. Auditory hallucinations are associated with sound and are more common in schizophrenia. Anxiety and agitation can be secondary to illusions.

CN: Physiological integrity; CNS: Physiological adaptation; CL: Analysis

36. Which neurologic change is an <u>expected</u> characteristic of aging?

1. Widening of the sulci
2. Depletion of neurotransmitters
3. Neurofibrillary tangles and plaques
4. Degeneration of the frontal and temporal lobes

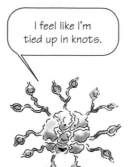

I feel like I'm tied up in knots.

36. 3. Aging isn't necessarily associated with significant decline, but neurofibrillary tangles and plaques are expected changes. These normal occurrences are sometimes referred to as benign senescent forgetfulness of age-associated memory impairment.

CN: Physiological integrity; CNS: Physiological adaptation; CL: Analysis

37. A major consideration in assessing memory impairment in an elderly individual includes which factor?

1. Allergies
2. Past surgery
3. Age at onset of symptoms
4. Social and occupational lifestyle

37. 4. Minor memory problems are distinguished from dementia by their minor severity and their lack of significant interference with the client's social or occupational lifestyle. Other options would be included in the history data but don't directly correlate with the client's lifestyle.

CN: Psychosocial integrity; CNS: None; CL: Analysis

38. During morning care, a nursing assistant asks a client with dementia, "How was your night?" The client replies, "My husband and I went out to dinner and a movie and had a wonderful evening!" Which state best describes the client's actions?
1. Delirium
2. Perseveration
3. Confabulation
4. Showing a sense of humor

38. 3. Confabulation is the process in which an individual makes up stories to answer questions. It's considered a defense tactic to protect the individual's self-esteem and prevent others from noticing the memory loss. Delirium is a state of mental confusion and excitement characterized by disorientation to time and place, often with hallucinations, incoherent speech, and a continual state of aimless physical activity. Perseveration is persistent repetition of the same word or idea in response to different questions. The client's response isn't meant to be humorous.
CN: Psychosocial integrity; CNS: None; CL: Application

39. A nursing assistant tells a nurse, "The client with amnesia looks fine but responds to questions in a vague, distant manner. What should I be doing for her?" Which response is the <u>most appropriate</u>?
1. "Give her lots of space to test her independence."
2. "Keep her busy and make sure she doesn't take naps during the day."
3. "Whenever you think she needs direction, use short, simple sentences."
4. "Spend as much time with her as you can, and ask questions about her recent life."

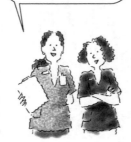

Teaching nursing assistants helps to improve the quality of care they provide.

39. 3. Disruptions in the ability to perform basic care, confusion, and anxiety are often apparent in clients with amnesia. Offering simple directions to promote daily functions and reduce confusion helps increase feelings of safety and security. Giving this client lots of space may make her feel insecure. Asking her many questions that she won't be able to answer just intensifies her anxiety level. There is no significant rationale for keeping her busy all day with no rest periods; the client may become more tired and less functional at other basic tasks.
CN: Safe, effective care environment; CNS: Management of care; CL: Application

40. With amnestic disorders, in which cognitive area is a change expected?
1. Speech
2. Concentration
3. Intellectual function
4. Recent short-term and long-term memory

40. 4. The primary area affected in amnesia is memory; all other areas of cognition are normal.
CN: Physiological integrity; CNS: Physiological adaptation; CL: Application

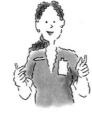

Question 41 is asking which action is best.

41. Which nursing action is the <u>best</u> way to help a client with mild Alzheimer's disease to remain functional?
1. Obtain a physician's order for a mild anxiolytic to control behavior.
2. Call attention to all mistakes so they can be quickly corrected.
3. Advise the client to move into a retirement center.
4. Maintain a stable, predictable environment and daily routine.

41. 4. Clients in the early stages of Alzheimer's disease remain fairly functional with familiar surroundings and a predictable routine. They become easily disoriented with surprises and social overstimulation. Anxiolytics can impair memory and worsen the problem. Calling attention to all the client's mistakes is nonproductive and serves to lower the client's self-esteem. Moving to an unfamiliar environment will heighten the client's agitation and confusion.
CN: Psychosocial integrity; CNS: None; CL: Application

CN: Client needs category   CNS: Client needs subcategory   CL: Cognitive level

42. The nurse is providing nursing care to a client with Alzheimer's-type dementia. Which nursing intervention takes top priority?
1. Establish a routine that supports former habits.
2. Maintain physical surroundings that are cheerful and pleasant.
3. Maintain an exact routine from day to day.
4. Control the environment by providing structure, boundaries, and safety.

43. The nurse finds a 78-year-old client with Alzheimer's-type dementia wandering in the hall at 3 a.m. The client has removed his clothing and says to the nurse, "I'm just taking a stroll through the park." What's the <u>best</u> approach to this behavior?
1. Immediately help the client back to his room and into some clothing.
2. Tell the client that such behavior won't be tolerated.
3. Tell the client it's too early in the morning to be taking a stroll.
4. Ask the client if he would like to go back to his room.

44. Which nursing diagnosis is appropriate for a client diagnosed with an amnestic disorder?
1. *Grieving*
2. *Ineffective denial*
3. *Ineffective coping*
4. *Risk for injury*

45. The nurse is planning care for a client who was admitted with dementia due to Alzheimer's disease. The family reports that the client has to be watched closely for wandering behavior at night. Which nursing diagnosis is the nurse's top priority?
1. *Disturbed sleep pattern*
2. *Insomnia*
3. *Risk for injury*
4. *Activity intolerance*

46. Which medical condition may be associated with an amnestic disorder?
1. Drug overdose
2. Cerebral anoxia
3. Medications (anticonvulsants)
4. Lead, mercury, and carbon dioxide toxins

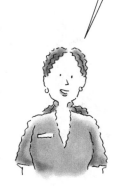

You need to determine which approach is best.

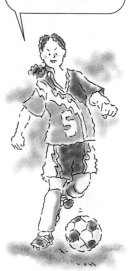

You've reached question 45. Now's the time to kick it into high gear!

42. 4. By controlling the environment and providing structure and boundaries, the nurse is helping to keep the client safe and secure, which is a top-priority nursing measure. Establishing a routine that supports former habits and maintaining cheerful, pleasant surroundings and an exact routine foster a supportive environment; however, keeping the client safe and secure takes priority.
CN: Safe, effective care environment; CNS: Management of care; CL: Application

43. 1. The nurse shouldn't allow the client to embarrass himself in front of others. Intervene as soon as the behavior is observed. Scolding the client isn't helpful because it isn't something the client can understand. Don't engage in social chatter. The interaction with this client should be concrete and specific. Don't ask the client to choose unnecessarily. The client may not be able to make appropriate choices.
CN: Psychosocial integrity; CNS: None; CL: Application

44. 4. Changes in cognitive ability place a client at high risk for injury. The client isn't aware of a loss and therefore doesn't grieve for it. The client isn't in denial but has an impaired ability to learn new information or to remember past information. The client isn't aware of a need to cope.
CN: Safe, effective care environment; CNS: Management of care; CL: Analysis

45. 3. Providing a safe, effective care environment takes priority with this client. *Disturbed sleep pattern*, *Insomnia*, and *Activity intolerance* are important but not the priority.
CN: Safe, effective care environment; CNS: Management of care; CL: Application

46. 2. A variety of medical conditions are related to amnestic disorders, such as head trauma, stroke, cerebral neoplastic disease, herpes simplex, encephalitis, poorly controlled insulin-dependent diabetes, and cerebral anoxia. The other three options are substance-induced.
CN: Physiological integrity; CNS: Physiological adaptation; CL: Application

47. Which laboratory evaluation is an <u>expected</u> part of the *initial* workup for an amnestic disorder?
1. Angiography
2. Cardiac catheterization
3. Electrocardiography
4. Metabolic and endocrine tests

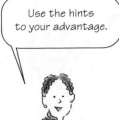

Use the hints to your advantage.

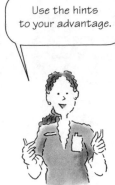

48. Which nursing intervention is appropriate for a client with memory impairment?
1. Speak to the client in a high-pitched tone.
2. Offer low-dose sedative-hypnotic drugs.
3. Ask a series of questions when obtaining information.
4. Identify yourself and look directly into the client's eyes.

49. Transient global amnesia is generally associated with which disorder?
1. Adjustment disorders
2. Cardiac anomalies
3. Cerebrovascular disease
4. Sleep disorders

50. During conversation with a client, the nurse observes that he shifts from one topic to the next on a regular basis. Which disorder is the client *most likely* to have?
1. Flight of ideas
2. Concrete thinking
3. Ideas of reference
4. Loose associations

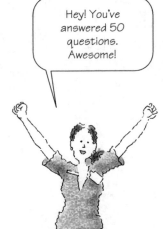

Hey! You've answered 50 questions. Awesome!

47. 4. An amnesic disorder is caused by either physiological effects of a medical condition or effects of a substance, medication, or toxin, so metabolic and endocrine tests should be done. The other options are diagnostic tests related to the cardiovascular system.
CN: Health promotion and maintenance; CNS: None; CL: Application

48. 4. Clients with memory impairments need to reestablish the nurse's identification constantly. High-pitched tones may create more anxiety. A low-dose sedative-hypnotic medication may be used to promote rapid-eye-movement sleep. Asking a series of questions may create confusion; ask only one question at a time.
CN: Safe, effective care environment; CNS: Management of care; CL: Application

49. 3. Transient global amnesia is usually associated with cerebrovascular disease that involves transient impairment in blood flow through the vertebrobasilar arteries. No correlation exists with the other options.
CN: Physiological integrity; CNS: Physiological adaptation; CL: Analysis

50. 4. Loose associations are conversations that constantly shift in topic. Loose associations don't necessarily start in a disorganized way; the conversations can begin cogently, then become loose. Flight of ideas is characterized by conversation that's disorganized from the onset. Concrete thinking implies highly definitive thought processes. Ideas of reference is characterized by a delusional belief that things irrelevant to the client, such as newspaper headlines, are referring to the client directly.
CN: Psychosocial integrity; CNS: None; CL: Application

CN: Client needs category   CNS: Client needs subcategory   CL: Cognitive level

51. For a client with dementia, which assessment finding indicates worsening of dementia?
1. The client resists logical explanations.
2. The client stops redirecting negative energy.
3. The client stops maintaining a nondefensive position.
4. The client becomes increasingly agitated.

52. For the family of a client with Alzheimer's disease, one goal is effective communication. Which outcome is successful for this goal?
1. Family members don't use humor with the client.
2. Family members speak to the client in a loud voice.
3. Family members give the client one-step commands.
4. Family members don't touch the client while speaking.

53. Immediately after visiting hours, a nurse identifies wandering behavior in a client with Alzheimer's disease. The client is showing which behavior?
1. The client may need to walk after eating a complete meal.
2. The client may feel tense because of an uncomfortable situation.
3. The client may be demonstrating several eccentric behaviors.
4. The client may have difficulty following directions.

54. For a client with dementia who lives in a long-term care facility, which outcome takes the highest nursing care <u>priority</u>?
1. Maintaining the client's optimal level of functioning
2. Identifying coping methods the client can use to handle stress
3. Facilitating client conversation with five people each day
4. Having the client use physical activity to work off aggressive energy

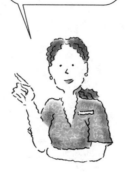

For effective communications, think clear and concise.

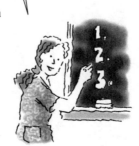

As a nurse, you will often need to prioritize!

51. 4. A client with dementia who becomes increasingly agitated may be unable to perform expected tasks. Communication must be clear and concise; giving logical explanations is inappropriate. This client may revert to old ways of coping, and trying to change the client rarely proves successful; the nurse should try to decrease the source of negativity. The client with dementia is rarely defensive.
CN: Psychosocial integrity; CNS: None; CL: Analysis

52. 3. Giving one-step commands keeps communication simple, clear, concise, and pleasant. Humor must be used judiciously so as not to confuse the client. Speaking in a loud voice may be interpreted as shouting and cause agitation. Depending on the situation, the use of touch may be appropriate, helping to reassure and soothe the client.
CN: Psychosocial integrity; CNS: None; CL: Application

53. 2. Tension and stress may cause a client with Alzheimer's disease to want to get away from an uncomfortable situation. Exercise is an important health promotion activity, but it doesn't help explain wandering behavior. Eccentric behaviors are rarely related to wandering. Many clients with dementia have difficulty following directions; however, wandering typically results from disorientation.
CN: Psychosocial integrity; CNS: None; CL: Application

54. 1. The highest nursing care priority is to maintain the client's optimal level of functioning. Reducing the client's stress is the nurse's responsibility. Having a conversation with five people each day is unrealistic for this client. Expecting a client with dementia to use physical activity to decrease aggressive energy is also unrealistic.
CN: Safe, effective care environment; CNS: Management of care; CL: Application

55. A nurse is assessing a client for dementia. What history would the nurse expect to find in a client with dementia? Select all that apply:

1. There's a slow progression of symptoms.
2. The client admits to feelings of sadness.
3. The client acts apathetic and pessimistic.
4. The family can't determine when the symptoms first appeared.
5. There are changes in the client's basic personality.
6. The client has great difficulty paying attention to others.

55. 1, 4, 5, 6. Common characteristics of dementia are a slow onset of symptoms, which makes it difficult to determine when they first occurred. It progresses to noticeable changes in the client's personality and impaired ability to pay attention to other people. Feelings of sadness, apathy, and pessimism are symptoms of depression.
CN: Health promotion and maintenance; CNS: None; CL: Analysis

56. A delusional client approaches a nurse, states, "I am the Easter Bunny," and insists that the nurse refer to him as such. Which nursing interventions should the nurse implement when working with this client? Select all that apply:

1. Consistently use the client's name in interaction.
2. Smile at the humor of the situation.
3. Agree that the client is the Easter Bunny.
4. Logically point out why the client could not be the Easter Bunny.
5. Provide as-needed medication.
6. Provide the client with structured activities.

56. 1, 6. Continued reality-based orientation is necessary, so it is appropriate to use the client's name in any interaction. Structured activities can help the client refocus and resolve his delusion. The nurse shouldn't contribute to the delusion by going along with the situation. Logical arguments and as-needed medication aren't likely to change the client's beliefs.
CN: Psychosocial integrity; CNS: None; CL: Analysis

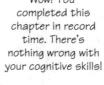

Wow! You completed this chapter in record time. There's nothing wrong with your cognitive skills!

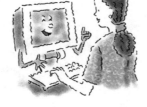

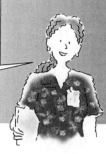

No, this chapter doesn't cover quirks of the rich and famous. It's all about mental disorders affecting the personality. Have a blast!

Chapter 17
Personality disorders

1. A client tells the nurse that her coworkers are sabotaging the computer. When the nurse asks questions, the client becomes argumentative. Which intervention would be most appropriate for the nurse to implement?
　1. Encourage the client to vent his anger about his coworkers.
　2. Tell the client that his coworkers haven't touched his computer.
　3. Use clear and consistent speech when talking to the client.
　4. Tell the client to go to his room and stay there until he calms down.

2. A nurse observes that a client is mistrustful and shows hostile behavior. Which type of personality disorder is the client <u>most likely</u> to have?
　1. Antisocial
　2. Avoidant
　3. Borderline
　4. Paranoid

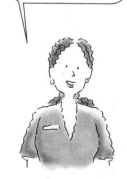

Understanding a client's traits will help you deal with him effectively.

3. The nurse is caring for a client with paranoid personality disorder. Which behavior is a common characteristic of this disorder?
　1. The client can't follow limits set on his behavior.
　2. The client is afraid another person will inflict harm.
　3. The client avoids responsibility for his health care.
　4. The client depends on others to make important decisions.

1. 3. Using clear and consistent speech when talking with the client helps him focus on reality and fosters a therapeutic relationship. Encouraging the client to vent his anger at his coworkers validates his suspicious thoughts and may make him more argumentative. Trying to convince him that his coworkers haven't touched his computer or telling him to go to his room may make him more defensive.
CN: Psychosocial integrity; CNS: None; CL: Analysis

2. 4. Paranoid individuals have a need to constantly scan the environment for signs of betrayal, deception, and ridicule, appearing mistrustful and hostile. They expect to be tricked or deceived by others. The extreme suspiciousness is lacking in antisocial personalities, who tend to be more arrogant and self-assured despite their vigilance and mistrust. Individuals with avoidant personality disorders are guarded, fearing interpersonal rejection and humiliation. Clients with borderline personality disorders behave impulsively and tend to manipulate others.
CN: Psychosocial integrity; CNS: None; CL: Application

3. 2. A client with paranoid personality disorder is afraid others will inflict harm. An individual with antisocial personality disorder won't be able to follow the limits set on behavior. An individual with an avoidant personality might avoid responsibility for health care because he tends to scan the environment for threatening things. A client with dependent personality disorder is likely to want others to make important decisions for him.
CN: Psychosocial integrity; CNS: None; CL: Analysis

4. Which statement is typical for a client diagnosed with paranoid personality disorder?
   1. "I understand you're to blame."
   2. "I must be seen first; it's not negotiable."
   3. "I see nothing humorous in this situation."
   4. "I wish someone would select the outfit for me."

5. Which characteristic is expected for a client with paranoid personality disorder who receives bad news?
   1. The client is overly dramatic after hearing the facts.
   2. The client focuses on self to not become overanxious.
   3. The client responds from a rational, objective point of view.
   4. The client doesn't spend time thinking about the information.

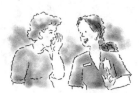

Pssst! Do you want to know the answer to this question?

6. A nurse is caring for a client with paranoid personality disorder. The nurse would expect to observe which of the following conditions?
   1. Exhibitionism
   2. Impulsiveness
   3. Secretiveness
   4. Self-destructiveness

7. Which type of behavior is expected from a client diagnosed with paranoid personality disorder?
   1. Eccentric
   2. Exploitative
   3. Hypersensitive
   4. Seductive

4. 3. Clients with paranoid personality disorder tend to be extremely serious and lack a sense of humor. Clients with borderline personality disorder tend to blame others for their problems. Clients with narcissistic personality disorders have a sense of self-importance and entitlement. Clients with dependent personality disorder want others to make their decisions.
CN: Psychosocial integrity; CNS: None; CL: Analysis

5. 3. Clients with paranoid personality disorder are affectively restricted, appear unemotional, and appear rational and objective. Clients with histrionic personality disorder are overly dramatic in response to stress. Clients with narcissistic personality disorder focus on themselves and don't spend time thinking about bad news. Clients with an obsessive-compulsive personality disorder are preoccupied with the fear of becoming very anxious and losing control.
CN: Psychosocial integrity; CNS: None; CL: Analysis

6. 3. Clients with paranoid personality disorder tend to be secretive. Clients with histrionic personality disorder tend to be exhibitionists, and those with borderline personality disorder tend to be impulsive and self-destructive.
CN: Psychosocial integrity; CNS: None; CL: Application

7. 3. People with paranoid personality disorders are hypersensitive to perceived threats. Schizotypal personalities appear eccentric and engage in activities others find perplexing. Clients with narcissistic personality disorder are interpersonally exploitative to enhance themselves or indulge their own desires. A client with histrionic personality disorder can be extremely seductive when in search of stimulation and approval.
CN: Psychosocial integrity; CNS: None; CL: Analysis

CN: Client needs category   CNS: Client needs subcategory   CL: Cognitive level

8. A client with paranoid personality disorder is discussing current problems with a nurse. Which nursing intervention has <u>priority</u> in the care plan?

1. Have the client look at sources of frustration.
2. Have the client focus on ways to interact with others.
3. Have the client discuss the use of defense mechanisms.
4. Have the client clarify thoughts and beliefs about an event.

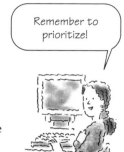

Remember to prioritize!

9. A client with a paranoid personality disorder makes an inappropriate and unreasonable report to a nurse. Which principle of good communication skills is important to use?

1. Use logic to address the client's concern.
2. Confront the client about the stated misperception.
3. Use nonverbal communication to address the issue.
4. Tell the client matter-of-factly that you don't share his interpretation.

10. Which short-term goal is <u>most appropriate</u> for a client with paranoid personality disorder who has impaired social skills?

1. Obtain feedback from other people.
2. Discuss anxiety-provoking situations.
3. Address positive and negative feelings about self.
4. Identify personal feelings that hinder social interaction.

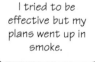

I tried to be effective but my plans went up in smoke.

11. Which intervention is important for a client with paranoid personality disorder taking olanzapine (Zyprexa)?

1. Explain effects of serotonin syndrome.
2. Teach the client to watch for extrapyramidal adverse reactions.
3. Explain that the drug is less effective if the client smokes.
4. Discuss the need to report paradoxical effects such as euphoria.

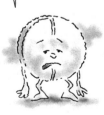

8. 4. Clarifying thoughts and beliefs helps the client avoid misinterpretations. Clients with a paranoid personality disorder tend to mistrust people and don't see interacting with others as a way to handle problems. They tend to be aggressive and argumentative rather than frustrated. The client's priority must be to interpret his thoughts and beliefs realistically, rather than discuss defensive mechanisms. A paranoid client will focus on defending self rather than acknowledging the use of defense mechanisms.
CN: Safe, effective care environment; CNS: Management of care; CL: Analysis

9. 4. Telling the client you don't share his interpretation helps the client differentiate between realistic and emotional thoughts and conclusions. When the nurse uses logic to respond to a client's inappropriate statement, the nurse risks creating a power struggle with the client. The use of nonverbal communication will probably be misinterpreted and arouse the client's suspicion. It's unwise to confront a client with a paranoid personality disorder as the client will immediately become defensive.
CN: Psychosocial integrity; CNS: None; CL: Analysis

10. 4. The client must address the feelings that impede social interactions before developing ways to address impaired social skills. Feedback can only be obtained after action is taken to improve or change the situation. Discussion of anxiety-provoking situations is important but doesn't help the client with impaired social skills. Addressing the client's positive and negative feelings about self won't directly influence impaired social skills.
CN: Psychosocial integrity; CNS: None; CL: Application

11. 3. Olanzapine is less effective for clients who smoke cigarettes. Serotonin syndrome occurs with clients who take a combination of antidepressant medications. Olanzapine doesn't cause euphoria, and extrapyramidal adverse reactions aren't a problem. However, the client should be aware of adverse effects such as tardive dyskinesia.
CN: Physiological integrity; CNS: Pharmacological and parenteral therapies; CL: Application

12. Which approach should be used with a client with paranoid personality disorder who misinterprets many things the health care team says?
 1. Limit interaction to activities of daily living.
 2. Address only problems and causes of distress.
 3. Explore anxious situations and offer reassurance.
 4. Speak in simple messages without details.

13. A client with paranoid personality disorder responds aggressively during a psychoeducational group therapy to something another client said about him. Which explanation is the most likely?
 1. The client doesn't want to participate in the group.
 2. The client took the statement as a personal criticism.
 3. The client is impulsive and was acting out of frustration.
 4. The client was attempting to handle emotional distress.

14. A client with a paranoid personality disorder tells a nurse of his decision to stop talking to his wife. Which area should be assessed?
 1. The client's doubts about the partner's loyalty
 2. The client's need to be alone and have time for self
 3. The client's decision to separate from the marital partner
 4. The client's fears about becoming too much like the partner

15. Which characteristic of a client with a paranoid personality disorder makes it difficult for a nurse to establish an interpersonal relationship?
 1. Dysphoria
 2. Hypervigilance
 3. Indifference
 4. Promiscuity

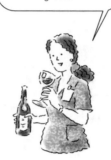

Cheers to you—you're doing great!

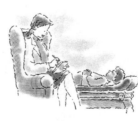

Try to establish a therapeutic relationship with the client.

12. 4. If the nurse speaks to the client with clear and simple messages, there's less chance information will be misinterpreted. Interaction can't be limited because it will interfere with working on identified treatment goals. Discussing complex topics creates a situation in which the client will have additional information to misinterpret. If the nurse addresses only problems and specific stressors, it will be difficult to establish a trust relationship.
CN: Psychosocial integrity; CNS: None; CL: Application

13. 2. Clients with paranoid personality disorder tend to be hypersensitive and take what other people say as a personal attack on their character. The client is driven by the suspicion that others will inflict harm. Group participation would be minimal because the client is directing energy toward emotional self-protection. Clients with a paranoid personality disorder tend to be rigid and guarded rather than expressive and acting out. The client with a paranoid personality disorder is acting to defend himself, not handle emotional distress.
CN: Psychosocial integrity; CNS: None; CL: Analysis

14. 1. Clients with paranoid personality disorder are preoccupied with the loyalty or trustworthiness of people, especially family and friends. People commonly withdraw from a client with paranoid personality disorder due to the difficulty in maintaining a healthy relationship. The client's need to be alone and have time for self isn't related to the decision to stop talking to a partner. These clients focus on the belief that others will harm them, not that they may become like a marital partner.
CN: Psychosocial integrity; CNS: None; CL: Application

15. 2. Clients with paranoid personality disorder think others will harm, deceive, or exploit them in some way, and they're often guarded and ready to defend themselves from actual or perceived attacks. They don't tend to be dysphoric, indifferent, or promiscuous.
CN: Psychosocial integrity; CNS: None; CL: Application

CN: Client needs category   CNS: Client needs subcategory   CL: Cognitive level

16. The wife of a client diagnosed with paranoid personality disorder tells the client she wants a divorce. When discussing this situation with the couple, which factor should help the nurse form a care plan for this couple?
1. Denied grief
2. Intense jealousy
3. Exploitation of others
4. Self-destructive tendencies

17. A client with a paranoid personality disorder tells a nurse that another nurse is out to get him. Which action by the nurse may cause this paranoid client distress?
1. Giving as-needed medication to another client
2. Taking the clients outside the unit for exercise
3. Checking vital signs of each person on the unit
4. Talking to another client in the corner of the lounge

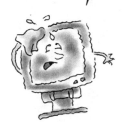

I wonder what they're saying about me?

18. Which statement made by a client with paranoid personality disorder shows that teaching about social relationships is effective?
1. "As long as I live, I won't abide by social rules."
2. "Sometimes I can see what causes relationship problems."
3. "I'll find out what problems others have so I won't repeat them."
4. "I don't have problems in social relationships; I never really did."

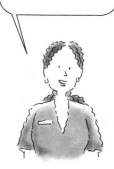

The word long-term is a clue to the correct choice.

19. Which long-term goal is appropriate for a client with paranoid personality disorder who is trying to improve peer relationships?
1. The client will verbalize a realistic view of self.
2. The client will take steps to address disorganized thinking.
3. The client will become appropriately interdependent on others.
4. The client will become involved in activities that foster social relationships.

16. 2. Clients with paranoid personality disorder are often extremely suspicious and jealous and make frequent accusations of partners and family members. Clients with paranoid personality disorder don't tend to struggle with the denial of grief. Clients with narcissistic personality disorder tend to exploit other people. Clients with borderline personality disorder have self-destructive tendencies.
CN: Psychosocial integrity; CNS: None; CL: Application

17. 4. Clients with paranoid personality disorder tend to interpret any discussion that doesn't include them as evidence of a plot against them. Giving medication to another client wouldn't alarm the client. Checking vital signs on each client on the unit or taking the clients outside for exercise probably wouldn't be seen as a threat to the client's well-being.
CN: Psychosocial integrity; CNS: None; CL: Application

18. 2. Progress is shown when the client addresses behaviors that negatively impact relationships. Clients with paranoid personality disorder tend to have impaired social relationships and are very uncomfortable in social settings. Clients with paranoid personality disorder struggle to understand and express their feelings about social rules. Knowing other people's problems isn't useful; the client must focus on his own issues. Not recognizing the problem indicates the client is in denial.
CN: Psychosocial integrity; CNS: None; CL: Application

19. 4. An appropriate long-term goal is for the client to increase interactions and social skills and make the commitment to become involved with others on a long-term basis. To verbalize a realistic view of self is a short-term goal. The client with a paranoid personality disorder doesn't tend to have disorganized thinking. A client with paranoid personality disorder won't allow himself to be interdependent on others.
CN: Psychosocial integrity; CNS: None; CL: Analysis

20. A family of a client with paranoid personality disorder is trying to understand the client's behavior. Which intervention should help the family?
1. Help the family find ways to handle stress.
2. Explore the possibility of finding respite care.
3. Help the family manage the client's eccentric action.
4. Encourage the family to focus on the client's strength.

21. A client with antisocial personality disorder is trying to convince a nurse that he deserves special privileges and that an exception to the rules should be made for him. Which response is the <u>most appropriate?</u>
1. "I believe we need to sit down and talk about this."
2. "Don't you know better than to try to bend the rules?"
3. "What you're asking me to do for you is unacceptable."
4. "Why don't you bring this request to the community meeting?"

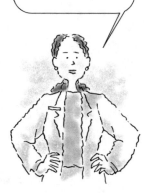

Therapeutic interventions must be appropriate for the client.

22. A client with antisocial personality disorder tells a nurse, "Life has been full of problems since childhood." Which situation or condition should the nurse explore in the assessment?
1. Birth defects
2. Distracted easily
3. Hypoactive behavior
4. Substance abuse

This is one of those further teaching questions. It asks you to identify a client behavior that signals the need for more teaching.

23. Which behavior by a client with antisocial personality disorder alerts the nurse to the need for teaching related to interaction skills?
1. Frequently crying
2. Having panic attacks
3. Avoiding social activities
4. Failing to follow social norms

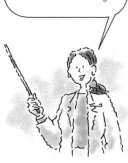

20. 3. The family needs to know how to handle the client's symptoms and eccentric behaviors. All people need to learn strategies for handling stress, but the focus must be on helping the family learn how to handle symptoms. There's no need to find respite care for a client with a paranoid personality disorder. Focusing on the client's strengths is a positive action, but the family in this situation must learn how to manage the client's behavior.
CN: Psychosocial integrity; CNS: None; CL: Application

21. 3. These clients often try to manipulate the nurse to get special privileges or make exceptions to the rules on their behalf. By informing the client directly when actions are inappropriate, the nurse helps the client learn to control unacceptable behaviors by setting limits. By sitting down to talk about the request, the nurse is telling the client there's room for negotiation when there is none. The second option humiliates the client. The client's behavior is unacceptable and shouldn't be brought to a community meeting.
CN: Psychosocial integrity; CNS: None; CL: Application

22. 4. Clients with antisocial personality disorder often engage in substance abuse during childhood. They don't have a higher incidence of birth defects than other people. Clients with antisocial personality disorder are often manipulative and are no more distracted from issues than others. They tend to be hyperactive, not hypoactive.
CN: Psychosocial integrity; CNS: None; CL: Application

23. 4. Failure to abide by social norms influences the client's ability to interact in a healthy manner with peers. Clients with antisocial personality disorders don't have frequent crying episodes or panic attacks. Avoiding social activities is more likely to be observed in avoidance personality style.
CN: Psychosocial integrity; CNS: None; CL: Analysis

CN: Client needs category   CNS: Client needs subcategory   CL: Cognitive level

24. When reviewing a client's chart, the nurse notes the progress note below. Which statement about the client's condition is <u>most</u> accurate?

Progress notes	
9/15/10	Client, age 28, admitted to unit with
1130	diagnosis of antisocial personality dis-
	order and suicide attempt after
	cutting his right wrist. Right wrist
	dressing appears dry and intact. Client
	states, @I don't want to be here and
	I'm not following your treatment plan
	or any of your rules. I'm going to tell
	everyone here not to follow your
	rules.@ ——— Barbara Jones, RN

1. The client requires psychotropic drugs to treat his condition, which he refuses.
2. The client manipulates other clients but not his family.
3. The client may not be motivated to change his behavior or his lifestyle.
4. The client could quickly make behavior changes if motivated.

25. Which intervention should be done <u>first</u> for a client who has an antisocial personality disorder and a history of polysubstance abuse?
1. Human immunodeficiency virus (HIV) testing
2. Electrolyte profile
3. Anxiety screening
4. Psychological testing

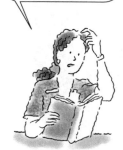

Which intervention should be done first?

26. Which short-term goal is appropriate for a client with an antisocial personality disorder who acts out when distressed?
1. Develop goals for personal improvement.
2. Identify situations that are out of the client's control.
3. Encourage the client to identify traumatic life events.
4. Learn to express feelings in a nondestructive manner.

24. 3. Clients with antisocial personality disorder feel nothing is wrong with their behavior and have no desire to change. These clients don't benefit from psychotropic drug therapy. They attempt to manipulate all people with whom they come in contact. A quick behavior change isn't realistic expectation for clients with this disorder.
CN: Psychosocial integrity; CNS: None; CL: Applicationv

25. 1. A client who engages in high-risk behaviors such as polysubstance abuse should undergo HIV testing. This client would benefit from an entire chemistry profile as part of a complete medical examination, rather than a singular test for electrolytes. An anxiety screen isn't needed for a client with antisocial personality disorder. Information from psychological testing is valuable when developing a treatment but isn't an immediate concern.
CN: Safe, effective care environment; CNS: Management of care; CL: Application

26. 4. By working on appropriate expression of feelings, the client learns how to talk about what's stressful, rather than hurt himself or others. The most pressing need is to learn to cope and talk about problems rather than act out. Developing goals for personal improvement is a long-term goal, not a short-term one. Although it's important to differentiate what is and isn't under the client's control, the most important goal for handling distress is to talk about feelings appropriately. The identification of traumatic life events will occur only after the client begins to express feelings appropriately.
CN: Psychosocial integrity; CNS: None; CL: Application

27. A nurse notices other clients on the unit avoiding a client diagnosed with antisocial personality disorder. When discussing appropriate behavior in group therapy, which comment is <u>expected</u> about this client by his peers?
1. Lack of honesty
2. Belief in superstitions
3. Show of temper tantrums
4. Constant need for attention

28. During a family meeting for a client with antisocial personality disorder, which statement is expected from an exasperated family member?
1. "Today I'm the enemy, but tomorrow I'll be a saint to him."
2. "When he's wrong, he never apologizes or even acts sorry."
3. "Sometimes I can't believe how he exaggerates about everything."
4. "There are times when his compulsive behavior is too much to handle."

29. Which goal is <u>most appropriate</u> for a client with antisocial personality disorder with a high risk for violence directed at others?
1. The client will discuss the desire to hurt others rather than act.
2. The client will be given something to destroy to displace the anger.
3. The client will develop a list of resources to use when anger escalates.
4. The client will understand the difference between anger and physical symptoms.

30. A client with antisocial personality disorder says, "I always want to blow things off." Which response is the most appropriate?
1. "Try to focus on what needs to be done and just do it."
2. "Let's work on considering some options and strategies."
3. "Procrastinating is a part of your illness that we'll work on."
4. "The best thing to do is decide on some useful goals to accomplish."

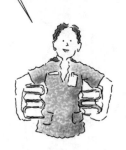

Read this question carefully. It seems to be asking you for a positive response, but it isn't.

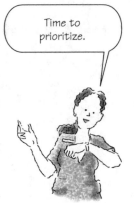

Time to prioritize.

27. 1. Clients with antisocial personality disorder tend to engage in acts of dishonesty, shown by lying. Clients with schizotypal personality disorder tend to be superstitious. Clients with histrionic personality disorders tend to overreact to frustrations and disappointments, have temper tantrums, and seek attention.
CN: Psychosocial integrity; CNS: None; CL: Application

28. 2. The client with antisocial personality disorder has no remorse. The client with borderline personality disorder shows splitting. The client with antisocial personality disorder doesn't tend to exaggerate about life events or be compulsive.
CN: Psychosocial integrity; CNS: None; CL: Analysis

29. 1. By discussing the desire to be violent toward others, the nurse can help the client get in touch with the pain associated with the angry feelings. It isn't helpful to have the client destroy something. The client needs to talk about strong feelings in a nonviolent manner, not refer to a list of crisis references. Helping the client understand the relationship between feelings and physical symptoms can be done after discussing the desire to hurt others.
CN: Psychosocial integrity; CNS: None; CL: Analysis

30. 2. By considering options or strategies, the client gains skills to overcome ineffective behaviors. The client tends to be irresponsible and needs guidance on what specifically to focus on to change behavior. Clients with an antisocial personality disorder don't tend to struggle with procrastination; instead, they show reckless and irresponsible behaviors. It's premature to decide on goals when the client needs to address the mental mind-set and work to change the irresponsible behavior.
CN: Psychosocial integrity; CNS: None; CL: Analysis

CN: Client needs category   CNS: Client needs subcategory   CL: Cognitive level

31. Which goal for the family of a client with antisocial disorder should the nurse stress in her teaching?
1. The family must assist the client to decrease ritualistic behavior.
2. The family must learn to live with the client's impulsive behavior.
3. The family must stop reinforcing inappropriate negative behavior.
4. The family must start to use negative reinforcement of the client's behavior.

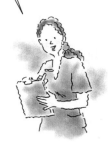

Teach the client skills to overcome ineffective behaviors.

31. 3. The family needs help learning how to stop reinforcing inappropriate client behavior. Negative reinforcement is an inappropriate strategy for the family to use to support the client. The family can set limits and reinforce consequences when the client shows short-sightedness and poor planning. Clients with antisocial personality disorder don't show ritualistic behaviors.
CN: Psychosocial integrity; CNS: None; CL: Analysis

32. Which nursing intervention has priority in the care plan for a client with antisocial personality disorder who shows defensive behaviors?
1. Help the client accept responsibility for his own decisions and behaviors.
2. Work with the client to feel better about himself by taking care of basic needs.
3. Teach the client to identify the defense mechanisms used to cope with distress.
4. Confront the client about the disregard of social rules and the feelings of others.

32. 1. Clients with antisocial personality disorder tend to blame other people for their behaviors and need to be taught how to take responsibility for their actions. Clients with antisocial personality disorder don't tend to have problems with self-care habits or meeting their basic needs. Clients with antisocial personality disorder will deny they're defensive or distressed. Most often, these clients feel justified with retaliatory behavior. To confront the client would only cause him to become even more defensive.
CN: Psychosocial integrity; CNS: None; CL: Analysis

33. A client with antisocial personality disorder is trying to manipulate the health care team. Which strategy is important for the staff to use?
1. Focus on how to teach the client more effective behaviors for meeting basic needs.
2. Help the client verbalize underlying feelings of hopelessness and learn coping skills.
3. Remain calm and don't emotionally respond to the client's manipulative actions.
4. Help the client eliminate the intense desire to have everything in life turn out perfectly.

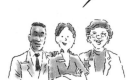

The staff must work together as a team.

33. 3. The best strategy to use with a client trying to manipulate staff is to stay calm and refrain from responding emotionally. Negative reinforcement of inappropriate behavior increases the chance it will be repeated. Later, it may be possible to address how to meet the client's basic needs. Clients with antisocial personality disorder don't tend to experience feelings of hopelessness or to desire life events to turn out perfectly. In most cases, these clients negate responsibility for their behavior.
CN: Psychosocial integrity; CNS: None; CL: Analysis

34. A client with dependent personality disorder is working to increase self-esteem. Which statement by the client shows teaching was successful?
1. "I'm not going to look just at the negative things about myself."
2. "I'm most concerned about my level of competence and progress."
3. "I'm not as envious of the things other people have as I used to be."
4. "I find I can't stop myself from taking over things others should be doing."

34. 1. As the client makes progress on improving self-esteem, self-blame and negative self-evaluations will decrease. Clients with dependent personality disorder tend to feel fragile and inadequate and would be extremely unlikely to discuss their level of competence and progress. These clients focus on self and aren't envious or jealous. Individuals with dependent personality disorders don't take over situations because they see themselves as inept and inadequate.
CN: Psychosocial integrity; CNS: None; CL: Application

35. A client is suspected of having antisocial personality disorder. Which finding <u>most</u> supports this diagnosis?
    1. The client has delusional thinking.
    2. The client has feelings of inferiority.
    3. The client has disorganized thinking.
    4. The client has multiple criminal charges.

36. A client with antisocial personality disorder talks about personal life changes that need to occur. Which client statement shows group therapy is having a <u>positive</u> therapeutic effect?
    1. "I'm not doing as bad as I thought I was."
    2. "I wish I could believe I can change, but it's probably too late."
    3. "I see all the problems, but I'm not sure there are good solutions."
    4. "I'm finally learning how to live my life without living on the edge."

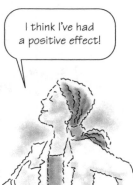

I think I've had a positive effect!

37. A nurse tells a client with a personality disorder that he must clean his room before he can go to the dayroom. The client asks if he can play one game of pool first. What's the most appropriate response by the nurse?
    1. "You can play one quick game. Then you have to clean your room."
    2. "No, you may not."
    3. "No, you may not play pool first. The rules were explained to you."
    4. "Yes, you may play a quick game. But don't tell the other clients about this."

38. A nurse determines that a client with antisocial personality disorder is beginning to practice several socially acceptable behaviors in the group setting. Which behavior is the nurse <u>most likely</u> to observe in this client?
    1. Fewer panic attacks
    2. Acceptance of reality
    3. Improved self-esteem
    4. Decreased physical symptoms

35. 4. Clients with antisocial personality disorder are commonly sent for treatment by the court after multiple crimes or for the use of illegal substances. Clients with antisocial personality disorder don't tend to have delusional thinking, feelings of inferiority, or disorganized thinking.
CN: Psychosocial integrity; CNS: None; CL: Application

36. 4. The client is becoming aware of risky behaviors and how problematic these behaviors are. The first option indicates denial, and the client is somewhat defensive about making a change. The second option indicates defeat, and the client seems to feel stuck. The third option indicates problem identification but also uncertainty and ambivalence about the client's ability to change.
CN: Psychosocial integrity; CNS: None; CL: Analysis

37. 3. This response is firm and reinforces the rules. Allowing the client to play one game before cleaning his room and telling him not to tell anyone else encourages manipulative behavior. Saying no to the client without an explanation doesn't outline or reinforce the rules.
CN: Psychosocial integrity; CNS: None; CL: Analysis

38. 3. When clients with antisocial personality disorder begin to practice socially acceptable behaviors, they also frequently experience a more positive sense of self-esteem. Clients with antisocial personality disorder don't tend to have panic attacks, somatic manifestations of their illness, or withdrawal or alteration in their perception of reality.
CN: Psychosocial integrity; CNS: None; CL: Application

CN: Client needs category   CNS: Client needs subcategory   CL: Cognitive level

39. A client with borderline personality disorder is admitted to the unit after slashing his wrist. Which goal is <u>most important</u> after promoting safety?
 1. Establish a therapeutic relationship with the client.
 2. Identify whether splitting is present in the client's thoughts.
 3. Talk about the client's acting out and self-destructive tendencies.
 4. Encourage the client to understand why he blames others.

40. Which nursing intervention is most appropriate in helping a client with a borderline personality disorder identify appropriate behaviors?
 1. Schedule a family meeting.
 2. Place the client in seclusion.
 3. Formulate a behavioral contract.
 4. Perform a mental status assessment.

41. Which statement is <u>typical</u> of a client with borderline personality disorder who has recurrent suicidal thoughts?
 1. "I can't believe how everyone has suddenly stopped believing in me."
 2. "I don't care what other people say, I know how badly I looked to them."
 3. "I might as well check out since my boyfriend doesn't want me anymore."
 4. "I won't stop until I've gotten revenge on all those people who blamed me."

42. The nurse is taking a health history on a client with borderline personality disorder. Which of the following findings would the nurse expect to observe?
 1. A negative sense of self
 2. A tendency to be compulsive
 3. A problem with communication
 4. An inclination to be philosophical

43. Which characteristic or situation is indicated when a client with borderline personality disorder has a crisis?
 1. Antisocial behavior
 2. Suspicious behavior
 3. Relationship problems
 4. Auditory hallucinations

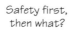
Safety first, then what?

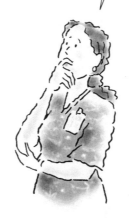

39. 1. After promoting client safety, the nurse establishes a rapport with the client to facilitate appropriate expression of feelings. A therapeutic relationship also must be established before working on the issue of splitting. At this time, the client isn't ready to address unhealthy behavior. A therapeutic relationship must be established before the nurse can effectively work with the client on self-destructive tendencies.
CN: Safe, effective care environment; CNS: Management of care; CL: Application

40. 3. The use of a behavioral contract establishes a framework for healthier functioning and places responsibility for actions back on the client. Seclusion will reinforce the fears of abandonment of clients with borderline personality. Performing a mental status assessment or scheduling a family meeting won't help the client identify appropriate behaviors.
CN: Psychosocial integrity; CNS: None; CL: Application

41. 3. This statement is typical for the borderline personality disorder client who is suicidal and reflects the tendency toward all-or-nothing thinking. The first option indicates the client has experienced a credibility problem, the second option indicates the client is extremely embarrassed, and the last option indicates the client has antisocial personality disorder. None of these is a characteristic of borderline personality disorder.
CN: Safe, effective care environment; CNS: Safety and infection control; CL: Application

42. 1. Clients with a borderline personality disorder have low self-esteem and a negative sense of self. They have little or no problem expressing themselves and communicating with others, and although they have a tendency to be impulsive, they aren't usually compulsive or philosophical.
CN: Psychosocial integrity; CNS: None; CL: Application

43. 3. Relationship problems can precipitate a crisis because they bring up issues of abandonment. Clients with borderline personality disorder aren't usually suspicious; they're more likely to be depressed or highly anxious. They don't have symptoms of antisocial behavior or auditory hallucinations.
CN: Psychosocial integrity; CNS: None; CL: Analysis

44. Which assessment finding is seen in a client diagnosed with borderline personality disorder?

  1. Abrasions in various healing stages
  2. Intermittent episodes of hypertension
  3. Alternating tachycardia and bradycardia
  4. Mild state of euphoria with disorientation

44. 1. Clients with borderline personality disorder tend to self-mutilate and have abrasions in various stages of healing. The other options don't tend to occur with this disorder.
CN: Psychosocial integrity; CNS: None; CL: Application

45. Which <u>short-term</u> goal is appropriate for a client with borderline personality disorder with low self-esteem?

  1. Write in a journal daily.
  2. Express fears and feelings.
  3. Stop obsessive-compulsive behaviors.
  4. Decrease dysfunctional family conflicts.

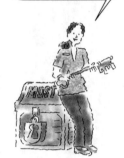

The word short-term is the key to the answer.

45. 2. Acknowledging fears and feelings can help the client identify parts of himself that are uncomfortable, and he can begin to work on developing a positive sense of self. Writing in a daily journal isn't a short-term goal to enhance self-esteem. A client with borderline personality disorder doesn't struggle with obsessive-compulsive behaviors. Decreasing dysfunctional family conflicts is a long-term goal.
CN: Psychosocial integrity; CNS: None; CL: Analysis

46. Which intervention is important to include in a teaching plan for a family with a member diagnosed with borderline personality disorder?

  1. Teach the family methods for handling the client's anxiety.
  2. Explore how the family reinforces the sick role with the client.
  3. Encourage the family to have the client express intense emotions.
  4. Help the family put pressure on the client to improve current behavior.

46. 1. The family needs to learn how to handle the client's intense stress and low tolerance for frustration. Family members don't want to reinforce the sick role; they're more concerned with preventing anxiety from escalating. Clients with borderline personality disorder already maintain intense emotions, and it isn't safe to encourage further expression of them. The family doesn't need to put pressure on the client to change behavior; this approach will only cause inappropriate behavior to escalate.
CN: Psychosocial integrity; CNS: None; CL: Application

47. In planning care for a client with borderline personality disorder, a nurse must be aware that this client is prone to develop which condition?

  1. Binge eating
  2. Memory loss
  3. Cult membership
  4. Delusional thinking

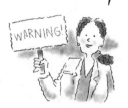

Clients with borderline personality disorder are likely to act out in self-destructive ways.

47. 1. Clients with borderline personality disorder are likely to develop dysfunctional coping and act out in self-destructive ways such as binge eating. They aren't prone to develop memory loss or delusional thinking. Becoming involved in cults may be seen in some clients with antisocial personality disorder.
CN: Psychosocial integrity; CNS: None; CL: Analysis

CN: Client needs category CNS: Client needs subcategory CL: Cognitive level

48. Which statement is expected from a client with borderline personality disorder with a history of dysfunctional relationships?
1. "I won't get involved in another relationship."
2. "I'm determined to look for the perfect partner."
3. "I've decided to learn better communication skills."
4. "I'm going to be an equal partner in a relationship."

48. 2. Clients with borderline personality disorder would decide to look for a perfect partner. This characteristic is a result of the dichotomous manner in which these clients view the world. They go from relationship to relationship without taking responsibility for their behavior. It's unlikely that an unsuccessful relationship will cause clients to make a change. They tend to be demanding and impulsive in relationships. There's no thought given to what one wants or needs from a relationship. Because they tend to blame others for problems, it's unlikely they would express a desire to learn communication skills.
CN: Psychosocial integrity; CNS: None; CL: Analysis

49. Which nursing intervention is most appropriate for a client with borderline personality disorder working on developing healthy relationships?
1. Have the client assess current behaviors.
2. Work with the client to develop outgoing behavior.
3. Limit the client's interactions to family members only.
4. Encourage the client to approach others for interactions.

Appropriate care considers the client's best interests.

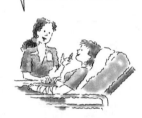

49. 1. Self-assessment of behavior enables the client to look at himself and identify social behaviors that need to be changed. It isn't useful to work on developing outgoing behavior. It's unrealistic to have clients with borderline personality disorder limit their interactions to family members only. Clients with borderline personality disorder don't tend to have difficulty approaching and interacting with other people; in fact, they tend to be demanding and the center of attention.
CN: Psychosocial integrity; CNS: None; CL: Analysis

50. Which defense mechanism is most likely to be seen in a client with borderline personality disorder?
1. Compensation
2. Displacement
3. Identification
4. Projection

50. 4. Clients with borderline personality disorder tend to blame and project their feelings and inadequacies onto others. They don't model themselves after other people or tend to use compensation to handle distress. Clients with borderline personality disorder are impulsive and tend to react immediately. It's unlikely they would displace their feelings onto others.
CN: Psychosocial integrity; CNS: None; CL: Analysis

51. What would be an important guideline for nurses working with clients with borderline personality disorder?
1. When behavioral problems emerge, calmly review the therapeutic goals and boundaries of treatment.
2. Try to prevent or reduce untoward effects of manipulation.
3. Remain neutral and avoid engaging in power struggles.
4. Respect a client's need for social isolation.

51. 1. Reminding the borderline client of the goals and boundaries of treatment helps the client to focus on therapy. Manipulation is an issue with antisocial personality clients. Power struggles are an issue for the narcissistic client and respecting the client's need for social isolation describes a client with schizotypal personality disorder.
CN: Safe, effective care environment; CNS: Safety & infection control; CL: Application

52. Which nursing intervention has <u>priority</u> for a client with borderline personality disorder?
1. Maintain consistent, realistic limits.
2. Give instructions for meeting basic self-care needs.
3. Engage in daytime activities to stimulate wakefulness.
4. Have the client attend group therapy on a daily basis.

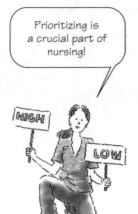

Prioritizing is a crucial part of nursing!

52. 1. Clients with borderline personality disorder who are needy, dependent, and manipulative will benefit greatly from maintaining consistent, realistic limits. They don't tend to have difficulty meeting their self-care needs and don't tend to have sleeping difficulties. They enjoy attending group therapy because they typically attempt to use the opportunity to become the center of attention.
CN: Safe, effective care environment; CNS: Management of care; CL: Application

53. Which outcome indicates individual therapy has been effective for a client with borderline personality disorder?
1. The client accepts that medication isn't a treatment of choice.
2. The client agrees to undergo hypnosis for suppression of memories.
3. The client understands the organic basis for the problematic behavior.
4. The client verbalizes awareness of the consequences for unacceptable behaviors.

53. 4. An indication of effective individual therapy for this client is his expressed awareness of consequences for unacceptable behaviors. Medications can control symptoms. However, monitoring for reckless use or abuse of drugs must be done for the client with borderline personality disorder. Hypnosis isn't a treatment used with a client with borderline personality disorder. There's no organic basis for the development of this disorder.
CN: Psychosocial integrity; CNS: None; CL: Application

54. Which action by a client with borderline personality disorder indicates adequate learning about personal behavior?
1. The client talks about intense anger.
2. The client smiles while making demands.
3. The client decides never to engage in conflict.
4. The client stops the family from controlling finances.

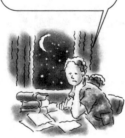

I know all about adequate learning.

54. 1. Learning has occurred when anger is discussed rather than acted out in unhealthy ways. The behavior to change would be the demands placed on others. Smiling while making these demands shows manipulative behavior. Not engaging in conflict is unrealistic. It's important to help this client slowly develop financial responsibility rather than just stopping the family from monitoring the client's overspending.
CN: Psychosocial integrity; CNS: None; CL: Application

55. A nurse is planning care for a client with borderline personality disorder who has been agitated. Which instruction is included for the client and family?
1. Encourage the rebuilding of family relationships.
2. Help the client handle anxiety before it escalates.
3. Have the client participate in a weekly support group.
4. Discuss the client's bad habits that need to be changed.

55. 2. The client needs help handling anxiety because escalating anxiety can trigger self-destructive behaviors in clients with borderline personality disorder. When a client with borderline personality disorder is agitated, it's difficult to communicate, let alone rebuild family relationships. Participation in a weekly support group won't be enough to help the client handle agitation. When a client is agitated, it isn't appropriate to discuss bad habits that need to be changed. This action may further agitate the client.
CN: Psychosocial integrity; CNS: None; CL: Application

CN: Client needs category   CNS: Client needs subcategory   CL: Cognitive level

56. A client with a borderline personality disorder isn't making progress on the identified goals. Which client factor should be <u>reevaluated?</u>
1. Memory
2. Motivation
3. Orientation
4. Perception

57. The nurse is performing an assessment on a client with dependent personality disorder. Which of the following characteristics would the nurse <u>most likely</u> assess in this client?
1. Abrasive to others
2. Indifferent to others
3. Manipulative of others
4. Overreliant on others

58. A client with dependent personality disorder is working on goals for self-care. Which short-term goal is <u>most important</u> to the client's activities of daily living?
1. Do all self-care activities independently.
2. Write a daily schedule for each day of the week.
3. Do self-care activities in a minimal amount of time.
4. Determine activities that can be performed without help.

59. A nurse is teaching the family of a client diagnosed with dependent personality disorder. Which information would be most appropriate for the nurse to include?
1. Stress-reduction techniques
2. Panic attack prevention
3. Exercise program development
4. Aggressive outburst reduction

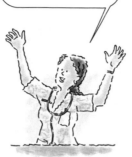
You've finished 56 questions. That should motivate you to keep going.

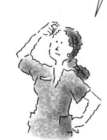
It's most important that I answer this question correctly.

56. 2. Clients with borderline personality disorders tend to be poorly motivated for treatment. They don't tend to have perception problems such as hallucinations or illusions, problems in orientation, or memory problems.
CN: Psychosocial integrity; CNS: None; CL: Analysis

57. 4. Clients with dependent personality disorder are extremely overreliant on other people; they aren't abrasive, assertive, or indifferent. They're clinging and demanding of others; they don't manipulate. People with dependent personality disorder rely on others and want to be taken care of.
CN: Psychosocial integrity; CNS: None; CL: Application

58. 4. By determining activities that can be performed without assistance, the client can then begin to practice them independently. If the nurse only encourages a client to perform self-care activities independently, nothing may change. Writing a daily schedule doesn't help the client focus on what needs to be done to promote self-care. The amount of time needed to perform self-care activities isn't important. If time pressure is put on the client, there may be more reluctance to perform self-care activities.
CN: Psychosocial integrity; CNS: None; CL: Application

59. 1. The family needs information about coping skills to help the client learn to handle stress. Clients with dependent personality disorder don't tend to have panic attacks or aggressive outbursts; they tend to be passive and submit to others. Exercise is a health promotion activity for all clients. Clients with dependent personality disorder wouldn't need exercise promoted more than other people.
CN: Safe, effective care environment; CNS: Management of care; CL: Application

60. Which strategy is appropriate for a client with dependent personality disorder?
1. Orient the client to current surroundings.
2. Reassure the client about personal safety.
3. Ask questions to help the client recall problems.
4. Differentiate between positive and negative feedback.

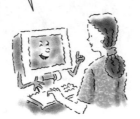

Think carefully. You know the answer to this one.

60. 4. Clients with dependent personality disorder tend to view all feedback as criticism; they frequently misinterpret another's remarks. Clients with dependent personality disorder don't need orientation to their surroundings. Personal safety isn't an issue because a person with dependent personality disorder typically isn't self-destructive. Memory problems aren't associated with this disorder, so asking questions to stimulate the client's memory isn't necessary.
CN: Psychosocial integrity; CNS: None; CL: Application

61. A client with dependent personality disorder is crying after a family meeting. Which statement by a family member is most likely the cause of upset to this client?
1. "You take advantage of people, especially the people in our family."
2. "You act like you love me one minute but hate me the next minute."
3. "You feel like you deserve everything, whether you work for it or not."
4. "You always agree to everything, but deep down inside you feel differently."

61. 4. The client was confronted by a family member about behavior that doesn't represent the client's true feelings. Clients are afraid they won't be taken care of if they disagree. Clients with a dependent personality disorder don't have a sense of entitlement and don't take advantage of other people, but they subordinate their needs to others. They don't show the defense mechanism of splitting, where a person is valued and then devalued.
CN: Psychosocial integrity; CNS: None; CL: Analysis

62. A client with dependent personality disorder is having trouble performing activities of daily living. Which nursing intervention should help facilitate the client's daily activities?
1. Have the client eat three meals a day.
2. Work with the client to establish a budget.
3. Make a chart to document hygiene practices.
4. Discuss how the client can obtain a driver's license.

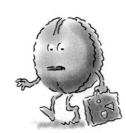

It takes me a while, but I'll get the job done.

62. 2. Clients with dependent personality disorder tend to withdraw from adult responsibilities. Managing money through the use of a budget is a first step toward assuming adult responsibilities. These clients don't tend to have problems with nutritional intake. Hygiene issues usually aren't a problem for clients with dependent personality disorder. Clients with a dependent personality disorder don't have any special reasons for not obtaining a driver's license.
CN: Psychosocial integrity; CNS: None; CL: Application

63. A client with a dependent personality disorder is taking fluoxetine (Prozac) for depression. Which instruction is included in client teaching?
1. Drink only wine and beer when taking this drug.
2. Add as-needed doses if depression becomes worse.
3. Expect 3 to 4 weeks to go by before effects are seen.
4. Be aware that alterations in usual sleep patterns, especially nightmares, may occur.

63. 3. The client must take the drug for 3 to 4 weeks before therapeutic effects are seen. The nurse must caution the client against the use of alcohol, including wine and beer, when taking fluoxetine. The client is to take the drug as prescribed. Additional doses must not be self-administered. Fluoxetine treats disruptions in sleep and doesn't cause nightmares.
CN: Physiological integrity; CNS: Pharmacological and parenteral therapies; CL: Application

CN: Client needs category   CNS: Client needs subcategory   CL: Cognitive level

64. Which behavior by a client with dependent personality disorder shows the client has made progress toward the goal of increasing problem-solving skills?
　　1. The client is courteous.
　　2. The client asks questions.
　　3. The client stops acting out.
　　4. The client controls emotions.

65. In planning care for a client with borderline personality disorder, the nurse must account for which behavioral trait?
　　1. An inability to make decisions independently
　　2. A propensity to act out when feeling afraid, alone, or devalued
　　3. A belief the client deserves special privileges not accorded to others
　　4. A display of inappropriately seductive appearance and behavior

66. Which <u>short-term</u> goal is appropriate for a client with dependent personality disorder experiencing excessive dependency needs?
　　1. Verbalize self-confidence in own abilities.
　　2. Decide relationships don't take energy to sustain.
　　3. Discuss feelings related to frequent mood swings.
　　4. Stop obsessive thinking that impedes daily social functioning.

67. A client with dependent personality disorder is thinking about getting a part-time job. Which nursing intervention will help this client when employment is obtained?
　　1. Help the client develop strategies to control impulses.
　　2. Explain that there are consequences for inappropriate behaviors.
　　3. Have the client work to sustain healthy interpersonal relationships.
　　4. Help the client decrease the use of regression as a defense mechanism.

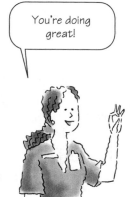

You're doing great!

64. 2. The client with dependent personality disorder is passive and tries to please others. By asking questions, the client is beginning to gather information, the first step of decision making. These clients don't tend to have emotional outbursts or to be impolite. They avoid expressing their feelings or acting out for fear of displeasing others.
CN: Psychosocial integrity; CNS: None; CL: Analysis

65. 2. Clients with borderline personality disorder have an intense fear of abandonment. These clients are able to make decisions independently. Feeling deserving of special privileges is characteristic of a person with narcissistic personality disorder. Inappropriate seductive appearance and behavior is characteristic of someone with histrionic personality disorder.
CN: Psychosocial integrity; CNS: None; CL: Application

66. 1. Individuals with dependent personalities believe they must depend on others to be competent for them. They need to gain more self-confidence in their own abilities. The client must realize that relationships take energy to develop and sustain. Clients with dependent personality disorder usually don't have obsessive thinking or mood swings to interfere with their socialization.
CN: Psychosocial integrity; CNS: None; CL: Application

67. 3. Sustaining healthy relationships will help the client be comfortable with peers in the job setting. Clients with dependent personality disorder don't usually use regression as a defense mechanism. It's common to see denial and introjection used. They don't usually have trouble with impulse control or offensive behavior that would lead to negative consequences.
CN: Psychosocial integrity; CNS: None; CL: Analysis

68. A client with dependent personality disorder has difficulty expressing personal concerns. Which communication technique is <u>best</u> to teach the client?
1. Questioning
2. Reflection
3. Silence
4. Touch

69. A nurse is evaluating the effectiveness of an assertiveness group that a client with dependent personality disorder attended. Which client statement indicates the group had therapeutic value?
1. "I can't seem to do the things other people do."
2. "I wish I could be more organized like other people."
3. "I want to talk about something that's bothering me."
4. "I just don't want people in my family to fight any more."

70. After a family visit, a client with dependent personality disorder becomes anxious. Which situation is a possible cause of the anxiety?
1. Sensitivity to criticism
2. Discussion of family rules
3. Being asked personal questions
4. Identification of eccentric behavior

71. A client with dependent personality disorder has a history of minor GI problems. Which goal has <u>priority</u>?
1. Get a referral to a specialist.
2. Consult with a dietitian regularly.
3. Arrange for a family support meeting.
4. Examine the client's present level of coping skills.

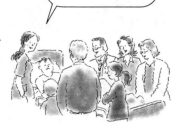

There are so many ways to communicate. How do I know which is the best?

A family visit can be upsetting to the client.

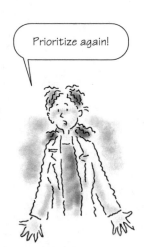

Prioritize again!

68. 1. Questioning is a way to learn to identify feelings and express self. The use of reflection isn't a communication technique that will help the client express personal feelings and concerns. Using silence won't help the client identify and discuss personal concerns. The use of touch to express feelings and personal concerns must be used very judiciously.

CN: Psychosocial integrity; CNS: None; CL: Application

69. 3. By asking to talk about a bothersome situation, the client has taken the first step toward assertive behavior. To smooth over or minimize troubling events isn't an assertive position. The first option reflects a lack of self-confidence; it's not an assertive statement. Statements that express the client's wishes aren't assertive statements.

CN: Psychosocial integrity; CNS: None; CL: Analysis

70. 1. Clients with dependent personality disorder are extremely sensitive to criticism and can become very anxious when they feel interpersonal conflict or tension. When they have discussions about family rules, they try to become submissive and please others rather than become anxious. When they're asked personal questions, they don't necessarily become anxious. Clients with dependent personality disorder don't tend to show eccentric behavior that causes them anxiety.

CN: Psychosocial integrity; CNS: None; CL: Application

71. 4. Many clients with GI discomfort tend to be anxious and need help developing coping skills. Before a referral is obtained, other factors that could cause GI upset must be addressed. A client with dependent personality disorder usually is overdependent on family members and doesn't tend to need a nurse to advocate for client support. Consulting with a dietitian wouldn't be a priority goal. A consultation would be initiated only after other variables were assessed and a need was identified.

CN: Safe, effective care environment; CNS: Management of care; CL: Application

CN: Client needs category   CNS: Client needs subcategory   CL: Cognitive level

72. Which emotional health problem may potentially coexist in a client with dependent personality disorder?
1. Psychotic disorder
2. Anxiety disorder
3. Alcohol-related disorder
4. Posttraumatic stress disorder

73. A nurse notices that a client with dependent personality disorder is depressed. Which factor is assessed as contributing to depression?
1. Unmet needs
2. Sense of smothering
3. Messy, unkempt appearance
4. Difficulty delaying gratification

74. A client with dependent personality disorder makes the following statement, "I'll never be able to take care of myself." Which response is best?
1. "How can you say that? You can function."
2. "Let's talk about what's making you feel so fearful."
3. "I think we need to work on identifying your strengths."
4. "Can we talk about this tomorrow at the family meeting?"

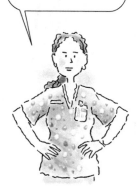

Keep in mind the type of personality this client has.

75. A client on your unit says the Mafia has a contract out on him. He refuses to leave his semiprivate room and insists on frisking his roommate before allowing him to enter. Which action should the nurse take first?
1. Transfer the client to a private room.
2. Acknowledge the client's fear when he refuses to leave his room or wants to frisk his roommate.
3. Transfer the roommate to another room.
4. Lock the client out of his room for a while each day so he can see he's safe.

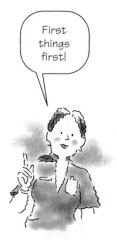

First things first!

72. 2. Because they've placed their own needs in the hands of others, clients with dependent personalities are extremely vulnerable to anxiety disorder. They don't tend to have coexisting problems of posttraumatic stress disorder, psychotic disorder, or alcohol-related disorder.
CN: Psychosocial integrity; CNS: None; CL: Analysis

73. 1. Having many unmet needs is a precursor to depression. Clients with dependent personality disorder don't experience a sense of smothering, a problem seen in clients with panic disorder. Poor hygiene is often a *manifestation, not* a cause, of depression. Clients with problems delaying gratification tend to have anxiety problems, not problems with depression.
CN: Psychosocial integrity; CNS: None; CL: Analysis

74. 2. The client with dependent personality disorder is afraid of abandonment and being unable to care for himself. Talking about his fears is a useful strategy. The first option is inappropriate because the nurse doesn't recognize the client's feelings. When the client makes a desperate statement, the nurse must respond to the client's feelings, rather than insert her opinion. Working on identifying a client's strengths will add to his feelings of not being strong enough to care for himself. Waiting to talk about his concern until the family meeting minimizes its importance.
CN: Psychosocial integrity; CNS: None; CL: Analysis

75. 2. Acknowledging underlying feelings may help defuse the client's anxiety without promoting his delusional thinking. This, in turn, may help the client distinguish between his emotional state and external reality. Transferring either client to another room would validate the client's delusional thinking. Locking the client out of his room may further escalate the client's anxiety and stimulate aggressive acting-out behavior.
CN: Psychosocial integrity; CNS: None; CL: Application

76. A client with schizotypal personality disorder is sitting in a puddle of urine. He's playing in it, smiling, and softly singing a child's song. Which action would be best?
1. Admonish the client for not using the bathroom.
2. Firmly tell the client that her behavior is unacceptable.
3. Ask the client whether she's ready to get cleaned up now.
4. Help the client to the shower, and change the bedclothes.

77. A client with avoidant personality disorder says occupational therapy (OT) is boring and he doesn't want to go. Which action would be best?
1. State firmly that you'll escort him to OT.
2. Arrange with OT for the client to do a project on the unit.
3. Ask the client to talk about why OT is boring.
4. Arrange for the client not to attend OT until he feels better.

78. A client with paranoid personality disorder works toward the goal of increasing social interaction. Which behavior indicates that the client is meeting this goal?
1. The client develops and follows a schedule of group activities.
2. The client verbalizes aggressive feelings to the nurse.
3. The client visits the consumer center to use the Internet.
4. The client explores somatic complaints with the staff.

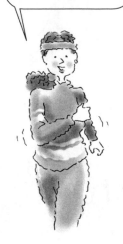

You've passed the 75 mark. Not too much more to go!

Which answer will help the client increase his social interaction?

76. 4. A client with a schizotypal personality disorder can experience high levels of anxiety and regress to childlike behaviors. This client may require help meeting self-care needs. The client may not respond to the other options or those options may generate more anxiety.
CN: Psychosocial integrity; CNS: None; CL: Application

77. 1. If given the chance, a client with avoidant personality disorder typically elects to remain immobilized. The nurse should insist that the client participate in OT. Arranging for the client to do a project on the unit validates and reinforces the client's desire to avoid going to OT. Addressing an invalid issue such as the client's perceived boredom avoids the real issue: the client's need for therapy. There's no indication that the client is incapable of participating in OT.
CN: Psychosocial integrity; CNS: None; CL: Application

78. 1. By developing and following a schedule of group activities, the client increases opportunities to use social skills and increase interactions with others. Verbalizing aggressive feelings doesn't give the client opportunities to increase social interaction. Using a computer at the consumer center is a solitary activity. Talking to the staff about somatic complaints doesn't provide opportunities for social interaction.
CN: Psychosocial integrity; CNS: None; CL: Application

79. A nurse works with the family of a client diagnosed with schizoid personality disorder, helping them to assist him in making decisions. Which outcome indicates the nurse's interventions have been successful?
 1. The family prevents the client from experiencing disappointments.
 2. The family encourages the client to talk about specific issues and concerns.
 3. The family removes alcohol and unnecessary prescription drugs from the house.
 4. The family doesn't let the client obtain secondary gains from illness.

80. A nurse discusses job possibilities with a client with schizoid personality disorder. Which suggestion by the nurse should be helpful?
 1. "You could work in a family restaurant part-time on the weekends and holidays."
 2. "Maybe your friend could get you that customer service job where you work only in the evenings."
 3. "Your idea of applying for the position of filing and organizing records is worth pursuing."
 4. "Being an introvert limits the employment opportunities you can pursue."

81. A client with borderline personality disorder is learning how to verbalize, rather than act on, the desire to hurt himself. Which intervention should the nurse use to help him recognize angry feelings?
 1. Explain how pain triggers intense anger and causes the client to act out.
 2. Determine how problems with the client's family cause her to act aggressively.
 3. Teach the client that being volatile is a normal reaction to unfair events.
 4. Have the client work on identifying speech and behavior that accompany anger.

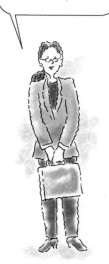

When trying to answer question 80, think about the type of activities this client prefers.

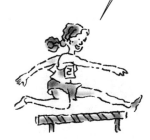

Three more hurdles...I mean questions...to go!

79. 2. A client with schizoid personality disorder typically is vague and has difficulty with self-expression; encouraging the client to talk about specific issues and concerns shows that the nurse's interventions were successful. It's neither realistic nor helpful for the family to protect the client from disappointments. Clients with schizoid personality disorder aren't at high risk for substance abuse and don't seek secondary gains from illness.
CN: Psychosocial integrity; CNS: None; CL: Application

80. 3. Clients with schizoid personality disorder prefer solitary activities, such as filing, to working with others. Working as a cashier or customer service representative would involve interacting with many people. Not all jobs require extensive interpersonal contact.
CN: Psychosocial integrity; CNS: None; CL: Analysis

81. 4. Aggressive speech and inappropriate behaviors indicate that the client is angry or upset; these feelings may trigger acting out. Pain rarely triggers intense anger or makes a client act out. Blaming one's family of origin for inappropriate handling of anger isn't helpful. Being volatile isn't a normal reaction to unfair life events. The client needs to express anger in safe and appropriate ways.
CN: Psychosocial integrity; CNS: None; CL: Analysis

82. A client with borderline personality disorder states that he doesn't know how to deal with his impulsive behavior. Which intervention should the nurse implement?
1. Teach the client that impulsive behavior is part of his illness.
2. Explore how depression influences impulsive situations.
3. Select an example of an impulsive situation and explore it.
4. Decrease interactions in which impulsive behavior occurs.

83. A nurse is monitoring a client who appears to be hallucinating. She notes paranoid content in the client's speech and that he appears agitated. The client is gesturing at a figure on the television. Which nursing interventions are appropriate? Select all that apply:
1. In a firm voice, instruct the client to stop the behavior.
2. Reinforce that the client is not in any danger.
3. Acknowledge the presence of the hallucinations.
4. Instruct other team members to ignore the client's behavior.
5. Immediately implement physical restraint procedures.
6. Use a calm voice and simple commands.

84. When assessing a client diagnosed with impulse control disorder, the nurse observes violent, aggressive, and assaultive behavior. Which assessment data is the nurse also likely to find? Select all that apply:
1. The client functions well in other areas of his life.
2. The degree of aggressiveness is out of proportion to the stressor.
3. The violent behavior is most often justified by the stressor.
4. The client has a history of parental alcoholism and chaotic, abusive family life.
5. The client has no remorse about the inability to control his behavior.

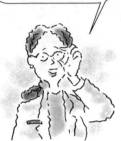

In question 82, focus on the client's impulsive behavior.

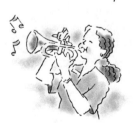

An incredible job! You've finished another big chapter! That's music to my ears!

82. 3. By selecting an impulsive situation to explore with the client, the nurse can help him begin to understand the causes and consequences of his behavior and learn how to modify it. Although impulsive behavior is part of borderline personality disorder, the nurse's intervention needs to address ways to handle it. Anxiety, not depression, is strongly related to impulsive behavior. Decreasing social interactions is unrealistic; it's more useful to address the impulsive behavior.
CN: Psychosocial integrity; CNS: None; CL: Analysis

83. 2, 3, 6. Using a calm voice, the nurse should reassure the client that he's safe. She shouldn't challenge the client; rather, she should acknowledge his hallucinatory experience. It's not appropriate to request that the client stop the behavior. Implementing restraints isn't warranted at this time. Although the client is agitated, no evidence exists that he is at risk for harming himself or others.
CN: Psychosocial integrity; CNS: None; CL: Application

84. 1, 2, 4. A client with an impulse control disorder who displays violent, aggressive, and assaultive behavior generally functions well in other areas of his life. The degree of aggressiveness is typically out of proportion with the stressor. Such a client commonly has a history of parental alcoholism and a chaotic family life, and often verbalizes sincere remorse and guilt for the aggressive behavior.
CN: Psychosocial integrity; CNS: None; CL: Application

CN: Client needs category   CNS: Client needs subcategory   CL: Cognitive level

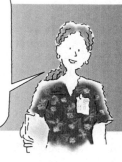

So I'm talking to Queen Elizabeth the other day, and she said you'd do spectacularly well on this chapter. (I'm kidding. What, do I look delusional?) Personally, I think you'll do even better than that. Go for it!

Chapter 18
Schizophrenic & delusional disorders

1. A schizophrenic client tells his primary nurse that he's scheduled to meet the King of Samoa at a special time, making it impossible for the client to leave his room for dinner. Which response by the nurse is <u>most appropriate</u>?
   1. "It's meal time. Let's go so you can eat."
   2. "The King of Samoa told me to take you to dinner."
   3. "Your physician expects you to follow the unit's schedule."
   4. "People who don't eat on this unit aren't being cooperative."

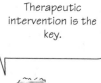

Therapeutic intervention is the key.

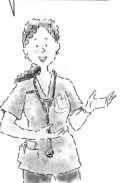

2. During breakfast, a client announces that he is still the President of the United States. What is the <u>best</u> response from the nurse?
   1. "How are you, Mr. President?"
   2. "The real president was on TV last night."
   3. "How is your breakfast?"
   4. "Is this the Oval Office then?"

3. A 40-year-old client with a diagnosis of chronic, undifferentiated schizophrenia lives in a rooming house that has a weekly nursing clinic. He scratches while he tells the nurse he feels creatures eating away at his skin. Which intervention should be done <u>first</u>?
   1. Talk about his hallucinations and fears.
   2. Refer him for anticholinergic adverse reactions.
   3. Assess for possible physical problems such as rash.
   4. Call his physician to get his medication increased to control his psychosis.

1. 1. A delusional client is so wrapped up in his false beliefs that he tends to disregard activities of daily living, such as nutrition and hydration. He needs clear, concise, firm directions from a caring nurse to meet his needs. The second option belittles and tricks the client, possibly evoking mistrust on the part of the client. The third option evades the issue of meeting his basic needs. The last option is demeaning and doesn't address the delusion.
CN: Health promotion and maintenance; CNS: None; CL: Application

2. 3. Asking about breakfast redirects the client and focuses him on a structured activity or reality-based task. The other responses focus attention on or support the client's delusion.
CN: Psychosocial integrity; CNS: None; CL: Application

3. 3. Clients with schizophrenia generally have poor visceral recognition because they live so fully in their fantasy world. They need to have an in-depth assessment of physical complaints that may spill over into their delusional symptoms. Talking with the client won't provide an assessment of his itching, and itching isn't an adverse reaction of antipsychotic drugs. Calling the physician to get the client's medication increased doesn't address his physical complaints.
CN: Safe, effective care environment; CNS: Management of care; CL: Application

CN: Client needs category   CNS: Client needs subcategory   CL: Cognitive level

4. A 22-year-old schizophrenic client was admitted to the psychiatric unit during the night. The next morning, he began to misidentify the nurse and call her by his sister's name. Which intervention is best?
1. Assess the client for potential violence.
2. Take the client to his room, where he'll feel safer.
3. Assume the misidentification makes the client feel more comfortable.
4. Correct the misidentification, and orient the client to the unit and staff.

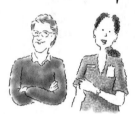

Orienting a new client to the staff and the surroundings can help him feel in control.

4. 4. Misidentification can contribute to anxiety, fear, aggression, and hostility. Orienting a new client to the hospital unit, staff, and other clients, along with establishing a nurse-client relationship, can decrease these feelings and help the client feel in control. Assessing for potential violence is an important nursing function for any psychiatric client, but a perceived supportive environment reduces the risk for violence. Withdrawing to his room, unless interpersonal relationships have become nontherapeutic for him, encourages the client to remain in his fantasy world.
CN: Psychosocial integrity; CNS: None; CL: Application

5. Which term describes an effect of isolation?
1. Delusions
2. Hallucinations
3. Lack of volition
4. Waxy flexibility

5. 2. Prolonged isolation can produce sensory deprivation, manifested by hallucinations. A delusion is a false, fixed belief that has no basis in reality. Lack of volition is a symptom associated with type I negative symptoms of schizophrenia. Waxy flexibility is a motor disturbance that's a predominant feature of catatonic schizophrenia.
CN: Psychosocial integrity; CNS: None; CL: Application

6. A client diagnosed with schizophrenia several years ago tells a nurse that he feels "very sad." The nurse observes that he's smiling when he says it. Which term best describes the nurse's observation?
1. Inappropriate affect
2. Extrapyramidal
3. Insight
4. Inappropriate mood

6. 1. Affect refers to behaviors such as facial expression that can be observed when a person is expressing and experiencing feelings. If the client's affect doesn't reflect the emotional content of the statement, the affect is considered inappropriate. Extrapyramidal symptoms are adverse effects of some categories of medication. Insight is a component of the mental status examination and is the ability to perceive oneself realistically and understand if a problem exists. Mood is an extensive and sustained feeling tone.
CN: Psychosocial integrity; CNS: None; CL: Application

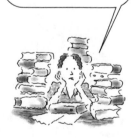

The word disorganized refers to a type of schizophrenia, and to me!

7. A disorganized schizophrenic's symptoms include the distressing triad of extreme social withdrawal, odd mannerisms, and other regressive behaviors. The nurse's most therapeutic intervention is which of the following?
1. Require the client to attend one group activity each day.
2. Suggest that the client keeps up with his same gender peer group.
3. Interact with the client often and briefly, in a friendly manner.
4. Allow the client to come out when he is ready.

7. 3. Interacting with the client often and in a friendly manner suggests planned, short, frequent, and undemanding interactions. Clients with disorganized schizophrenia require one-on-one non-threatening activities and should not remain in social isolation.
CN: Psychosocial integrity; CNS: None; CL: Application

CN: Client needs category   CNS: Client needs subcategory   CL: Cognitive level

8. A client on the psychiatric unit is copying and imitating the movements of his primary nurse. During recovery, he says, "I thought the nurse was my mirror. I felt connected only when I saw my nurse." This behavior is known by which term?
   1. Modeling
   2. Echopraxia
   3. Ego-syntonicity
   4. Ritualism

9. The teenage son of a father with schizophrenia is worried that he might have schizophrenia as well. Which behavior would be an indication that he should be evaluated for signs of the disorder?
   1. Moodiness
   2. Preoccupation with his body
   3. Spending more time away from home
   4. Changes in sleep patterns

10. The nurse is teaching the family of a client with a psychiatric disorder about <u>traditional</u> antipsychotic drugs and their effect on symptoms. Which of the following symptoms would be most responsive to these types of drugs?
   1. Apathy
   2. Delusions
   3. Social withdrawal
   4. Attention impairment

Pay attention to the key word in questions 10 and 11.

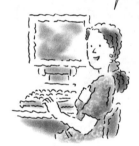

11. A client was hospitalized after his son filed a petition for involuntary hospitalization for safety reasons. The son seeks out the nurse because his father is angry and refuses to talk with him. He's frustrated and feeling very guilty about his decision. Which response to this client is the most <u>empathic</u>?
   1. "Your father is here because he needs help."
   2. "He'll feel differently about you as he gets better."
   3. "It sounds like you're feeling guilty about leaving your father here."
   4. "This is a stressful time for you, but you'll feel better as he gets well."

8. 2. Echopraxia is the copying of another's behaviors and is the result of the loss of ego boundaries. Modeling is the conscious copying of someone's behaviors. Ego-syntonicity refers to behaviors that correspond with the individual's sense of self. Ritualistic behaviors are repetitive and compulsive.
CN: Psychosocial integrity; CNS: None; CL: Application

9. 4. In conjunction with other signs, changes in sleep patterns are distinctive initial signs of schizophrenia. Other signs include changes in personal care habits and social isolation. Moodiness, preoccupation with the body, and spending more time away from home are normal adolescent behaviors.
CN: Health promotion and maintenance; CNS: None; CL: Application

10. 2. Positive symptoms, such as delusions, hallucinations, thought disorder, and disorganized speech, respond to traditional antipsychotic drugs. The other options are part of the category of negative symptoms, including affective flattening, restricted thought and speech, apathy, anhedonia, asociality, and attention impairment, and are more responsive to the new atypical antipsychotics, such as clozapine (Clozaril), risperidone (Risperdal), and olanzapine (Zyprexa).
CN: Physiological integrity CNS: Pharmacological and parenteral therapies; CL: Application

11. 3. This response focuses on the son and helps him discuss and deal with his feelings. Unresolved feelings of guilt, shame, isolation, and loss of hope impact on the family's ability to manage the crisis and be supportive to the client. The other options offer premature reassurance and cut off the opportunity for the son to discuss his feelings.
CN: Psychosocial integrity; CNS: None; CL: Application

12. A client followed her antipsychotic medication regimen for a number of years. Her physician treats her urinary tract infection with antibiotic therapy. Which action is a nursing responsibility?
1. Arrange for possible hospitalization.
2. Have a visiting nurse give the medication.
3. Give instructions on the medication, possible adverse effects, and a return demonstration for teaching effectiveness.
4. Develop a psychoeducational program to address the client's emotional and physical problems arising from physiologic problems.

13. Which sign indicates tardive dyskinesia?
1. Involuntary movements
2. Blurred vision
3. Restlessness
4. Sudden fever

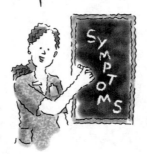

Signs and symptoms are big on NCLEX examinations. Better know them cold.

14. A client approaches a nurse and tells her that he hears voices telling him that he's evil and deserves to die. Which response by the nurse is most appropriate?
1. "The voices aren't real, so ignore them."
2. "I don't see anyone in the room."
3. "I don't hear any voices, but I understand that you do."
4. "Tell the voices you won't listen to them."

15. A 49-year-old client is admitted to the emergency department frightened and reporting that he's hearing voices telling him to do bad things. Which intervention should be the nurse's <u>priority</u>?
1. Tell the client he's safe and that the voices aren't real.
2. Tell the client he's safe now and promise the staff will protect him.
3. Assess the nature of the commands by asking the client what the voices are saying.
4. Administer a neuroleptic medication.

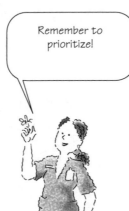

Remember to prioritize!

12. 3. The client has been successful and reliable in carrying out her current medication regimen. The nurse should assume the competency includes self-administration of antibiotics if the instructions are understood. No evidence exists that the client is having a relapse as a result of the infection, so she wouldn't need a psychoeducational program or hospitalization. Having a community nurse give the medication encourages dependency as opposed to self-care.
CN: Safe, effective care environment; CNS: Management of care; CL: Application

13. 1. Symptoms of tardive dyskinesia include tongue protrusion, lip smacking, chewing, blinking, grimacing, choreiform movements of limbs and trunk, and foot tapping. Blurred vision is a common adverse reaction of antipsychotic drugs and usually disappears after a few weeks of therapy. Restlessness is associated with akathisia. Sudden fever is a symptom of a malignant neurologic disorder.
CN: Physiological integrity; CNS: Reduction of risk potential; CL: Application

14. 3. The nurse should let the client know that although she can't hear the voices, she understands that they are real to him. She should keep communication open and encourage him to talk. Telling the client that the voices aren't real may make him hold tighter to his belief and doesn't promote trust. Telling him to talk back to the voices validates their reality.
CN: Psychosocial integrity; CNS: None; CL: Application

15. 3. Safety is the priority. The nurse should directly ask the client about the nature of the auditory commands to adequately assess the safety of the client and staff. The nurse should never make promises to the client that she may not be able to fulfill. The physician may order a neuroleptic, but the nurse's priority is to address safety.
CN: Safe, effective care environment; CNS: Management of care; CL: Application

16. Which pair of numbers of members in a therapy group is ideal?
1. 1 to 4
2. 4 to 7
3. 7 to 10
4. 10 to 15

16. 3. The ideal number of members in an in-patient group is 7 to 10. Having fewer than 7 members provides inadequate interaction and material for successful group process. Having more than 10 members doesn't allow for adequate time for individual participation.
CN: Psychosocial integrity; CNS: None; CL: Application

17. A client admitted to an inpatient unit approaches a nursing student saying he descended from a long line of people of a "superrace." Which action is correct?
1. Smile and walk into the nurse's station.
2. Challenge the client's false belief.
3. Listen for hidden messages in themes of delusion, indicating unmet needs.
4. Introduce yourself, shake hands, and sit down with the client in the day room.

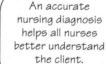

Teach nursing students the importance of genuine interest and concern for client's needs.

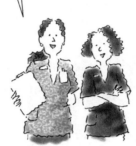

17. 4. The first goal is to establish a relationship with the client, which includes creating psychological space for the creation of trust. The student should sit and make herself available, reflecting concern and interest. Walking into the nurse's station would indicate disinterest and lack of concern about the client's feelings. After establishing a relationship and lessening the client's anxiety, the student can orient the client to reality, listen to his concerns and fears, and try to understand the feelings reflected in the delusions. Delusions are firmly maintained false beliefs, and attempts to dismiss them don't work.
CN: Safe, effective care environment; CNS: Management of care; CL: Application

18. Which nursing diagnosis is most appropriate for a client with acute schizophrenic reaction?
1. *Social isolation related to impaired ability to trust*
2. *Impaired physical mobility related to fear of hostile impulses*
3. *Disturbed sleep patterns related to impaired thinking ability*
4. *Risk for other-directed violence related to perceptual distortions*

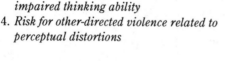

An accurate nursing diagnosis helps all nurses better understand the client.

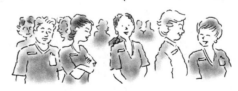

18. 1. Clients with schizophrenia are mistrustful, which results in withdrawal and social isolation. Mobility isn't a common problem for persons with schizophrenia. Sleep disturbance may be present but isn't the most common symptom. Contrary to popular belief, persons with schizophrenia usually aren't violent.
CN: Safe, effective care environment; CNS: Management of care; CL: Analysis

19. A nurse is assisting with morning care when a client suddenly throws off the covers and starts shouting, "My body is changing and disintegrating because I'm not of this world." Which term best describes this behavior?
1. Depersonalization
2. Ideas of reference
3. Looseness of association
4. Paranoid ideation

19. 1. Depersonalization is a state in which the client feels unreal or believes parts of the body are being distorted. Ideas of reference are beliefs unrelated to situations and hold special meaning for the individual. The term loose associations refers to sentences that have vague connections to each other. Paranoid ideations are beliefs that others intend to harm the client in some way.
CN: Psychosocial integrity; CNS: None; CL: Analysis

20. A 16-year-old client with a diagnosis of undifferentiated schizophrenia has become very clingy and begins sucking her thumb while interacting with the nurse. The nurse understands that these behaviors indicate which defense mechanism?
1. Repression
2. Regression
3. Rationalization
4. Projection

21. Which assessment technique is best when interviewing a client with paranoia?
1. Using indirect questions
2. Using direct questions
3. Using lead-in remarks
4. Using open-ended sentences

22. A nurse on a psychiatric unit observes a client in the corner of the room moving his lips as if he were talking to himself. Which action is the <u>most appropriate</u>?
1. Ask him why he's talking to himself.
2. Leave him alone until he stops talking.
3. Tell him it isn't good for him to talk to himself.
4. Invite him to join in a card game with the nurse.

23. A client makes vague statements with no logical connections. He asks whether the nurse understands. Which response is best?
1. "Why don't we wait until later to talk about it?"
2. "You're not making sense, so I won't talk about this topic."
3. "Yes, I understand the overall sense of the logical connections from the idea."
4. "I want to understand what you're saying, but I'm having difficulty following you."

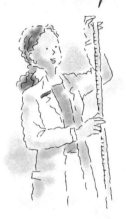

Any way you measure it, you're doing great.

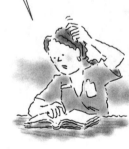

I'm trying to understand but sometimes it's difficult.

20. 2. Regression, a return to earlier behavior in order to reduce anxiety, is the basic defense mechanism in schizophrenia. Repression is the blocking of unacceptable thoughts or impulses from the consciousness. Rationalization is a defense mechanism used to justify one's behavior. Projection is a defense mechanism in which one blames others and attempts to justify actions.
CN: Psychosocial integrity; CNS: None; CL: Application

21. 2. Direct questioning is the most appropriate technique to use when interviewing a client with paranoid schizophrenia. Specific questions, such as "Are you hearing voices right now?" provide the nurse useful information. The other forms of communication may be misunderstood by the client and his responses may be vague.
CN: Psychosocial integrity; CNS: None; CL: Application

22. 4. Being with the nurse provides stimulation that competes with the hallucinations. The client doesn't think he's talking to himself, he's responding only to the voices he hears. Being alone keeps the client in his fantasy world. Telling the client that he shouldn't talk to himself fails to understand how real his fantasy world and hallucinations are.
CN: Psychosocial integrity; CNS: None; CL: Application

23. 4. The nurse needs to communicate that she wants to understand without blaming the client for the lack of understanding. Asking the client to wait because he's too confused cuts off an attempt to communicate and asks the client to do what he can't at present. Telling the client that he isn't making sense is judgmental and could impair the therapeutic relationship. Pretending to understand is a violation of trust and can damage the therapeutic relationship.
CN: Psychosocial integrity; CNS: None; CL: Application

CN: Client needs category   CNS: Client needs subcategory   CL: Cognitive level

24. A client asks a nurse if she hears the voice of the nonexistent man speaking to him. Which response is best?
1. "No one is in your room except you."
2. "Yes, I hear him, but I won't listen to him."
3. "What has he told you? Is it helpful advice?"
4. "No, I don't hear him, but I know you do. What is he saying?"

25. Which instruction is correct for a client taking chlorpromazine?
1. Reduce the dosage if you feel better.
2. Occasional social drinking isn't harmful.
3. Stop taking the drug immediately if adverse reactions develop.
4. Schedule routine medication checks.

26. A 34-year-old male client is referred to a mental health clinic by the court. The client harassed a couple next-door to him with charges that the wife was in love with him. He wrote love notes and called her on the telephone throughout the night. The client is employed and has had no problems in his job. Which disorder is suspected?
1. Major depression
2. Paranoid schizophrenia
3. Delusional disorder
4. Bipolar affective disorder

27. A homebound client taking clozapine (Clozaril) tells the nurse he has been feeling tired for 5 days. His temperature is 99.6° F; pulse, 110 beats/minute; and respirations, 20 breaths/minute. Which instruction is correct?
1. Take the medication with milk.
2. Stop the medication at once, and see the physician immediately.
3. Understand that the symptoms will disappear as soon as he gets more rest.
4. Stop the medication gradually, and see the physician next week.

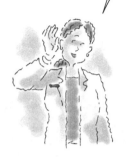

Do you hear what I hear?

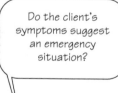

Do the client's symptoms suggest an emergency situation?

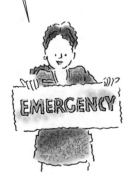

24. 4. This response points out reality and shows concern and support. Attempting to argue the client out of the belief might entrench him more firmly in his belief, making him feel more out of control because of the negative and fearful nature of hallucinations. The other two options violate the trust of the therapeutic relationship.
CN: Safe, effective care environment; CNS: Management of care; CL: Application

25. 4. Ongoing assessment by a primary health care provider is important to assess for adverse reactions and continued therapeutic effectiveness. The dosage should be changed only after checking with the primary care provider. Alcoholic beverages are contraindicated while taking an antipsychotic drug. Adverse reactions should be reported immediately to determine if the drug should be discontinued.
CN: Physiological integrity; CNS: Pharmacological and parenteral therapies; CL: Application

26. 3. The client has a delusional disorder with erotomanic delusions as his primary symptom and believes he's loved intensely by a married person showing no interest in him. No symptoms of major depression exist. The client doesn't believe someone is trying to harm him, the hallmark characteristic of paranoia. Bipolar affective disorder is characterized by cycles of extreme emotional highs (mania) and lows (depression).
CN: Psychosocial integrity; CNS: None; CL: Application

27. 2. He should stop the medication and see his physician immediately because fever can be a sign of agranulocytosis, which is a medical emergency. Taking antipsychotic medication with milk, nicotine, and caffeine will decrease the effectiveness. Rest will have no effect on this client's symptoms. Drowsiness and fatigue usually disappear with continued therapy.
CN: Physiological integrity; CNS: Pharmacological and parenteral therapies; CL: Application

28. A client who is delusional approaches the nurse and states, "You are my aunt and you live with my family." Which statement by the nurse would be the most therapeutic?
1. "I'm not your aunt."
2. "I don't live here."
3. "I'm honored."
4. "This is my name. What is your aunt's name?"

28. 4. By the nurse stating her name and asking the name of the client's aunt, the nurse acknowledges the client is speaking of family, while basing it in a realistic interaction. The other responses all focus on and respond directly to the client's fixed delusional system.
CN: Psychosocial integrity; CNS: None; CL: Application

29. A client tells the nurse that he can only drink bottled water since the water from his sink has been poisoned. The nurse understands that the client is exhibiting which behavior?
1. Paranoia
2. Auditory hallucinations
3. Delusions of grandeur
4. Perseveration

29. 1. This client is exhibiting extreme suspiciousness and distrust of others. Auditory hallucinations occur when a client hears voices that are often threatening or violent. Delusions of grandeur are an exaggerated sense of self-importance. A client with perseveration involuntarily repeats words.
CN: Psychosocial integrity; CNS: None; CL: Application

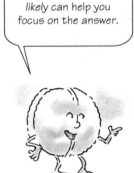

The words most likely can help you focus on the answer.

30. A client with a diagnosis of paranoid-type schizophrenia is receiving an antipsychotic medication. His physician has just prescribed benztropine (Cogentin). The nurse realizes that this medication was <u>most likely</u> prescribed in response to which possible adverse reaction?
1. Tardive dyskinesia
2. Hypertensive crisis
3. Acute dystonia
4. Orthostatic hypotension

30. 3. Benztropine is used as adjunctive therapy in parkinsonism and for all conditions and medications that produce extrapyramidal symptoms except tardive dyskinesia. Its anticholinergic effect reduces the extrapyramidal effects associated with antipsychotic drugs. Hypertensive crisis and orthostatic hypotension aren't associated with extrapyramidal symptoms.
CN: Psychosocial integrity; CNS: Pharmacological and parenteral therapies; CL: Analysis

31. Which action by a nurse is an appropriate therapeutic intervention for a client experiencing hallucinations?
1. Confine him in his room until he feels better.
2. Provide a competing stimulus that distracts from the hallucinations.
3. Discourage attempts to understand what precipitates his hallucinations.
4. Support perceptual distortions until he gives them up of his own accord.

31. 2. Providing competing stimuli acknowledges the presence of the hallucination and teaches ways to decrease the frequency of hallucinations. The other options support and maintain hallucinations or deny their existence.
CN: Psychosocial integrity; CNS: None; CL: Application

32. A client with schizophrenia reports that her hallucinations have decreased in frequency. Which intervention would be appropriate to begin addressing the client's problem with social isolation?
1. Have the client join in a group game.
2. Name the client as the leader of the client support group.
3. Have the client play solitaire.
4. Ask the client to participate in a group sing-along.

33. A single 24-year-old client is admitted with acute schizophrenic reaction. Which method is appropriate therapy for this type of schizophrenia?
1. Counseling to produce insight into behavior
2. Biofeedback to reduce agitation associated with schizophrenia
3. Drug therapy to reduce symptoms associated with acute schizophrenia
4. Electroconvulsive therapy to treat the mood component of schizophrenia

34. A client tells a nurse voices are telling him to do "terrible things." Which action is part of the initial therapy?
1. Find out what the voices are telling him.
2. Let him go to his room to decrease his anxiety.
3. Begin talking to the client about an unrelated topic.
4. Tell the client the voices aren't real.

35. A client is preoccupied with his belief that the CIA has been planning to take him away to save the agency from his influence. These delusions are a defense against which underlying feeling?
1. Aggression
2. Guilt
3. Inferiority
4. Persecution

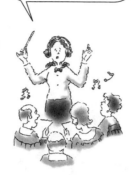

Music can be very therapeutic.

32. 4. Having the client participate in a non-competitive group activity that doesn't require individual participation won't present a threat to the client. Games can become competitive and lead to anxiety or hostility. The client probably lacks sufficient social skills to lead a group at this time. Playing solitaire doesn't encourage socialization.

CN: Psychosocial integrity; CNS: None; CL: Application

33. 3. Drug therapy is usually successful in normalizing behavior and reducing or eliminating hallucinations, delusions, thought disorder, affect flattening, apathy, and asociality. Counseling isn't appropriate at this time. Electroconvulsive therapy might be considered for schizoaffective disorder, which has a mood component, and is a treatment of choice for clinical depression. Biofeedback reduces anxiety and modifies behavioral responses but isn't the major component in the treatment of schizophrenia.

CN: Psychosocial integrity; CNS: None; CL: Application

34. 1. For safety purposes, the nurse must find out whether the voices are directing the client to harm himself or others. Further assessment can help identify appropriate therapeutic interventions. Isolating a person during this intense sensory confusion often reinforces the psychosis. Changing the topic indicates that the nurse isn't concerned about the client's fears. Dismissing the voices shuts down communication between the client and the nurse.

CN: Psychosocial integrity; CNS: None; CL: Application

35. 3. The delusional system contains grandiose ideation that allows the client to feel important rather than inferior. Feelings of aggression will appear as violent or hostile thoughts. Guilt results in beliefs that the person deserves to be punished. Persecution is the fear that others are trying to harm you.

CN: Psychosocial integrity; CNS: None; CL: Application

36. A client has started taking haloperidol (Haldol). Which instruction is <u>most appropriate</u> for a client taking haloperidol?
  1. You should report feelings of restlessness or agitation at once.
  2. Use a sunscreen outdoors on a year-round basis.
  3. Be aware you'll feel increased energy taking this drug.
  4. This drug will indirectly control essential hypertension.

37. A 45-year-old client experiencing delusions has been admitted to the crisis center. When assessing the content of the delusions, the nurse should look for which aspect of the delusions?
  1. Logic
  2. Religious beliefs
  3. Themes
  4. True experiences

38. The nurse is caring for a 58-year-old male client diagnosed with paranoid schizophrenia. When the client says, "The earth and the roof of the house rule the political structure with particles of rain," the nurse recognizes this as which type of expression?
  1. Tangentiality
  2. Perseveration
  3. Loose association
  4. Thought blocking

39. Which symptom indicates that schizophrenia is a thought disorder?
  1. Faulty logic
  2. Distorted but organized thinking
  3. Organized but disruptive thoughts
  4. Appropriate perception, but difficulty responding appropriately to people and events

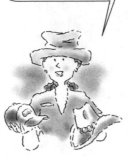

Which hat do you think is *most appropriate*?

36. 1. Agitation and restlessness are adverse effects of haloperidol and can be treated with anticholinergic drugs. Haloperidol isn't likely to cause photosensitivity or control essential hypertension. Although the client may experience increased concentration and activity, these effects are due to a decrease in symptoms, not the drug itself.
CN: Physiological integrity; CNS: Pharmacological and parenteral therapies; CL: Application

37. 3. Understanding the themes inherent in the client's psychotic symptoms may help the nurse learn what stresses trigger the symptoms. A delusion is a false, fixed belief that misrepresents perceptions or experiences and isn't open to rational argument. Assessing for logic, religious beliefs, or true experiences draws the nurse into the delusional thinking and therefore isn't therapeutic.
CN: Psychosocial integrity; CNS: None; CL: Analysis

38. 3. Loose association refers to changing ideas from one unrelated theme to another, as exhibited by the client. Tangentiality is the wandering from topic to topic. Perseveration is involuntary repetition of the answer to a question in response to a new question. Thought blocking is having difficulty articulating a response or stopping midsentence.
CN: Psychosocial integrity; CNS: None; CL: Application

39. 1. Thought disorders are characterized by problems in the form and organization of thinking. They appear as loose associations, word salad, tangentiality, illogicality, circumstantiality, pressure of speech, and poverty of speech that impairs communication. Thinking is disorganized and perceptions are often misinterpreted. The other options are inaccurate characteristics of schizophrenia.
CN: Psychosocial integrity; CNS: None; CL: Analysis

CN: Client needs category CNS: Client needs subcategory CL: Cognitive level

40. A client with schizophrenia tells the nurse that the President consults with him before making major decisions. Which is the best response by the nurse?
  1. "How long have you known the President?"
  2. "You're fortunate to know the President."
  3. "How will you speak with the President from the hospital?"
  4. "You must feel important. Now let's make your bed."

41. A client is admitted after being found on a highway, hitting at cars and yelling at motorists. When approached by the nurse, the client shouts, "You're the one who stole my husband from me!" Which term describes the client's condition?
  1. Hallucinatory experience
  2. Delusional experience
  3. Disorientation to the environment
  4. Phobic experience

42. The nurse is teaching the family of a client with schizophrenia about symptoms of remission. Which of the following responses would be the most accurate?
  1. The disease is in the prodromal phase.
  2. The client no longer has prominent psychotic symptoms.
  3. The client is free from all signs of illness and is no longer on medication.
  4. The client is free from all signs of illness whether or not he's on medication.

43. A client with schizophrenia is huddled on the floor and appears to be interacting with someone underneath the bed. The nurse notes that the client appears afraid. Which assessment by the nurse is most likely correct?
  1. The client is having hallucinations.
  2. The client is having suicidal ideations.
  3. The client is having nightmares.
  4. The client is having delusions.

I'd be remiss if I didn't advise you to read this question carefully.

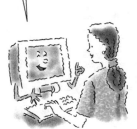

40. 4. Acknowledging that the client feels important addresses the underlying reason for the delusion. The other options reinforce the reality of the delusion.
CN: Psychosocial integrity; CNS: None; CL: Analysis

41. 2. A delusion is a false, fixed belief manufactured without appropriate or sufficient evidence to support it. The client's statements don't represent hallucinations because they aren't perceptual disorders. No information in the question addresses orientation. The client's statements don't represent a phobia because they don't represent an irrational fear.
CN: Psychosocial integrity; CNS: None; CL: Application

42. 2. Schizophrenia is a chronic disorder with periods of remission and exacerbation. The prodromal phase is the precursor to an exacerbation. Clients aren't usually cured but are treated over time with case management, medication, symptom management skills, social skill training, network support, vocational training, and health-promoting practices.
CN: Psychosocial integrity; CNS: None; CL: Application

43. 1. The client appears to be having auditory hallucinations and is hearing voices that he perceives to be coming from under the bed. There is no evidence that the client is having suicidal ideations, nightmares, or delusions.
CN: Psychosocial integrity; CNS: None; CL: Analysis

44. A nurse on an inpatient unit is having a discussion with a client with schizophrenia about his schedule for the day. The client comments that he was highly active at home and then explains the volunteer job he held. Which term describes the client's thinking?
1. Circumstantiality
2. Loose associations
3. Referential
4. Tangentiality

45. While talking to a client with schizophrenia, a nurse notes the client frequently uses unrecognizable words with no common meaning. Which term describes this?
1. Echolalia
2. Clang association
3. Neologisms
4. Word salad

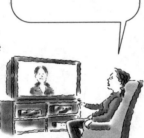

Are you talking to me?

46. While caring for a hospitalized client diagnosed with schizophrenia, a nurse observes the client watching television. The client tells the nurse the television is speaking directly to him. Which term describes this belief?
1. Autistic thinking
2. Concrete thinking
3. Paranoid thinking
4. Referential thinking

47. A nurse is talking with a family of a client diagnosed with schizophrenia. The mother asks, "What causes this disorder?" Which explanation is the <u>most widely accepted</u>?
1. Prenatal or postpartum central nervous system damage
2. Bacterial infections in the mother during pregnancy or delivery
3. A biological predisposition exacerbated by environmental stressors
4. Lack of bonding and attachment during infancy, which leads to depression in later life

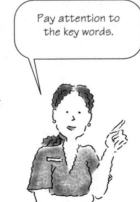

Pay attention to the key words.

44. 4. Tangentiality describes thought patterns loosely connected but not directly related to the topic. In circumstantiality, the person digresses with unnecessary details. Loose associations are rapid shifts in the expression of ideas from one subject to another in an unrelated manner. Referential thinking is when an individual incorrectly interprets neutral incidents and external events as having a particular or special meaning for him.
CN: Psychosocial integrity; CNS: None; CL: Application

45. 3. Neologisms are newly coined words with personal meanings to the client with schizophrenia. Echolalia is parrotlike echoing of spoken words or sounds. Clang association is the linking of words by sound rather than meaning. A word salad is stringing words in sequence that have no connection to one another.
CN: Psychosocial integrity; CNS: None; CL: Application

46. 4. Referential, or primary process thinking, is a belief that incidents and events in the environment have special meaning for the client. Autistic thinking is a disturbance in thought due to the intrusion of a private fantasy world, internally stimulated, resulting in abnormal responses to people. Concrete thinking is the literal interpretation of words and symbols. Paranoid thinking is the belief that others are trying to harm you.
CN: Psychosocial integrity; CNS: None; CL: Application

47. 3. The holistic theory, currently the most widely accepted theory of its type, states that an interaction between biological predisposition and environmental stressors is the cause of schizophrenia. The biological explanation states that schizophrenia is caused by a brain disease, a bacterial infection in utero, or early brain damage. The psychoanalytic perspective involves the belief that the mother-infant bond is the source of the schizophrenia.
CN: Physiological integrity; CNS: Physiological adaptation; CL: Application

48. Which action should a nurse implement when caring for a client who is having a delusion?
1. Ask the client to describe his delusion.
2. Explain to the client that the delusion isn't real.
3. Act as if the delusion is real to reduce the client's anxiety.
4. Engage the client in an organized activity.

49. During the initial interview, a schizophrenic client states to the nurse, "I don't enjoy things anymore. I used to love to read mystery books, but even that isn't enjoyable now." The nurse correctly identifies the client is experiencing which of the following conditions?
1. Avolition
2. Anhedonia
3. Alogia
4. Flat affect

50. In preparation for discharge, a client diagnosed with schizophrenia was taught self-symptom management as part of a relapse prevention program. Which statement indicates the client understands symptom monitoring?
1. "When I hear voices, I become afraid I'll relapse."
2. "My parents aren't involved enough to be aware if I begin to relapse."
3. "My family is more protected from stress if I keep them out of my illness process."
4. "When I'm feeling stressed, I go to a quiet room by myself and do imagery."

51. A client diagnosed with schizophrenia has been taking haloperidol (Haldol) for 1 week when a nurse observes that the client's eyeball is fixated on the ceiling. Which <u>specific</u> condition is the client exhibiting?
1. Akathisia
2. Neuroleptic malignant syndrome
3. Oculogyric crisis
4. Tardive dyskinesia

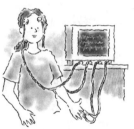

Feedback alerts you to a lack of understanding.

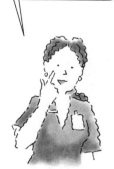

Keep your eye on question 51. It's asking for a specific condition.

48. 4. Engaging the client in an organized activity reinforces reality. Asking the client to describe the delusion and acting as if the delusion is real reinforce the delusion's reality. Explaining that the delusion isn't real won't help and may make the client hold tighter to the delusion.
CN: Psychosocial integrity; CNS: Physiological adaptation; CL: Application

49. 2. Anhedonia is the loss of pleasure in things that are usually pleasurable. Avolition is the lack of motivation. Alogia, also called poverty of speech, is a decrease in the amount of richness of speech. A flat affect is the absence of emotional expression.
CN: Physiological integrity; CNS: None; CL: Application

50. 4. This statement indicates the client has learned a technique for coping with stress with the use of imagery technique. The other options don't show an understanding of self-symptom monitoring and may result in symptom intensification and possible relapse.
CN: Psychosocial integrity; CNS: None; CL: Application

51. 3. An oculogyric crisis involves a fixed positioning of the eyes, typically in an upward gaze. Neuroleptic malignant syndrome causes increased body temperature, muscle rigidity, and altered consciousness. Akathisia is a restlessness that can cause pacing and tapping of the fingers or feet. Stereotyped involuntary movements (tongue protrusion, lip smacking, chewing, blinking, and grimacing) characterize tardive dyskinesia.
CN: Physiological integrity; CNS: Pharmacological and parenteral therapies; CL: Application

52. A client taking antipsychotic medications shows dystonic reactions, including *torticollis* and *oculogyric crisis*. Which medication is given?
1. Benztropine (Cogentin)
2. Chlordiazepoxide (Librium)
3. Diazepam (Valium)
4. Fluoxetine (Prozac)

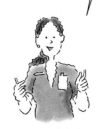

For question 53, you're looking for the *most appropriate* action.

53. A 50-year-old schizophrenic client becomes agitated and confronts the nurse with clenched fists. Which would be the <u>most appropriate</u> intervention by the nurse?
1. Take the client by the hand and lead him to the activity room for cards.
2. Step up to the client and tell him his behavior is inappropriate.
3. Call for security to take him to a seclusion room.
4. Speak to him in a quiet voice and offer him medication to help him calm down.

54. A 20-year-old client has been diagnosed with schizophrenia. He presently lives by himself, doesn't bathe, doesn't dress himself, and is erratic with eating, drinking, and taking prescribed medications. Which nursing diagnosis for this client has <u>priority</u>?
1. *Ineffective role performance related to isolation*
2. *Activity intolerance related to perceptual distortions*
3. *Ineffective coping*
4. *Imbalanced nutrition: Less than body requirements related to symptoms of schizophrenia*

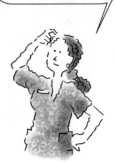

They're all important, but which one takes priority?

55. As a nurse approaches the nursing station, a client with the diagnosis of delusional disorder raises his voice and says, "You're following me. What do you want?" To prevent escalating fear and anger, the nurse takes a nonthreatening posture and makes which response in a calm voice?
1. "Are you frightened?"
2. "You know I'm not following you."
3. "You'll have to go into seclusion if you continue to threaten me."
4. "I'm sorry if I frightened you. I was returning to the nursing station after going out for lunch."

CN: Client needs category   CNS: Client needs subcategory   CL: Cognitive level

52. 1. Benztropine and trihexyphenidyl are anticholinergic drugs used to counteract the dystonic reactions and adverse reactions of antipsychotic drugs. The antihistamine diphenhydramine is also effective in treating extrapyramidal symptoms. Fluoxetine is an antidepressant, and diazepam and chlordiazepoxide are benzodiazepines.
CN: Physiological integrity; CNS: Pharmacological and parenteral therapies; CL: Application

53. 4. Always use the least restrictive means to calm a client. Never touch an agitated client; touch can be misinterpreted as a threat and can further escalate the situation. Stepping up to an agitated client can be seen as an aggressive act. Seclusion is a last resort.
CN: Physiological integrity; CNS: Reduction of risk potential; CL: Application

54. 4. The deterioration of the client undergoing a schizophrenic crisis is manifested in multiple self-care deficits. Adequate nutrition in these instances is the primary concern of the nurse. The other problems can be addressed after the client has been stabilized.
CN: Safe, effective care environment; CNS: Management of care; CL: Application

55. 4. Being clear in communication, remaining calm, and showing concern increases the chance the client will cooperate, lessening potential for violence. The first option tries to identify the client's feelings but doesn't convey warmth and concern. The second option isn't empathic and shows no indication of trying to reach the client at a level beyond content of communication. The third option may increase the client's anxiety, fear, and mistrust when the nurse engages in a power struggle and triggers competitiveness within the client.
CN: Psychosocial integrity; CNS: None; CL: Application

56. Which action by a client with stable schizophrenia is <u>most important</u> for preventing relapse?
1. Attending group therapy sessions
2. Participating in family support meetings
3. Attending social skills training sessions
4. Consistently taking prescribed medications

57. A client approaches the nurse and points at the sky, showing her where the men would be coming from to get him. Which response is <u>most therapeutic?</u>
1. "Why do you think the men are coming here?"
2. "You're safe here, we won't let them harm you."
3. "It seems like the world is pretty scary for you, but you're safe here."
4. "There are no bad men in the sky because no one lives that close to earth."

58. A client is brought to the crisis response center by his family. During evaluation, he reports being depressed for the last month and complains about voices constantly whispering to him. Which diagnosis is the <u>most likely?</u>
1. Catatonic schizophrenia
2. Disorganized schizophrenia
3. Paranoid schizophrenia
4. Schizoaffective disorder

59. Which nursing intervention is <u>most appropriate</u> for use with a client with paranoid schizophrenia?
1. Defend yourself when the client is verbally hostile toward you.
2. Provide a warm approach by touching the client.
3. Explain everything you're doing before you do it.
4. Clarify the content of the client's delusions.

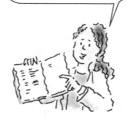

The words *most important* in question 56 indicate the need to prioritize. As a matter of fact, there's lots of prioritizing on this page.

56. 4. Although all of the choices are important for preventing relapse, compliance with the medication regimen is central to the treatment of schizophrenia, a brain disease.
CN: Safe, effective care environment; CNS: Management of care; CL: Application

57. 3. This response acknowledges the client's fears, listens to his feelings, and offers a sense of security as the nurse tries to understand the concerns behind the symbolism. She reflects these concerns to the client, along with reassurance of safety. The first option validates the delusion, not the feelings and fears, and doesn't orient the client to reality. The second option gives false reassurance. Because the nurse isn't sure of the symbolism, she can't make this promise. The last option rejects the client's feelings and doesn't address the client's fears.
CN: Safe, effective care environment; CNS: Management of care; CL: Application

58. 4. A client with major depressive episode who begins to hear voices and at times thinks someone is after him is most likely schizoaffective. The client who repeats phrases and shows waxy flexibility or stupor with prominent grimaces is most likely catatonic. The client with disorganized speech and behavior and a flat or inappropriate affect most likely has disorganized schizophrenia. The client who expresses thoughts of people spying on him, attributes ulterior motives to others, and has a flat affect is most likely paranoid schizophrenic.
CN: Psychosocial integrity; CNS: None; CL: Analysis

59. 3. Explaining everything you do will prevent misinterpretation of your actions. A non-defensive stance provides an atmosphere in which the client's angry feelings can be explored. Touching the paranoid client should be avoided because it can be interpreted as threatening. The content of delusions should not be the focus of your care because the content is illogical.
CN: Psychosocial integrity; CNS: None; CL: Analysis

60. The nurse is interviewing a client with a delusional disorder. Which of the following conditions would the nurse expect from this client?
1. Bizarre behavior
2. Agitation
3. Impaired short-term memory
4. Apparently normal functioning

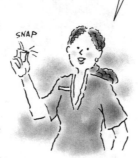

You've finished 60 questions. The rest of this test should be a snap.

SNAP

60. 4. The psychosocial functioning of the person with a delusional disorder may be relatively unimpaired. Another common characteristic of the client with a delusional disorder is the apparent normality of his behavior and appearance when his delusional ideas aren't being discussed or acted on. The client with delusional disorder doesn't have such symptoms as concrete thinking, bizarre or agitated behavior, and impaired memory, typical of a client with schizophrenia who functions at a lower level.
CN: Psychosocial integrity; CNS: None; CL: Application

61. A client is admitted to a psychiatric unit for a delusional disorder. He explains to a nurse that he made a contract with God to be the best minister on earth. Now that he has achieved the goal, most of his friends have stopped seeing him out of envy. On mental status examination, there is little impairment in psychosocial functioning. Which condition is expected?
1. Nonbizarre delusions
2. Fragmentary delusions
3. Regressive behavior
4. Regressive delusions

61. 1. The essential feature of delusional disorder is the presence of one or more nonbizarre delusions that persist for at least 1 month. The most common delusions by subtypes are erotomanic, grandiose, jealousy, persecutory, and somatic. Bizarre delusions are patently absurd beliefs with absolutely no foundation in reality. Fragmentary delusions are unconnected delusions not organized around a coherent theme. Regressive behaviors revert back to a less mature state and aren't associated with a mental disorder.
CN: Psychosocial integrity; CNS: None; CL: Application

62. Which statement made by a client taking fluphenazine tells the nurse that the client understands his discharge instructions?
1. "I need to stay out of the sun."
2. "I need to drink plenty of fluids."
3. "I can't eat cheese."
4. "I need to plan rest periods throughout the day."

62. 1. Fluphenazine is an antipsychotic drug that can cause photosensitivity and sunburn. Clients taking this drug don't need to increase fluid intake, avoid cheeses, or plan rest periods.
CN: Physiological integrity; CNS: Pharmacological and parenteral therapies; CL: Analysis

63. The nurse is teaching the family of a client who has been prescribed thiothixene (Navane). Which of the following adverse reactions concerning this medication would be the <u>most</u> accurate for the nurse to discuss?
1. Akinesia
2. Hypotension
3. Sedation
4. Weight gain

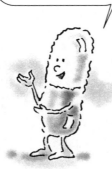

I didn't intend to cause any adverse reactions.

63. 1. Thiothixene is a high-potency agent with a high affinity for the dopamine-2 receptors, resulting in the increased likelihood of akinesia, a form of extrapyramidal symptoms. Although thiothixene targets other neurotransmitters responsible for hypotension, sedation, and weight gain, their affinity to these receptors is weak and more likely to occur with low-potency psychotropics.
CN: Physiological integrity; CNS: Pharmacological and parenteral therapies; CL: Application

64. Inability to carry out daily responsibilities typically occurs during the prodromal phase of schizophrenia. Which symptom may also occur during this phase?
1. Increased energy and motivation
2. Increased social interaction
3. Impaired role functioning and neglect of personal hygiene
4. Heightened work performance

65. The daughter of a client with schizophrenia states, "I'm afraid I may develop this disease, too." The nurse should teach the daughter that schizophrenia is linked to which factor?
1. Sexual abuse
2. A combination of genetic and other factors
3. Both parents having schizophrenia
4. Emotional trauma during childhood

66. A nurse teaches a class of caregivers about the positive and negative behaviors of schizophrenia. Positive behaviors include:
1. limited spontaneous speech.
2. inability to initiate and persist in goal-directed activities.
3. misinterpretation of experiences and altered sensory input.
4. extremely brief replies to questions.

67. A nurse is facilitating a group of schizophrenic clients when one client says, "I like to drive my car, bar, tar, far." This pattern of speech is known as which disorder?
1. Clang association
2. Echolalia
3. Echopraxia
4. Neologisms

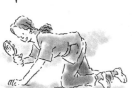

Families often search for the link to their loved one's disease.

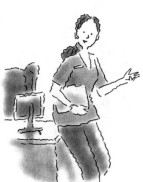

Which pattern of speech is the client using?

64. 3. Prodromal (early) signs and symptoms of schizophrenia can occur 1 month to 1 year before the first psychotic break and represent a clear deterioration in functioning. They may include impaired role functioning and neglect of personal hygiene as well as social withdrawal and depression. Increases in energy and social interaction and heightened work performance don't occur during the prodromal phase.
CN: Psychosocial integrity; CNS: None; CL: Application

65. 2. Experts believe schizophrenia results from a combination of genetic, environmental, and other factors—such as viruses, birth injuries, and nutritional factors. Schizophrenia incidence is higher among relatives of persons with the disease. It can occur even if both parents don't have schizophrenia. Emotional trauma during childhood hasn't been linked to schizophrenia.
CN: Psychosocial integrity; CNS: None; CL: Application

66. 3. Positive behaviors of schizophrenia include attention-getting behaviors, which can result from misinterpretation of experiences and altered sensing input (such as hallucinations, delusions, and bizarre behavior). Negative behaviors are those that render the client inert and unmotivated, such as lack of spontaneous speech, poverty of thought, apathy, and poor social functioning.
CN: Psychosocial integrity; CNS: None; CL: Application

67. 1. Linking together words based on their sounds rather than their meanings is called clang association. Echolalia is the involuntary parrotlike repetition of words spoken by others. Echopraxia refers to meaningless imitation of others' motions. Neologisms are new words that a person invents.
CN: Psychosocial integrity; CNS: None; CL: Application

68. A schizophrenic client who's receiving antipsychotic medication paces, fidgets, and can't seem to stay still. The nurse recognizes these behaviors as which disorder?
1. Tardive dyskinesia
2. Dystonia
3. Akathisia
4. Akinesia

68. 3. Akathisia is an extrapyramidal adverse effect of some antipsychotic medications, manifested by restlessness and an inability to stay still. Tardive dyskinesia refers to involuntary abnormal movements of the mouth, tongue, face, and jaw. Dystonia refers to difficulty with movement. Akinesia is absence of movement.
CN: Physiological integrity; CNS: Pharmacological and parenteral therapies; CL: Analysis

69. Which nursing diagnosis is <u>most appropriate</u> for a client diagnosed with schizophrenia, disorganized type?
1. *Feeding self-care deficit*
2. *Disturbed sleep pattern*
3. *Impaired verbal communication*
4. *Social isolation*

69. 3. Schizophrenia, disorganized type, is characterized by disorganized speech, disorganized behavior, and inappropriate or flat affect. *Feeding self-care deficit*, *Disturbed sleep pattern*, and *Social isolation* aren't classic manifestations of this type of schizophrenia.
CN: Psychosocial integrity; CNS: None; CL: Analysis

70. A client with paranoid schizophrenia tells the nurse that two people talking in the hall are planning to kidnap and kill him. The client's thought pattern reflects which disorder?
1. Auditory hallucinations
2. Delusions of grandeur
3. Ideas of reference
4. Echolalia

70. 3. A client with ideas of reference mistakenly believes that other people's thoughts, speech, and behaviors refer to the client. Auditory hallucinations are sounds that aren't based in reality. Delusions of grandeur are false beliefs that arise without appropriate external stimuli. Echolalia refers to involuntary repetition of words spoken by others.
CN: Psychosocial integrity; CNS: None; CL: Application

71. A client with schizophrenia is taking the atypical antipsychotic medication clozapine (Clozaril). Which signs and symptoms indicate the presence of adverse effects associated with this medication? Select all that apply:
1. Sore throat
2. Pill-rolling movements
3. Polyuria
4. Fever
5. Polydipsia
6. Orthostatic hypotension

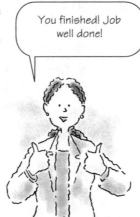

You finished! Job well done!

71. 1, 4. Sore throat, fever, and sudden onset of other flulike symptoms are signs of agranulocytosis. The condition is caused by a lack of sufficient granulocytes (a type of white blood cell), which causes the client to be susceptible to infection. The client's white blood cell count should be monitored at least weekly throughout the course of treatment. Pill-rolling movements can occur in those experiencing extrapyramidal adverse effects associated with antipsychotic medication that has been prescribed for a much longer time frame than clozapine. Polydipsia (excessive thirst) and polyuria (increased urine output) are common adverse effects of lithium. Orthostatic hypotension is an adverse effect of tricyclic antidepressants.
CN: Physiological integrity; CNS: Pharmacological and parenteral therapies; CL: Application

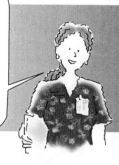

About the only substance of abuse this chapter *doesn't* cover is my personal weakness—chocolate mousse! Think of me as you work through this chapter. I'll be the one with chocolate smudges on her fingers. Tee-hee!

Chapter 19
Substance-related disorders

1. Family members of a client who abuses alcohol asks a nurse to help them intervene. Which action is essential for a successful intervention?
  1. All family members must tell the client they're powerless.
  2. All family members must describe how the addiction affects them.
  3. All family members must come up with their share of financial support.
  4. All family members must become caregivers during the detoxification period.

2. A client who abuses alcohol tells a nurse, "I'm sure I can become a social drinker." Which response is <u>most appropriate?</u>
  1. "When do you think you can become a social drinker?"
  2. "What makes you think you'll learn to drink normally?"
  3. "Does your alcohol use cause major problems in your life?"
  4. "How many alcoholic beverages can a social drinker consume?"

3. A client asks a nurse not to tell his parents about his alcohol problem. Which response is most appropriate?
  1. "How can you not tell them? Is that being honest?"
  2. "Don't you think you'll need to tell them someday?"
  3. "Do alcohol problems run in either side of your family?"
  4. "What do you think will happen if you tell your parents?"

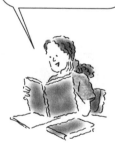

The words most appropriate help clarify the correct answer.

1. 2. After the family is taught about addiction, they must write down examples of how the addiction has affected each of them and use this information during the intervention. It isn't necessary to tell the client the family is powerless. The family is empowered through this intervention experience. In many cases, a third-party payer will help with treatment costs. Doing an intervention doesn't make family members responsible for financial support or providing care and support during the detoxification period.
CN: Psychosocial integrity; CNS: None; CL: Analysis

2. 3. This question may help the client recall the problematic results of using alcohol and the reasons the client began treatment. Asking when he believes he can become a social drinker will only encourage the addicted person to deny the problem and develop an unrealistic, self-defeating goal. Asking how many alcoholic beverages a social drinker can consume and why the client thinks he can drink normally will encourage the addicted person to defend himself and deny the problem.
CN: Psychosocial integrity; CNS: None; CL: Application

3. 4. Clients who struggle with addiction problems often believe people will be judgmental, rejecting, and uncaring if they are told that the client is recovering from alcohol abuse. The first option challenges the client and will put him on the defensive. The second option will make the client defensive and construct rationalizations as to why his parents don't need to know. The third option is a good assessment question, but it isn't an appropriate question to ask a client who's afraid to tell others about his addiction.
CN: Psychosocial integrity; CNS: None; CL: Analysis

CN: Client needs category   CNS: Client needs subcategory   CL: Cognitive level

4. A nurse assesses a client with alcohol withdrawal. Which finding is of <u>most</u> concern to the nurse?

　1. Hallucinations
　2. Nervousness
　3. Diaphoresis
　4. Nausea

5. The nurse is assessing a client with prolonged, chronic alcohol intake. Which of the following findings would the nurse expect to find?

　1. Enlarged liver
　2. Nasal irritation
　3. Muscle wasting
　4. Limb paresthesia

6. A client has an order for chlordiazepoxide (Librium) to be given as needed for signs and symptoms of alcohol withdrawal. Which symptoms indicate that the client needs this medication?

　1. Mild tremors, hypertension, tachycardia
　2. Bradycardia, hyperthermia, sedation
　3. Hypotension, decreased reflexes, drowsiness
　4. Hypothermia, mild tremors, slurred speech

7. A client who abuses alcohol tells a nurse, "Alcohol helps me sleep." Which information about alcohol use and sleep is <u>most accurate</u>?

　1. Alcohol doesn't help promote sleep.
　2. Continued alcohol use causes insomnia.
　3. One glass of alcohol at dinnertime can induce sleep.
　4. Sometimes alcohol can make one drowsy enough to fall asleep.

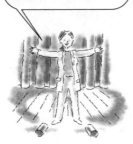

A disease can have many "stages," each with its own symptoms.

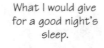

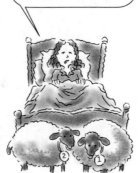

What I would give for a good night's sleep.

4. 1. Hallucinations are a sign of late alcohol withdrawal. The nurse should stay with the client, have someone notify the physician, and institute seizure precautions. Nervousness, diaphoresis, and nausea are signs of early withdrawal.
CN: Physiological integrity; CNS: Reduction of risk potential; CL: Analysis

5. 1. A major effect of alcohol on the body is liver impairment, and an enlarged liver is a common physical finding. Nasal irritation is commonly seen with clients who snort cocaine. Muscle wasting and limb paresthesia don't tend to occur with clients who abuse alcohol.
CN: Physiological integrity; CNS: Physiological adaptation; CL: Application

6. 1. Chlordiazepoxide is given during alcohol withdrawal. Symptoms that indicate a need for this drug include tremors, hypertension, tachycardia, and elevated body temperature. Bradycardia, sedation, hypotension, decreased reflexes, hypothermia, and slurred speech aren't symptoms of alcohol withdrawal.
CN: Physiological integrity; CNS: Pharmacological and parenteral therapies; CL: Application

7. 1. Alcohol use may initially promote sleep, but with continued use, it causes insomnia. Evidence shows that alcohol doesn't facilitate sleep. One glass of alcohol at dinnertime won't induce sleep. The last option doesn't give information about how alcohol affects sleep. It makes the client think alcohol use to induce sleep is an appropriate strategy to try.
CN: Physiological integrity; CNS: Physiological adaptation; CL: Analysis

CN: Client needs category　CNS: Client needs subcategory　CL: Cognitive level

8. A client withdrawing from alcohol is given lorazepam (Ativan). The nurse teaches the client's family about the drug. Which response by a family member indicates that the nurse's teaching has been successful?
1. "Short-term use of lorazepam can lead to dependence."
2. "The lorazepam will reduce the symptoms of withdrawal."
3. "The lorazepam will make him forget about symptoms of withdrawal."
4. "The lorazepam will also help with his heart disease."

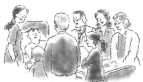

It's important to teach the family and the client.

9. A client who abuses alcohol tells a nurse everyone in his family has an alcohol problem and nothing can be done about it. Which response is the most appropriate?
1. "You're right, it's much harder to become a recovering person."
2. "This is just an excuse for you so you don't have to work on becoming sober."
3. "Sometimes nothing can be done, but you may be the exception in this family."
4. "Alcohol problems can occur in families, but you can decide to take the steps to become and stay sober."

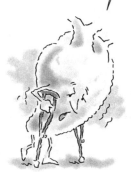

I feel like I'm failing fast.

10. A client with chronic alcoholism may be predisposed to develop which of the following conditions?
1. Arteriosclerosis
2. Heart failure
3. Heart valve damage
4. Pericarditis

11. Which assessment finding is commonly associated with the abuse of alcohol in a young, depressed adult woman?
1. Defiant responses
2. Infertility
3. Memory loss
4. Sexual abuse

8. 2. Lorazepam is a short-acting benzodiazepine usually given for 1 week to help the client in alcohol withdrawal. Long-term (not short-term) use of lorazepam can lead to dependence. The medication isn't given to help forget the experience; it lessens the symptoms of withdrawal. It isn't used to treat coexisting cardiovascular problems.
CN: Physiological integrity; CNS: Pharmacological and parenteral therapies; CL: Application

9. 4. This statement challenges the client to become proactive and take the steps necessary to maintain a sober lifestyle. The first option agrees with the client's denial and isn't a useful response. The second option confronts the client and may make him more adamant in defense of this position. The third option agrees with the client's denial and isn't a useful response.
CN: Psychosocial integrity; CNS: None; CL: Application

10. 2. Heart failure is a severe cardiac consequence associated with long-term alcohol use. Arteriosclerosis, heart valve damage, and pericarditis aren't medical consequences of alcoholism.
CN: Physiological integrity; CNS: Reduction of risk potential; CL: Application

11. 4. Many women diagnosed with substance abuse problems also have a history of physical or sexual abuse. Alcohol abuse isn't a common finding in a young woman showing defiant behavior or experiencing infertility. Memory loss isn't a common finding in a young woman experiencing alcohol abuse.
CN: Psychosocial integrity; CNS: None; CL: Analysis

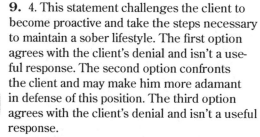

12. A nurse determines that a client who abused alcohol has nutritional problems. Which strategy is <u>best</u> for addressing the client's nutritional needs?
1. Encourage the client to eat a diet high in calories.
2. Help the client recognize and follow a balanced diet.
3. Have the client drink liquid protein supplements daily.
4. Have the client monitor the calories consumed each day.

13. A client with a history of alcohol abuse refuses to take vitamins. Which statement is most appropriate for explaining why vitamins are important?
1. "It's important to take vitamins to stop your craving."
2. "Prolonged use of alcohol can cause vitamin depletion."
3. "For every vitamin you take, you'll help your liver heal."
4. "By taking vitamins, you don't need to worry about your diet."

14. Which statement by a client who abuses alcohol indicates a need for nutritional teaching?
1. "I should avoid foods high in fat."
2. "I should eat only one balanced meal per day."
3. "I should take vitamin and mineral supplements."
4. "I should eat large portions of food containing fiber."

15. A client tells a nurse, "I've been drinking ever since they told me I had learning disabilities." Which rationale does this client's statement indicate?
1. The client is self-medicating.
2. The client has an excuse to drink.
3. The client isn't a productive person.
4. The client will be unable to stop drinking.

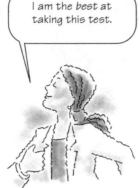

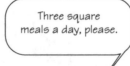
Three square meals a day, please.

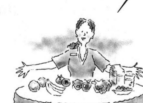

12. 2. Clients who abuse alcohol are usually malnourished and need help to follow a balanced diet. Increasing calories may cause the client to just eat empty calories. The client must be involved in the decision to supplement the daily dietary intake. The nurse can't force the client to drink liquid protein supplements. Having the client monitor calorie intake could be done only after the client recognizes the need to maintain a balanced diet. Calorie counts usually aren't needed in most recovering clients who begin to eat from the basic food groups.
CN: Physiological integrity; CNS: Basic care and comfort; CL: Application

13. 2. Chronic alcoholism interferes with the metabolism of many vitamins. Vitamin supplements can prevent deficiencies from occurring. Taking vitamins won't stop a person from craving alcohol or help a damaged liver heal. A balanced diet is *essential* in addition to taking multivitamins.
CN: Health promotion and maintenance; CNS: None; CL: Application

14. 2. If the client eats only one adequate meal each day, there will be a deficit of essential nutrients. It's appropriate for the client to take vitamin and mineral supplements to prevent deficiency in these nutrients. Avoiding foods high in fat content and consuming large portions of foods containing fiber indicate the client has good knowledge about nutrition.
CN: Health promotion and maintenance; CNS: None; CL: Analysis

15. 1. A client with learning disabilities may experience frustration, depression, or overall feelings of low self-esteem and may self-medicate with alcohol. Many people with learning disabilities don't resort to alcohol but develop other coping skills to handle the disability. People with learning disabilities can be very productive. A person with a learning disability can successfully recover from alcohol addiction.
CN: Psychosocial integrity; CNS: None; CL: Application

16. A nurse is caring for a client undergoing treatment for acute alcohol dependence. The client tells the nurse, "I don't have a problem. My wife made me come here." Which defense mechanism is the client using?
1. Projection and suppression
2. Denial and rationalization
3. Rationalization and repression
4. Suppression and denial

17. A nurse has a meeting with a family of a recovering client. The client tells a family member, "You made it easy for me to use alcohol. You always made excuses for my behavior." Which important issue should the family be encouraged to address?
1. Giving up enabling behaviors
2. Managing the client's self-care
3. Dealing with negative behaviors
4. Evaluating the home environment

18. Which short-term goal should be a <u>priority</u> for a client with a knowledge deficit about the effects of alcohol on the body?
1. Test blood chemistries daily.
2. Verbalize the results of substance use.
3. Talk to a pharmacist about the substance.
4. Attend a weekly aerobic exercise program.

19. A client recovering from alcohol abuse tells a nurse, "I feel so depressed about what I've done to my family that I feel like giving up." Assessment of which area is a <u>priority</u>?
1. Family support
2. A plan for self-harm
3. A sponsor for the client
4. Other ambivalent feelings

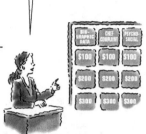

I'll take "Defense mechanisms" for $200, Alex.

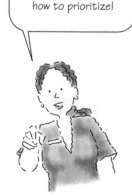

You need to know how to prioritize!

16. 2. The client is using denial and rationalization. Denial is the unconscious disclaimer of unacceptable thoughts, feelings, needs, or certain external factors. Rationalization is the unconscious effort to justify intolerable feelings, behaviors, and motives. The client isn't using projection, suppression, or repression.
CN: Psychosocial integrity; CNS: None; CL: Application

17. 1. Enabling the behaviors of family members allows the client to continue the addiction by rationalizing, denying, or otherwise excusing the problem. Managing the client's self-care isn't an issue that needs to be addressed based on the client's statement. Dealing with negative behaviors and evaluating the home environment don't address the client's statement about the family's enabling behavior.
CN: Psychosocial integrity; CNS: None; CL: Application

18. 2. It's important for the client to talk about the health consequences of the continued use of alcohol. Testing blood chemistries daily gives the client minimal knowledge about the effects of alcohol on the body and isn't the most useful information in a teaching plan. A pharmacist isn't the appropriate health care professional to educate the client about the effects of alcohol use on the body. Although exercise is an important goal of self-care, it doesn't address the client's knowledge deficit about the effects of alcohol on the body.
CN: Safe, effective care environment; CNS: Management of care; CL: Application

19. 2. When a client talks about giving up, the nurse must explore the potential for suicidal behavior. Although questioning the client about family support, the availability of a sponsor, or ambivalent feelings are important, the priority action is to assess for suicide.
CN: Psychosocial integrity; CNS: None; CL: Application

20. A client withdrawing from alcohol says he's worried about periodic hallucinations. Which intervention is best for this client's problem?
1. Point out that the sensation doesn't exist.
2. Allow the client to talk about the experience.
3. Encourage the client to wash the body areas well.
4. Determine if the client has a cognitive impairment.

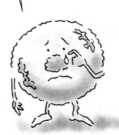

Alcohol can make me more susceptible to infections.

21. A client who has been drinking alcohol for 30 years asks a nurse if permanent damage has occurred to his immune system. Which response is the best?
1. "There is often less resistance to infections."
2. "Sometimes the body's metabolism will increase."
3. "Put your energies into maintaining sobriety for now."
4. "Drinking puts you at high risk for disease later in life."

22. A client experiencing alcohol withdrawal is upset about going through detoxification. Which goal is a <u>priority</u>?
1. The client will commit to a drug-free lifestyle.
2. The client will work with the nurse to remain safe.
3. The client will drink plenty of fluids on a daily basis.
4. The client will make a personal inventory of strengths.

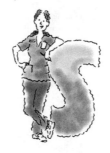

In this case, the "S" stands for "safety."

23. A client recovering from alcohol abuse needs to develop effective coping skills to handle daily stressors. Which intervention is most useful to the client?
1. Determine the client's level of verbal skills.
2. Help the client avoid areas that cause conflict.
3. Discuss examples of successful coping behavior.
4. Teach the client to accept uncomfortable situations.

20. 2. The client needs to talk about the periodic hallucinations to prevent them from becoming triggers to acting out behaviors and possible self-injury. The client's experience of sensory-perceptual alterations must be acknowledged; therefore, denying that the client's hallucinations exist isn't a helpful strategy. Determining if the client has a cognitive impairment and encouraging the client to wash the body areas well don't address the problem of periodic hallucinations.
CN: Psychosocial integrity; CNS: None; CL: Application

21. 1. Chronic alcohol use depresses the immune system and causes increased susceptibility to infections. A nutritionally well-balanced diet that includes foods high in protein and B vitamins will help develop a strong immune system. The potential damage to the immune system doesn't increase the body's metabolism. The third option negates the client's concern and isn't an appropriate or caring response. Drinking alcohol may put the client at risk for immune system problems at any time in life.
CN: Psychosocial integrity; CNS: None; CL: Analysis

22. 2. The priority goal is for client safety. Although drinking enough fluids, identifying personal strengths, and committing to a drug-free lifestyle are important goals, the nurse's first priority must be to promote client safety.
CN: Safe, effective care environment; CNS: Management of care; CL: Application

23. 3. The client needs help to identify successful coping behavior and develop ways to incorporate that behavior into daily functioning. There are many skills for coping with stress, and determining the client's level of verbal skills may not be important. Encouraging the client to avoid conflict prevents him from learning skills to handle daily stressors.
CN: Psychosocial integrity; CNS: None; CL: Analysis

CN: Client needs category   CNS: Client needs subcategory   CL: Cognitive level

24. A client is struggling with alcohol dependence. Which <u>communication strategy</u> would be most effective?
1. Speak briefly and directly.
2. Avoid blaming or preaching to the client.
3. Confront feelings and examples of perfectionism.
4. Determine if nonverbal communication will be more effective.

25. A nurse is working with a client on recognizing the relationship between alcohol abuse and interpersonal problems. Which intervention has <u>priority?</u>
1. Help the client identify personal strengths.
2. Help the client decrease compulsive behaviors.
3. Examine the client's use of defense mechanisms.
4. Have the client work with peers who can serve as role models.

26. A client recovering from alcohol addiction has limited coping skills. Which characteristic would indicate relationship problems?
1. The client is prone to panic attacks.
2. The client doesn't pay attention to details.
3. The client has poor problem-solving skills.
4. The client ignores the need to relax and rest.

27. A nurse suggests to a client struggling with alcohol addiction that keeping a journal may be helpful. The journal helps the client:
1. identify stressors and responses to them.
2. understand the diagnosis.
3. help others by reading the journal to them.
4. develop an emergency plan for use in a crisis.

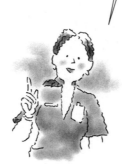

Remember to prioritize!

24. 2. Blaming or preaching to the client causes negativity and prevents the client from hearing what the nurse has to say. Speaking briefly to the client may not allow time for adequate communication. Perfectionism doesn't tend to be an issue. Determining if nonverbal communication will be more effective is better suited for a client with cognitive impairment.
CN: Psychosocial integrity; CNS: None; CL: Analysis

25. 3. Defense mechanisms can impede the development of healthy relationships and cause the client pain. After identifying barriers to relationship problems, it would be appropriate to identify or clarify personal strengths. Compulsive behavior doesn't tend to be a problem for alcoholic clients who struggle with interpersonal problems. Working with peers who are role models would be useful after the client recognizes and gains some insight into the problems. It isn't the priority intervention.
CN: Safe, effective care environment; CNS: Management of care; CL: Analysis

26. 3. To have satisfying relationships, a person must be able to communicate and problem solve. Relationship problems don't predispose people to panic attacks more than other psychosocial stressors. Paying attention to details isn't a major concern when addressing the client's relationship difficulties. Although ignoring the need for rest and relaxation is unhealthy, it shouldn't pose a major relationship problem.
CN: Psychosocial integrity; CNS: None; CL: Analysis

27. 1. Keeping a journal enables the client to identify problems and patterns of coping. From this information, the difficulties the client faces can be addressed. A journal isn't necessarily kept to promote better understanding of the client's illness, but it helps the client understand himself better. Journals aren't read to other people unless the client wants to share a particular part. Journals aren't typically used for identifying an emergency plan for use in a crisis.
CN: Psychosocial integrity; CNS: None; CL: Application

28. Which information is <u>most important</u> to use in a teaching plan for a client who abused alcohol?
1. Personal needs
2. Illness exacerbation
3. Cognitive distortions
4. Communication skills

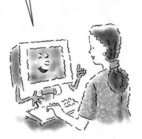

It is most important that you read this question carefully.

28. 4. Addicted clients typically have difficulty communicating their needs in an appropriate way. Learning appropriate communication skills is a major goal of treatment. Next, behavior that focuses on the self and meeting personal needs will be addressed. The identification of cognitive distortions would be difficult if the client has poor communication skills. Teaching about illness exacerbation isn't a skill, but it is essential for relaying information about relapse.
CN: Psychosocial integrity; CNS: None; CL: Analysis

29. Which assessment must be done before starting a teaching session with a client who abuses alcohol?
1. Sleep patterns
2. Decision making
3. Note-taking skills
4. Readiness to learn

29. 4. It's important to know if the client's current situation helps or hinders the potential to learn. Decision making and sleep patterns aren't factors that must be assessed before teaching about addiction. Note-taking skills aren't a factor in determining whether the client will be receptive to teaching.
CN: Psychosocial integrity; CNS: None; CL: Application

30. A nurse is developing strategies to prevent relapse with a client who abuses alcohol. Which client intervention is important?
1. Avoid taking over-the-counter medications.
2. Limit monthly contact with the family of origin.
3. Refrain from becoming involved in group activities.
4. Avoid people, places, and activities from the former lifestyle.

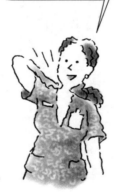

Congratulations! You've finished 30 questions!

30. 4. Changing the client's old habits is essential for sustaining a sober lifestyle. Certain over-the-counter medications that don't contain alcohol will probably need to be used by the client at certain times. It's unrealistic to have the client abstain from all such medications. Contact with the client's family of origin may not be a trigger to relapse, so limiting contact wouldn't be useful. Refraining from group activities isn't a good strategy to prevent relapse. Going to Alcoholics Anonymous and other support groups will help prevent relapse.
CN: Psychosocial integrity; CNS: None; CL: Analysis

31. A client recovering from alcohol abuse tells the nurse, "I get nothing out of Alcoholics Anonymous (AA) meetings." Which response is most appropriate?
1. "What were you told about going to AA meetings?"
2. "What do you want to get out of the AA meetings?"
3. "When do you think you'll stop going to the meetings?"
4. "Do you think you can control what happens in a meeting?"

31. 2. This response puts some of the responsibility for staying sober on the client and encourages the client to take a more active role. Asking what the client was told about AA meetings opens up a discussion that allows the client to continue to discuss disappointments rather than taking a proactive stand to support the value of AA meetings. The third option condones the client's desire to stop going to the meetings. The fourth option changes the issue from being responsible for staying sober to focusing on what the client can't control.
CN: Psychosocial integrity; CNS: None; CL: Analysis

CN: Client needs category   CNS: Client needs subcategory   CL: Cognitive level

32. A client asks a nurse, "Why does it matter if I talk to my peers in group therapy?" Which response is <u>most appropriate</u>?
1. "Group therapy lets you see what you're doing wrong in your life."
2. "Group therapy acts as a defense against your disorganized behavior."
3. "Group therapy provides a way to ask for support as well as to support others."
4. "In group therapy, you can vent your frustrations and others will listen."

33. A family meeting is held with a client who abuses alcohol. While listening to the family, which unhealthy communication pattern might be identified?
1. Use of descriptive jargon
2. Disapproval of behaviors
3. Avoidance of conflicting issues
4. Unlimited expression of nonverbal communication

34. A client addicted to alcohol begins individual therapy with a nurse. Which intervention should be a priority?
1. Learn to express feelings.
2. Establish new roles in the family.
3. Determine strategies for socializing.
4. Decrease preoccupation with physical health.

35. A client recovering from alcohol addiction asks a nurse how to talk to his children about the impact of his addiction on them. Which response is most appropriate?
1. "Try to limit references to the addiction, and focus on the present."
2. "Talk about all the hardships you've had in working to remain sober."
3. "Tell them you're sorry, and emphasize that you're doing so much better now."
4. "Talk to them by acknowledging the difficulties and pain your drinking caused."

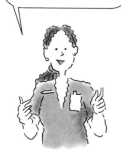

All answers may seem right, but choose the most appropriate one.

32. 3. The best response addresses how group therapy provides opportunities to communicate, learn, and give and get support. Group members will give a client feedback, not just point out what a client is doing wrong. Group therapy isn't a defense against disorganized behavior. People can express all kinds of feelings and discuss a variety of topics in group therapy. Interactions are goal oriented and not just vehicles to vent one's frustrations.
CN: Psychosocial integrity; CNS: None; CL: Application

33. 3. The interaction pattern of a family with a member who abuses alcohol often revolves around denying the problem, avoiding conflict, or rationalizing the addiction. Health care providers are more likely to use jargon. The family might have problems setting limits and expressing disapproval of the client's behavior. Nonverbal communication often gives the nurse insight into family dynamics.
CN: Psychosocial integrity; CNS: None; CL: Analysis

34. 1. The client must address issues, learn ways to cope effectively with life stressors, and express his needs appropriately. After the client establishes sobriety, the possibility of taking on new roles can become a reality. Determining strategies for socializing isn't the priority intervention for an addicted client. Usually, these clients need to change former socializing habits. Clients addicted to alcohol don't tend to be preoccupied with physical health problems.
CN: Safe, effective care environment; CNS: Management of care; CL: Analysis

35. 4. Part of the healing process for the family is to acknowledge the pain, embarrassment, and overall difficulties the client's drinking problem caused family members. The first option facilitates the client's ability to deny the problem. The second option prevents the client from acknowledging the difficulties the children endured. The third option leads the client to believe only a simple apology is needed. The addiction must be addressed and the children's pain acknowledged.
CN: Psychosocial integrity; CNS: None; CL: Application

36. A client with a diagnosis of alcohol dependency is being discharged from the hospital. Which goal will be a *priority* for successful outpatient therapy?
1. Find a way to drink socially.
2. Allow self to grieve recent losses.
3. Work to bring others into treatment.
4. Develop relapse-prevention strategies.

37. A client addicted to alcohol tells a nurse, "Making friends used to be hard for me." Which statement by the client indicates that client teaching about relationships was successful?
1. "I've set limits on my behaviors toward others."
2. "I need to be judgmental of others."
3. "I won't become intimately involved with others."
4. "I can't bear to see myself hurt again in a relationship."

38. A client who abused alcohol for more than 20 years is diagnosed with cirrhosis of the liver. Which statement by the client shows that teaching has been effective?
1. "If I decide to stop drinking, I won't kill myself."
2. "If I watch my blood pressure, I should be okay."
3. "If I take vitamins, I can undo some liver damage."
4. "If I use nutritional supplements, I won't have problems."

39. A client tells a nurse, "I'm not going to have problems from smoking marijuana." Which response is most appropriate?
1. "Evidence shows it can cause major health problems."
2. "Marijuana can cause reproductive problems later in life."
3. "Smoking marijuana isn't as dangerous as smoking cigarettes."
4. "Some people have minor or no reactions to smoking marijuana."

> Your client teaching stems in part from an understanding of the severity of disease.

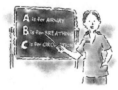

36. 4. The primary goal for a client in outpatient treatment is to focus on strategies that prevent relapse. Finding ways to drink socially and working to bring others into treatment aren't goals of outpatient therapy. Allowing self to grieve the losses the addiction caused is a part of the early work of inpatient therapy and may be continued in outpatient therapy.
CN: Safe, effective care environment; CNS: Management of care; CL: Analysis

37. 1. When the client can set personal limits and maintain boundaries, the ability to have successful interpersonal relationships can occur. Being judgmental is contraindicated if a client wants to have successful relationships. Setting arbitrary limits on relationships indicates the client needs to learn more interpersonal relationship skills. The universal truth about relationships is that they bring both joy and pain. The last statement indicates a need to learn more about relationships.
CN: Psychosocial integrity; CNS: None; CL: Application

38. 1. This statement reflects the client's perception of the severity of the condition and the life-threatening complications that can result from continued use of alcohol. Aggressive treatment is required, not merely watching one's blood pressure. At this point in the illness, there is little likelihood that liver damage from cirrhosis can be altered. The fourth option denies the severity of the problem and negates the life-threatening complications common with a diagnosis of cirrhosis.
CN: Psychosocial integrity; CNS: None; CL: Analysis

39. 2. Marijuana causes cardiac, respiratory, immune, and reproductive health problems. Most people who smoke marijuana don't have major health problems. All people who smoke marijuana have symptoms of intoxication. The residues from marijuana are more toxic than those from cigarettes.
CN: Psychosocial integrity; CNS: None; CL: Application

40. During an assessment of a client with a history of polysubstance abuse, which information is a <u>priority</u> to obtain after the names of the drugs?
1. Oral administration of any drug
2. Time of last use of each drug
3. How the drug was obtained
4. The place the drug was used

41. A client says, "I started using cocaine as a recreational drug, but now I can't seem to control the use." The nurse knows that the client's statement is *most* consistent with which drug behavior?
1. Toxic dose
2. Dual diagnosis
3. Cross-tolerance
4. Compulsive use

42. A client says he used amphetamines to be productive at work. Which symptom <u>commonly</u> occurs when the drug is abruptly discontinued?
1. Severe anxiety
2. Increased yawning
3. Altered perceptions
4. Amotivational syndrome

43. A 20-year-old client is admitted with bone marrow depression. He tells the nurse he's been abusing drugs since age 13. Which drug should the nurse expect to find in his history?
1. Amphetamines
2. Cocaine
3. Inhalants
4. Marijuana

44. Which reason best explains why it's important to monitor behavior in a client who has stopped using phencyclidine (PCP)?
1. Fatigue can cause feelings of being overwhelmed.
2. Agitation and mood swings can occur during withdrawal.
3. Bizarre behavior can be a precursor to a psychotic episode.
4. Memory loss and forgetfulness can cause unsafe conditions.

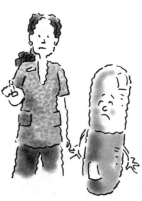

Remember to prioritize!

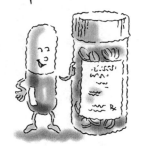

You should know which drugs cause which adverse effects!

40. 2. The time of last use gives information about expected withdrawal symptoms of the drugs and what immediate treatment is necessary. How the drugs were obtained and the places the drugs were used aren't essential information for treatment, nor is oral administration.
CN: Psychosocial integrity; CNS: None; CL: Application

41. 4. Compulsive drug use involves taking a substance for a period of time significantly longer than intended. A toxic dose is the amount of a drug that causes a poisonous effect. Dual diagnosis is the coexistence of a drug problem and a mental health problem. Cross-tolerance occurs when the effects of a drug are decreased and the client takes larger amounts to achieve the desired drug effect.
CN: Psychosocial integrity; CNS: None; CL: Application

42. 1. When amphetamines are abruptly discontinued, the client may experience severe anxiety or agitation. Increased yawning is a symptom of opioid withdrawal. Altered perceptions occur when a client is withdrawing from hallucinogens. Amotivational syndrome is seen with clients using marijuana.
CN: Psychosocial integrity; CNS: None; CL: Application

43. 3. Inhalants cause severe bone marrow depression. Marijuana, cocaine, and amphetamines don't cause bone marrow depression.
CN: Physiological integrity; CNS: Pharmacological and parenteral therapies; CL: Application

44. 3. Bizarre behavior and speech are associated with PCP withdrawal and can indicate psychosis. Fatigue isn't necessarily a problem when a client stops using PCP. Agitation, mood swings, memory loss, and forgetfulness don't tend to occur when a client has stopped using PCP.
CN: Psychosocial integrity; CNS: None; CL: Analysis

45. A client experiencing amphetamine withdrawal may commonly experience which of the following symptoms?
1. Disturbed sleep
2. Increased yawning
3. Psychomotor agitation
4. Inability to concentrate

46. Which condition can occur in a client who has just used cocaine?
1. Tachycardia
2. Hyperthermia
3. Hypotension
4. Bradypnea

47. Which information is most important in teaching a client who abuses prescription drugs?
1. Herbal substitutes are safer to use.
2. Medication should be used only for the reason prescribed.
3. The client should consult a physician before using a drug.
4. Consider if family members influence the client to use drugs.

48. The family of an adolescent who smokes marijuana asks a nurse if the use of marijuana leads to abuse of other drugs. Which response is <u>best</u>?
1. "Use of marijuana is a stage your child will go through."
2. "Many people use marijuana and don't use other street drugs."
3. "Use of marijuana can lead to abuse of more potent substances."
4. "It's difficult to answer that question as I don't know your child."

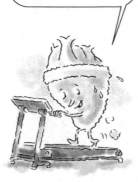

Somebody slow this thing down, please!

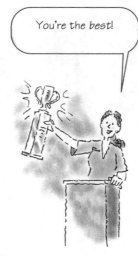

You're the best!

45. 1. It's common for a person withdrawing from amphetamines to experience disturbed sleep and unpleasant dreams. Increased yawning is seen with clients withdrawing from opioids. Psychomotor agitation is seen in cocaine withdrawal, and the inability to concentrate is seen in caffeine withdrawal.
CN: Psychosocial integrity; CNS: None; CL: Application

46. 1. Tachycardia is common because cocaine increases the heart's demand for oxygen. Cocaine doesn't cause hyperthermia (elevated temperature), hypotension (decreased blood pressure), or bradypnea (decreased respiratory rate).
CN: Psychosocial integrity; CNS: None; CL: Application

47. 2. People often take prescribed drugs for reasons other than those intended, primarily to self-medicate or experience a sense of euphoria. The safety and efficacy of most herbal remedies hasn't been established. Sometimes over-the-counter medications are necessary for minor problems. There may be a family history of substance abuse, but it isn't a priority when planning nursing care.
CN: Psychosocial integrity; CNS: None; CL: Application

48. 3. Marijuana is considered a "gateway drug" because it tends to lead to the abuse of more potent drugs. People who use marijuana tend to use or at least experiment with more potent substances. Marijuana isn't a part of a developmental stage that adolescents go through. It isn't important that the nurse knows the child.
CN: Psychosocial integrity; CNS: None; CL: Application

CN: Client needs category CNS: Client needs subcategory CL: Cognitive level

49. A pregnant client is thinking about stopping cocaine use. Which statement by the client indicates effective teaching about pregnancy and drug use?
1. "Right after birth, I'll give the baby up for adoption."
2. "I'll help the baby get through the withdrawal period."
3. "I don't want the baby to have withdrawal symptoms."
4. "It's scary to think the baby may have Down syndrome."

49. 3. Neonates born to mothers addicted to cocaine have withdrawal symptoms at birth. If the client says she'll give the baby up for adoption after birth or help the baby get through the withdrawal period, the teaching was ineffective because the mother doesn't see the impact of her drug use on the child. Use of cocaine during pregnancy doesn't contribute to the baby having Down syndrome.
CN: Psychosocial integrity; CNS: None; CL: Analysis

50. Which test might be ordered for a client with a history of cocaine abuse who exhibits behavior changes following a return from an inpatient treatment facility?
1. Antibody screen
2. Glucose screen
3. Hepatic screen
4. Urine screen

50. 4. A urine toxicology screen would show the presence of cocaine in the body. Glucose, hepatic, or antibody screening wouldn't show the presence of cocaine in the body.
CN: Psychosocial integrity; CNS: None; CL: Application

51. A nurse is assessing a client with a history of substance abuse who has pinpoint pupils, a heart rate of 56 beats/minute, a respiratory rate of 6 breaths/minute, and temperature of 96.4° F. Which substance should the nurse determine is the most likely cause of the client's symptoms?
1. Opioids
2. Amphetamines
3. Cannabis
4. Alcohol

51. 1. Opioids, such as morphine and heroin, can cause pinpont pupils and a reduced heart rate, respiratory rate, and body temperature with intoxication. Amphetamine intoxication can lead to tachycardia, euphoria, and irritability. Cannabis (marijuana) intoxication can cause slowed reflexes, lethargy, and tachycardia. Alcohol intoxication leads to slurred speech, unsteady gait, and uncoordination.
CN: Psychosocial integrity; CNS: None; CL: Application

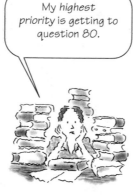

My *highest* priority is getting to question 80.

52. Which intervention is the <u>highest priority</u> in planning care for a client recovering from cocaine use?
1. Skin care
2. Suicide precautions
3. Frequent orientation
4. Nutrition consultation

52. 2. Clients recovering from cocaine use are prone to "postcoke depression" and have a likelihood of becoming suicidal if they can't take the drug. Frequent orientation and skin care are routine nursing interventions but aren't the most immediate considerations for this client. Nutrition consultation isn't the most pressing intervention for this client.
CN: Safe, effective care environment; CNS: Management of care; CL: Analysis

53. Which clinical condition is frequently seen with substance abuse clients who repeatedly use cocaine?
1. Panic attacks
2. Bipolar cycling
3. Attention deficits
4. Expressive aphasia

53. 2. Clients who frequently use cocaine will experience the rapid cycling effect of excitement and then severe depression. They don't tend to experience panic attacks, expressive aphasia, or attention deficits.
CN: Psychosocial integrity; CNS: None; CL: Analysis

54. A client who uses cocaine finally admits he also abused other drugs to <u>equalize the effect</u> of cocaine. Which substance might be included in the client's pattern of polysubstance abuse?
1. Alcohol
2. Amphetamines
3. Caffeine
4. Phencyclidine

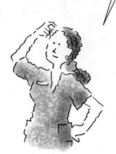

What would have the opposite effect?

54. 1. A cocaine addict will commonly use alcohol to decrease or equalize the stimulating effects of cocaine. Caffeine, phencyclidine, and amphetamines aren't used to equalize the stimulating effects of cocaine.
CN: Psychosocial integrity; CNS: None; CL: Application

55. A group of teenagers tell the school nurse they used cocaine because they were bored. Which short-term goal is the <u>most important</u> for the nurse to immediately initiate?
1. Prepare a drug lecture.
2. Restrict school privileges.
3. Establish an activity schedule.
4. Report the incident to their parents.

55. 3. Having an activity schedule enables the adolescents to develop coping skills to make better choices about what to do with their free time. Preparing a drug lecture or restricting school privileges won't be seen as useful by the adolescents and may inadvertently contribute to their inappropriate behavior. As the nurse works with the adolescents, it would be more effective to have the children talk to their parents about their drug use.
CN: Psychosocial integrity; CNS: None; CL: Application

56. Which statement by a client indicates teaching about cocaine use has been effective?
1. "I wasn't using cocaine to feel better about myself."
2. "I started using cocaine more and more until I couldn't stop."
3. "I'm not addicted to cocaine because I don't use it every day."
4. "I'm not going to be a chronic user, I only use it on holidays."

Don't panic now. Just attack this question with your eyes wide open.

56. 2. This statement reflects the trajectory or common pattern of cocaine use and indicates successful teaching. The first option reflects the client's denial. People gravitate to the drug and continue its use because it gives them a sense of well-being, competency, and power. Cocaine abusers tend to be binge users and can be drug-free for days or weeks between use, but they still have a drug problem. The fourth option indicates the client is in denial about the drug's potential to become a habit. Effective teaching didn't occur.
CN: Psychosocial integrity; CNS: None; CL: Analysis

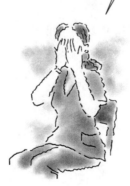

57. A client who formerly used lysergic acid diethylamide (LSD) is seeking counseling. Which characteristic or condition in the mental health history would be seen in this client?
1. Lack of trust
2. Panic attacks
3. Recurrent depression
4. Loss of ego boundaries

57. 2. Clients who used LSD typically have a history of panic attacks or psychotic behavior. This is often referred to as a "bad trip." Loss of ego boundaries, recurrent depression, and lack of trust don't tend to be problems for this type of client.
CN: Psychosocial integrity; CNS: None; CL: Analysis

CN: Client needs category   CNS: Client needs subcategory   CL: Cognitive level

58. A nurse is writing a nursing care plan for a client who has been using phencyclidine (PCP). Assessment for which emergency should be included?
1. Cardiac arrest
2. Seizure disorder
3. Violent behavior
4. Delirium reaction

59. A client who smoked marijuana daily for 10 years tells a nurse, "I don't have any goals, and I just don't know what to do." Which communication technique is the <u>most useful</u> when talking to this client?
1. Focus the interaction.
2. Use nonverbal methods.
3. Use reflection techniques.
4. Ask open-ended questions.

60. A nurse is assessing a client who uses heroin to determine if there are physical health problems. Which medical consequence of heroin use frequently occurs?
1. Hepatitis
2. Peptic ulcers
3. Hypertension
4. Chronic pharyngitis

61. The family of a client in rehabilitation following heroin withdrawal asks a nurse why the client is receiving naltrexone (ReVia). Which response is correct?
1. To help reverse withdrawal symptoms
2. To keep the client sedated during withdrawal
3. To take the place of detoxification with methadone
4. To decrease the client's memory of the withdrawal experience

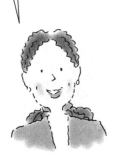

You're almost at question 60. That should motivate you to keep moving!

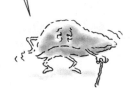

I feel so abused.

58. 3. When a client is using phencyclidine, an acute psychotic reaction can occur. The client is capable of sudden, explosive, violent behavior. Phencyclidine doesn't tend to cause cardiac arrest or a seizure disorder. Delirium is associated with inhalant intoxication.
CN: Physiological integrity; CNS: Reduction of risk potential; CL: Application

59. 1. A client with amotivational syndrome from chronic use of marijuana tends to talk in tangents and needs the nurse to focus the conversation. Nonverbal communication or reflection techniques wouldn't be useful as this client must focus and learn to identify and accomplish goals. Using only open-ended questions won't allow the client to focus and establish specific goals.
CN: Psychosocial integrity; CNS: None; CL: Application

60. 1. Hepatitis is the most common medical complication of heroin abuse. Peptic ulcers are more likely to be a complication of caffeine use, hypertension is a complication of amphetamine use, and chronic pharyngitis is a complication of marijuana use.
CN: Physiological integrity; CNS: Physiological adaptation; CL: Application

61. 1. Naltrexone is an opioid antagonist and helps the client stay drug-free. Keeping the client sedated during withdrawal isn't the reason for giving this drug. The drug doesn't decrease the client's memory of the withdrawal experience and isn't used in place of detoxification with methadone.
CN: Psychosocial integrity; CNS: None; CL: Application

62. Which nursing intervention has <u>priority</u> in a care plan for a client recovering from cocaine addiction?
1. Help the client find ways to be happy and competent.
2. Foster the creative use of self in community activities.
3. Teach the client to handle stresses in the work setting.
4. Help the client acknowledge the current level of dependency.

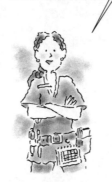

Maybe we should be called priority engineers instead of nurses.

62. 1. The major component of a treatment program for a client with cocaine addiction is to have the client feel happy and competent. Cocaine addiction is difficult to treat because the drug actions reinforce its use. There are often perceived positive effects. Clients often credit the drug with giving them creative energy instead of looking within themselves. Fostering the creative use of self may inadvertently reinforce the client's drug use. Teaching the client to handle stresses is appropriate but isn't the most immediate nursing action. Examining the client's level of dependency isn't the immediate choice, as the client needs to work on remaining drug free.
CN: Safe, effective care environment; CNS: Management of care; CL: Application

63. A client tells a nurse, "I've been clean from drugs for the past 5 years, but my life really hasn't changed." Which concept should be explored with this client?
1. Further education
2. Conflict resolution
3. Career development
4. Personal development

63. 4. True recovery involves changing the client's distorted thinking and working on personal and emotional development. Before the client pursues further education, career development, or conflict resolution skills, it's imperative the client devotes energy to emotional and personal development.
CN: Psychosocial integrity; CNS: None; CL: Analysis

64. A client discusses how drug addiction has made life unmanageable. Which information will help the client cope with the drug problem?
1. How peers have committed to sobriety
2. How to accomplish family of origin work
3. The addiction process and tools for recovery
4. How environmental stimuli serve as drug triggers

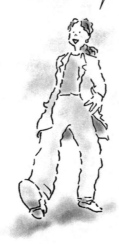

A journey of a thousand miles starts with one step.

64. 3. When the client admits life has become unmanageable, the best strategy is to teach about the addiction, how to obtain support, and how to develop new coping skills. Information about how peers committed to sobriety would be shared with the client as the treatment process begins. Identification of how environmental stimuli serve as drug triggers would be a later part of the treatment process and family of origin work. Initially, the client must commit to sobriety and learn skills for recovery.
CN: Psychosocial integrity; CNS: None; CL: Analysis

65. A nurse is collecting data from a client with a history of cocaine abuse. Which condition might <u>typically</u> be found with this client?
1. Glossitis
2. Pharyngitis
3. Bilateral ear infections
4. Perforated nasal septum

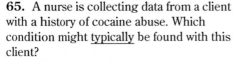

65. 4. When cocaine is snorted frequently, the client often develops a perforated nasal septum. Bilateral ear infections, pharyngitis, and glossitis aren't common physical findings for a client with a history of cocaine abuse.
CN: Psychosocial integrity; CNS: None; CL: Application

CN: Client needs category   CNS: Client needs subcategory   CL: Cognitive level

66. A client recovering from cocaine abuse is participating in group therapy. Which statement by the client indicates the client has benefited from the group?
1. "I think the laws about drug possession are too strict in this country."
2. "I'll be more careful about talking about my drug use to my children."
3. "I finally realize the short high from cocaine isn't worth the depression."
4. "I can't understand how I could get all these problems that we talked about in group."

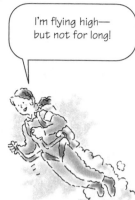

I'm flying high—but not for long!

67. A family expresses concern that a member who stopped using amphetamines 3 months ago is acting paranoid. Which explanation is the best?
1. A person gets symptoms of paranoia with polysubstance abuse.
2. When a person uses amphetamines, paranoid tendencies may continue for months.
3. Sometimes family dynamics and a high suspicion of continued drug use make a person paranoid.
4. Amphetamine abusers may have severe anxiety and paranoid thinking.

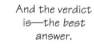

And the verdict is—the best answer.

68. A nurse is trying to determine if a client who abuses heroin has any drug-related legal problems. Which assessment question is the best to ask the client?
1. When did your spouse become aware of your use of heroin?
2. Do you have a probation officer that you report to periodically?
3. Have you experienced any legal violations while being intoxicated?
4. Do you have a history of frequent visits with the employee assistance program manager?

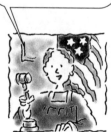

69. The severity of withdrawal symptoms for a client addicted to heroin may depend on which factor?
1. Ego strength
2. Liver function
3. Seizure history
4. Kidney function

66. 3. This is a realistic appraisal of a client's experience with cocaine and how harmful the experience is. The first option indicates the client was distracting self from personal issues and isn't working on goals in the group setting. Talking about drugs to children must be reinforced with nonverbal behavior, and not talking about drugs may give children the wrong message about drug use. The fourth option indicates the client is in denial about the consequences of cocaine use.
CN: Psychosocial integrity; CNS: None; CL: Analysis

67. 2. After a client uses amphetamines, there may be long-term effects that exist for months after use. Two common effects are paranoia and ideas of reference. Even with polysubstance abuse, the paranoia comes from the chronic use of amphetamines. The third option blames the family when the paranoia comes from the drug use. Severe anxiety isn't typically manifested in paranoid thinking.
CN: Psychosocial integrity; CNS: None; CL: Analysis

68. 3. This question focuses on obtaining direct information about drug-related legal problems. When a spouse becomes aware of a partner's substance abuse, the first action isn't necessarily to institute legal action. Even if the client reports to a probation officer, the offense isn't necessarily a drug-related problem. Asking if the client has a history of frequent visits with the employee assistance program manager isn't useful. It assumes any visit to the employee assistance program manager is related to drug issues.
CN: Psychosocial integrity; CNS: None; CL: Analysis

69. 2. Liver function status is an important variable that can be used to indicate the severity of a client's drug withdrawal. Ego strength, seizure history, and kidney function aren't variables that can be used to predict the severity of withdrawal symptoms.
CN: Physiological integrity; CNS: Reduction of risk potential; CL: Analysis

70. A client who uses cocaine denies that drug use is a problem. Which intervention strategy would be best to confront the client's denial?
1. State ways to cope with stress.
2. Repeat the drug facts as needed.
3. Identify the client's ambivalence.
4. Use open-ended, factual questions.

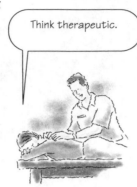

Think therapeutic.

70. 4. The use of open-ended, factual questions will help the client acknowledge that a drug problem is present. Stating ways to cope with stress and identifying the client's ambivalence won't be effective for breaking through a client's denial. Repeating drug facts won't be effective, as the client will perceive it as preaching or nagging.
CN: Psychosocial integrity; CNS: None; CL: Application

71. A nurse is working with parents of an adolescent client who abuses inhalants. Which information about consequences is best to include in a teaching plan?
1. Consequences must be enforceable.
2. Everything can become a consequence.
3. When setting consequences, be verbally forceful.
4. Consequences are seldom needed with adolescents.

71. 1. Consequences must be specific and enforceable. Sometimes parents are prone to make consequences that are too difficult to enforce or that actually become a punishment for the parents. Everything can't be made into a consequence. Being verbally forceful isn't appropriate because the consequence can occur in a civil tone of voice. A consequence can be used with every person regardless of developmental stage.
CN: Psychosocial integrity; CNS: None; CL: Analysis

72. A nurse is caring for a client undergoing treatment for cocaine abuse. The nurse should expect the client to make which statement if the client is pessimistic about treatment?
1. "I'll never get better. This is useless."
2. "I don't think I want to see my family anymore. They're not supportive."
3. "I'm fatigued all the time. My energy is low."
4. "I want to get better now. Can't we rush the treatment?"

72. 1. Clients withdrawing from drugs such as cocaine frequently experience depression. It's common for drug-addicted clients to experience fatigue without becoming pessimistic. Being impulsive or having feelings of estrangement aren't necessarily related to a client becoming pessimistic about treatment.
CN: Psychosocial integrity; CNS: None; CL: Analysis

73. A nurse is working with a client addicted to cocaine who is in denial. Which approach is most useful for dealing with the client's denial?
1. Ask whether the client sees the drug use as a problem.
2. Focus on the pain the client is having during withdrawal.
3. Reinforce the connection between drug use and harmful results.
4. Help the client recognize reality by pointing out withdrawal symptoms.

Only a handful of questions to go!

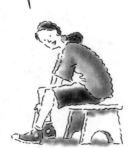

73. 3. To deal with the client's denial, the nurse must confront the drug use and point out the results of the behavior. Asking if the client sees the drug use as a problem will only reinforce the client's denial and provide a forum to intellectualize the problem or provide excuses for it. Pain isn't associated with withdrawal from cocaine. Pointing out withdrawal symptoms may not be the most effective strategy, as the client often downplays the significance of the problem.
CN: Psychosocial integrity; CNS: None; CL: Analysis

CN: Client needs category CNS: Client needs subcategory CL: Cognitive level

74. A client who uses cocaine is admitted to an intensive outpatient rehabilitation program. During cocaine withdrawal, which finding should the nurse expect when assessing the client?
1. GI distress
2. Blurred vision
3. Perceptual distortions
4. Increased appetite

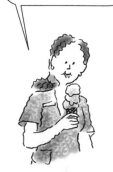

Which finding should you expect in question 74?

74. 4. Increased appetite is typical during cocaine or nicotine withdrawal. GI distress (especially nausea and vomiting) occurs during alcohol or opioid withdrawal. Blurred vision isn't typical in cocaine withdrawal. Perceptual distortions are common during withdrawal from phencyclidine (PCP, or "angel dust"), amphetamines, and hallucinogens.
CN: Physiological integrity; CNS: Physiological adaptation; CL: Application

75. A client who abuses alcohol is admitted to an outpatient drug and alcohol treatment facility. What's the most objective assessment method for determining if the client is still using alcohol?
1. Having the client walk a straight line
2. Smelling the client's breath
3. Giving the client a breath alcohol test
4. Asking the client if he has been drinking

75. 3. A breath alcohol test is the most objective way to determine if the client is still using alcohol. Having him walk a straight line and smelling his breath aren't objective tests. Asking him if he has been drinking may not elicit an honest answer (many clients who abuse alcohol deny alcohol use).
CN: Psychosocial integrity; CNS: None; CL: Application

76. During nicotine withdrawal, which client statement is typical?
1. "I sometimes feel like I'm seeing things."
2. "I feel lousy, and I'm grumpy with everybody."
3. "I can't believe I feel fine after just having stopped smoking."
4. "I'm always yawning now."

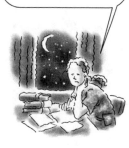

This isn't one of my better moments.

76. 2. During nicotine withdrawal, the client is typically irritable and nervous. Seeing things (hallucinations) isn't linked to nicotine withdrawal. A client going through nicotine withdrawal is unlikely to "feel fine." Yawning is associated with withdrawal from opioids, not nicotine.
CN: Physiological integrity; CNS: Physiological adaptation; CL: Application

77. A polyaddicted client is hospitalized for withdrawal complications. During his stay in a medical step-down unit, which immediate short-term goal takes highest priority?
1. The client will remain safe during the detoxification period.
2. The client will develop an accurate perception of his drug problem.
3. The client will abstain from mood-altering drugs.
4. The client will learn coping strategies to help him stop relying on drugs.

77. 1. Client safety takes highest priority during detoxification. During this time, it's unrealistic to expect clients to perceive their drug problems accurately; typically, they experience cognitive impairment or deny their addiction. In the hospital, the client usually doesn't have access to drugs and should be drug-free; the goal of abstaining from mood-altering drugs takes highest priority after discharge. Learning coping strategies is an appropriate goal immediately after withdrawal and when medical care is completed.
CN: Safe, effective care environment; CNS: Management of care; CL: Application

78. A client with an alcohol addiction requests a prescription for disulfiram (Antabuse). To determine the client's ability to take this drug appropriately, the nurse should focus on which factor?
1. Whether the client will take a prescription drug
2. Whether the client's family accepts the use of this treatment strategy
3. Whether the client is willing to follow the necessary dietary restrictions
4. Whether the client is motivated to stay sober

78. 4. A client with a strong craving for alcohol (and a lack of impulse control) isn't a good candidate for disulfiram therapy. Disulfiram is a prescription drug. Accepting the treatment strategy is a decision that the client and health care provider make; although family input may be welcome, family members don't make the final decision. Significant dietary restrictions aren't necessary during disulfiram therapy (except for alcohol and foods prepared or cooked in it).
CN: Psychosocial integrity; CNS: None; CL: Analysis

79. A nurse has developed a relationship with a client who has an addiction problem. Which information should indicate that the therapeutic interaction is in the working stage? Select all that apply:
1. The client addresses how the addiction has contributed to family distress.
2. The client reluctantly shares the family history of addiction.
3. The client verbalizes difficulty identifying personal strengths.
4. The client discusses financial problems related to the addiction.
5. The client expresses uncertainty about meeting with the nurse.
6. The client acknowledges the addiction's effects on the children.

79. 1, 3, 6. These statements are indicative of the nurse-client working phase, in which the client explores, evaluates, and determines solutions to identified problems. The remaining statements address what happens during the introductory phase of the nurse-client interaction.
CN: Psychosocial integrity; CNS: None; CL: Analysis

80. A client is receiving chlordiazepoxide (Librium) to control the symptoms of alcohol withdrawal. The chlordiazepoxide has been ordered as needed. Which symptoms may indicate the need for an additional dose of the medication? Select all that apply:
1. Tachycardia
2. Mood swings
3. Elevated blood pressure and temperature
4. Piloerection
5. Tremors
6. Increasing anxiety

80. 1, 3, 5, 6. Benzodiazepines are usually administered based on elevations in heart rate, blood pressure, and temperature as well as on the presence of tremors and increasing anxiety. Mood swings are expected during the withdrawal period and are not an indication for further medication administration. Piloerection is not a symptom of alcohol withdrawal.
CN: Physiological integrity; CNS: Pharmacological and parenteral therapies; CL: Analysis

You've finished chapter 19. You deserve a standing ovation!

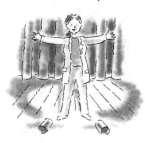

CN: Client needs category   CNS: Client needs subcategory   CL: Cognitive level

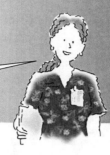

For more information on dissociative disorders, check this independent Web site: www.mentalhealth.com.

Chapter 20
Dissociative disorders

1. When taking a history from a client with dissociative identity disorder (DID), the nurse should expect the client to make which statement?
　1. "My father wasn't around much."
　2. "I feel good about myself."
　3. "I can recall many traumatic events from childhood."
　4. "My father loved me one day and hit me the next day."

2. A nursing care plan for a client with dissociative identity disorder (DID) should address which factor?
　1. Ritualistic behavior
　2. Out-of-body experiences
　3. History of severe childhood abuse
　4. Ability to give a thorough personal history

3. Which nursing diagnosis is most appropriate for a client with dissociative identity disorder (DID)?
　1. *Disturbed personal identity related to delusional ideations*
　2. *Risk for self-directed violence related to suicidal ideations or gestures*
　3. *Deficient diversional activity related to lack of environmental stimulation*
　4. *Disturbed sensory perception: visual hallucinations related to altered sensory reception of visual stimulation*

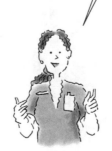

Nursing diagnoses standardize client care.

1. 4. Repeated exposure to a childhood environment that alternates between highly stressful and then loving and supportive can be a factor in the development of DID. Many children grow up in a household without a father but don't develop DID. Clients with DID commonly have low self-esteem. Because of dissociation from the trauma, a client with DID usually can't recall childhood traumatic events.
CN: Psychosocial integrity; CNS: None; CL: Application

2. 3. DID is theorized to develop as a protective response to such traumatic experiences as severe child abuse. Ritualistic behavior is seen with obsessive-compulsive disorders. Out-of-body experiences are more commonly associated with depersonalization disorder. Because of the dissociative response to personal experiences, people with DID are usually unable to give a thorough personal history.
CN: Psychosocial integrity; CNS: None; CL: Application

3. 2. A common reason clients with DID are admitted to a psychiatric facility is because one of the alter personalities is trying to kill another personality. Hallucinations, delusions, and personal identity disturbances are commonly associated with schizophrenic disorders. Because of the assortment of alter personalities controlling the client with DID, diversional activity deficit is rarely a problem.
CN: Safe, effective care environment; CNS: Management of care; CL: Application

CN: Client needs category　　CNS: Client needs subcategory　　CL: Cognitive level

4. Which nursing intervention is important for a client with dissociative identity disorder (DID)?
1. Give antipsychotic medications as prescribed.
2. Maintain consistency when interacting with the client.
3. Confront the client about the use of alter personalities.
4. Prevent the client from interacting with others when one of the alter personalities is in control.

5. A nurse notes a change in voice and mannerisms of a client with dissociative identity disorder (DID) after he learns that his wife has filed for a divorce. Which nursing intervention is <u>most appropriate?</u>
1. Avoid discussing the client's feelings.
2. Force the client to discuss his feelings.
3. Offer encouragement to the client that he'll be able to cope with the divorce.
4. Encourage the client to verbalize his feelings about the divorce.

6. A nurse determines therapeutic interactions have been successful when a client with dissociative identity disorder (DID) shows which behavior or reaction?
1. Confronts the abuser
2. Attends the unit's milieu meetings
3. Prevents alter personalities from emerging
4. Reports no longer having feelings of anger about childhood traumas

7. Which of the following behaviors is indicative of a client with dissociative identity disorder (DID)?
1. Complaining of physical health problems with no organic basis
2. Being unable to account for certain times on a day-to-day basis
3. Participating in discussions about abusive incidents that occurred in the past
4. Being able to form a therapeutic relationship with the nurse after meeting twice

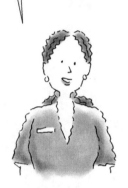

Understanding the client's problem allows you to provide more effective care.

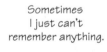

Sometimes I just can't remember anything.

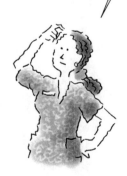

4. 2. Establishing trust and support is important when interacting with a client with DID. Many of these clients have had few healthy relationships. Medication hasn't proven effective in the treatment of DID. Confronting the client about the alter personalities would be ineffective because the client has little, if any, knowledge of the presence of these other personalities. Isolating the client wouldn't be therapeutically beneficial.
CN: Safe, effective care environment; CNS: Management of care; CL: Analysis

5. 4. Encouraging a client with DID to verbalize his feelings will help him cope with his anxieties. Forcing the client to discuss his feelings can increase his level of anxiety. Avoiding discussion of feelings doesn't reduce anxiety and avoids the issue. Offering encouragement that the client will be able to cope with the divorce gives false reassurance and can erode the client's trust in the nurse.
CN: Psychosocial integrity; CNS: None; CL: Analysis

6. 2. Attending milieu meetings decreases feelings of isolation and shows the client has begun to trust the nurse. Often the abuser was a part of the client's childhood, and confrontation in adulthood may not be possible or therapeutic. The client is often unaware of an alter personality and thus can't prevent these alter personalities from emerging. Clients with DID have dissociated from painful experiences, so the host personality often doesn't have negative feelings about such experiences.
CN: Psychosocial integrity; CNS: None; CL: Analysis

7. 2. When alter personalities are in control, periods of amnesia are common for clients with DID. Complaining of physical health problems with no organic basis describes clients with somatoform disorder. The client doesn't have memories of the abusive episodes, so he's unable to participate in discussions. These clients typically are slow in forming trusting relationships because many past relationships have been hurtful.
CN: Psychosocial integrity; CNS: None; CL: Application

CN: Client needs category   CNS: Client needs subcategory   CL: Cognitive level

8. A nurse is caring for a client with a dissociative disorder. Which intervention should the nurse include in the care plan?
1. Plan activities in which the client will be successful.
2. Offer praise whether or not the client has been successful.
3. Have the client engage in repetitive activities to reduce stress.
4. Encourage the client to keep a journal to recognize unsuccessful coping strategies.

9. A hospitalized client with dissociative identity disorder (DID) reports hearing voices. Which nursing intervention is <u>most appropriate</u>?
1. Tell the client to lie down and rest.
2. Give an as-needed dose of haloperidol (Haldol).
3. Encourage the client to continue with his daily activities.
4. Notify the physician that the client is having a psychotic episode.

10. Which goal would be the <u>most</u> important for a client with dissociative identity disorder (DID)?
1. Learning how to control periods of mania.
2. Learning how to integrate all the alternate personalities.
3. Developing coping strategies to deal with the traumatic childhood.
4. Determining what is causing them to feel they have periods of "lost time."

11. A client with dissociative identity disorder reports hearing voices and asks the nurse if that means he's "crazy." Which response would be the <u>most appropriate</u>?
1. "What do the voices tell you?"
2. "Why would you think you're crazy?"
3. "Clients with DID often report hearing voices."
4. "Hearing voices is often a symptom of schizophrenia."

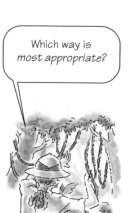

Which way is *most appropriate?*

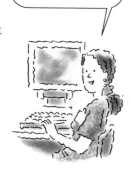

Think *therapeutic here.*

8. 1. The care plan should include activities that will help the client be successful and feel a sense of accomplishment. Offering false praise can harm the nurse–client relationship and erode any sense of trust that develops. Repetitive activities and keeping a journal aren't appropriate therapeutic interventions for this client.
CN: Psychosocial integrity; CNS: None; CL: Application

9. 3. Because many clients with DID hear voices, it's appropriate to have the client continue with daily activities. Having the client lie down and rest would have no therapeutic value. The voices the client hears are probably alter personalities communicating. This doesn't indicate a psychotic episode, so the physician wouldn't be notified to prescribe such antipsychotic medication as haloperidol.
CN: Safe, effective care environment; CNS: Management of care; CL: Application

10. 4. The initial symptom many clients with DID experience, prompting them to seek health care, is the sensation of lost time. These are times the alter personalities are in control. Before therapeutic interventions, clients with DID may not even be aware of childhood trauma because of dissociation from the event. Initially, the client with DID isn't aware of the presence of alternate personalities. Depression, not mania, may be another early symptom of clients with DID.
CN: Psychosocial integrity; CNS: None; CL: Application

11. 3. The most therapeutic answer is to give correct information. Asking what the voices tell the client would be changing the topic without answering the question. Asking "why" questions can put the client on the defensive. Schizophrenia isn't the only cause of hearing voices, and this response suggests the client may be schizophrenic.
CN: Psychosocial integrity; CNS: None; CL: Analysis

12. A nurse is preparing to admit a client with dissociative identity disorder (DID) to the inpatient psychiatric unit. Which intervention is most appropriate for this client?
1. Arrange to have staff check on the client every 15 to 30 minutes.
2. Prevent all family from visiting until the third day of hospitalization.
3. Make sure the staff understands the client will be on seizure precautions.
4. Place the client in a quiet room away from the noise of the nurse's station.

13. A client is being treated at a community mental health clinic. A nurse has been instructed to observe for any behaviors indicating dissociative identity disorder (DID). Which behavior would be included?
1. Delusions of grandeur
2. Reports of often being very tired
3. Changes in dress, mannerisms, and voice
4. Refusal to make a follow-up appointment

14. Which statement made by a client with dissociative identity disorder (DID) indicates an understanding of the nurse's teaching plan?
1. "I will never marry."
2. "I won't get better, even with treatment."
3. "I need to take my pills for anxiety."
4. "I need to attend my therapy sessions faithfully."

15. When interacting with a client with a dissociative identity disorder, a nurse observes that one of the alter personalities is in control. Which intervention is the <u>most appropriate</u>?
1. Give recognition to the alter personality.
2. Notify the physician.
3. Immediately stop interacting with the client.
4. Ignore the alter personality, and ask to speak to the host personality.

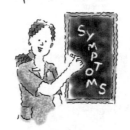

It helps to know what symptoms to watch for.

Stay focused on therapeutic interventions.

12. 1. A common reason for clients with DID to be hospitalized is for suicidal ideations or gestures. For the client's safety, frequent checks should be done. Family interactions might be therapeutic for the client, and the family may be able to provide a more thorough history because of the client's dissociation from traumatic events. Seizure activity isn't an expected symptom of DID. Because of the possibility of suicide, the client's room should be close to the nurse's station.
CN: Psychosocial integrity; CNS: None; CL: Application

13. 3. When alter personalities are in control, the person will have complete personality changes. Delusions of grandeur are more frequently associated with disorders such as manic states and schizophrenia. Complaints of fatigue aren't a main symptom of DID. The refusal to make a follow-up appointment could indicate many problems, including noncompliance.
CN: Psychosocial integrity; CNS: None; CL: Application

14. 4. Most clients with DID can be successfully treated with long-term therapy. For many of the conditions, pharmacologic therapy has little effect. Many clients with DID marry.
CN: Psychosocial integrity; CNS: None; CL: Application

15. 1. By giving recognition to the alter personalities, the nurse conveys to the client that she believes the alter personalities exist. The physician doesn't need to be notified because this is an expected occurrence. Asking to speak to the host personality or immediately stopping interaction with the client won't stop the client from being controlled by alter personalities.
CN: Psychosocial integrity; CNS: None; CL: Application

CN: Client needs category   CNS: Client needs subcategory   CL: Cognitive level

16. A client with dissociative identity disorder (DID) indicates that he understands the need to continue therapy when he makes which statement?
1. "Therapy will help eliminate my family problems."
2. "I must continue going to outpatient treatment for the next 2 months."
3. "I understand that I need to integrate all my alter personalities into one."
4. "Once therapy is complete, I won't have the traits of my alter personalities."

16. 3. The main goal of therapy for clients with DID is to integrate, not eliminate, the alter personalities. Therapy is often long-term. Through therapy, the client can learn how to cope with family problems.
CN: Psychosocial integrity; CNS: None; CL: Application

17. A family member of a client with dissociative identity disorder (DID) asks a nurse if hypnotic therapy might help the client. Which response would be <u>most appropriate</u>?
1. "What would make you think that?"
2. "No, hypnosis is rarely used in the treatment of psychiatric conditions."
3. "Yes, but this treatment is used only after other types of therapy have failed."
4. "Yes, often the client doesn't have conscious awareness of alter personalities."

17. 4. Because of dissociation from painful events, hypnosis is often very effective in the treatment of clients with DID. It may be under hypnosis that alter personalities start to emerge. Hypnosis is used in a variety of psychiatric conditions. The first option could place the family member on the defensive. Hypnosis is often a first-line treatment for the client with DID.
CN: Psychosocial integrity; CNS: None; CL: Application

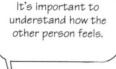

It's important to understand how the other person feels.

18. Which intervention is appropriate when caring for a client with dissociative identity disorder?
1. Remind the alter personalities they're part of the host personality.
2. Interact with the client only when the host personality is in control.
3. Establish an empathetic relationship with each emerging personality.
4. Provide positive reinforcement to the client when calm alter personalities are present instead of angry ones.

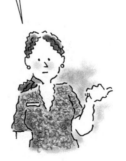

18. 3. Establishing an empathetic relationship with each emerging personality provides a therapeutic environment to care for the client. Interacting with the client only when the host personality is in control would be useless because the client has limited, if any, control or awareness when alter personalities are in control.
CN: Psychosocial integrity; CNS: None; CL: Application

19. While interacting with a client with dissociative identity disorder (DID), a nurse observes one of the alter personalities take over. The client goes from being very calm to angry and shouting. Which response would be most appropriate?
1. "Is one of you upset?"
2. "Why have you become angry?"
3. "Tell me what you're feeling right now."
4. "Let me speak to someone who isn't angry."

19. 3. This response encourages integration and discourages dissociation. When interacting with clients with DID, the nurse always wants to remind the client that the alter personalities are a component of one person. Responses reinforcing interaction with only one alter personality instead of trying to interact with the individual as a single person aren't appropriate. Asking "why" questions can put the client on the defensive and impede further communication.
CN: Psychosocial integrity; CNS: None; CL: Application

20. A client with dissociative identity disorder has been in therapy for 2 years and just learned her father passed away. Her father sexually abused her throughout her childhood. Which intervention would be most appropriate?
1. Have the client seek inpatient therapy.
2. Encourage the client's verbalization of feelings of anger and guilt.
3. Encourage the client's alter personalities to emerge during this stressful time.
4. Stress to the client that the death of the abuser should be very helpful in her healing process.

21. Which activity is <u>most</u> appropriate for a client with dissociative identity disorder (DID)?
1. Group therapy with only clients who have DID
2. Inpatient therapy groups led by a psychologist
3. Support group with adult survivors of child abuse
4. Group therapy with clients who have a variety of diagnoses

22. A nurse observes that the alter personality of a client with a dissociative identity disorder is in control. The client is sitting in the dayroom, interacting with others. His voice becomes louder and more intense and he's tearful and confused. Which action would be most appropriate?
1. Allow the client to continue interacting with clients in the dayroom.
2. Ask to speak to one of the adult alter personalities of the host personality.
3. Remove the client from the dayroom, and allow the client to play with toys.
4. Remove the client from the dayroom, and reorient him that he's in a safe place.

23. A nurse on the psychiatric unit is caring for a 51-year-old male client who's suicidal. Which nursing intervention takes <u>priority</u>?
1. Discouraging sleep except at bedtime
2. Making a verbal contract with the client to notify the staff of suicidal thoughts
3. Limiting time spent alone by encouraging the client to participate in group activities
4. Creating a safe physical and interpersonal environment

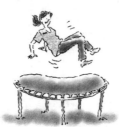

Keep it up, you're doing great!

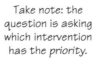

Take note: the question is asking which intervention has the *priority.*

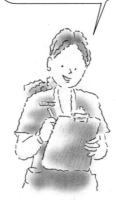

20. 2. The death of the abuser may cause the client to experience feelings of anger and guilt. Unless the client becomes suicidal or rapidly deteriorates, inpatient treatment won't be necessary. Encouraging the client's alter personalities to emerge could result in further dissociation. The death of the abuser can be a very stressful event and can leave the client with unresolved feelings.
CN: Health promotion and maintenance; CNS: None; CL: Analysis

21. 1. Homogenous group therapy has proven to be the most beneficial for clients with DID. In other groups, the members may find interacting on such an intimate level with a client with DID overwhelming and frightening. Not all victims of child abuse develop DID. Unless the client with DID is suicidal, hospitalization isn't required.
CN: Psychosocial integrity; CNS: None; CL: Application

22. 4. Removing the client at this time may protect him from future embarrassment. Asking to speak to an alter personality encourages dissociation. Allowing the client to play with toys also reinforces and encourages dissociation. Reorienting the client discourages dissociation and encourages integration.
CN: Safe, effective care environment; CNS: Safety and infection control; CL: Analysis

23. 4. Creating a safe environment, including removing obvious hazards, recognizing non-obvious hazards, maintaining close observation, serving as a client advocate in interpersonal situations, and communicating concern to the client in verbal and non-verbal ways, is the nurse's highest priority. Other interventions, such as discouraging sleep except at bedtime, making a verbal contract, and encouraging participation in group activities, should be included in the client's plan, but these don't have top priority.
CN: Psychosocial integrity; CNS: None; CL: Application

CN: Client needs category   CNS: Client needs subcategory   CL: Cognitive level

24. A 14-year-old client is admitted to an inpatient adolescent unit. The treatment team believes he has dissociative identity disorder (DID). Based on this information, which intervention should the nurse anticipate using?
1. Request a social work consultation.
2. Institute elopement precautions.
3. Confront the parents about the staff's suspicion of child abuse.
4. Prevent the client from interacting with other clients on the unit.

25. Which behavior reported by a family member of a client with dissociative identity disorder (DID) indicates that the client's therapy is effective?
1. The client is forgetful.
2. The client sleeps through the night.
3. The client has had several unsuccessful relationships.
4. The client hears voices.

26. A client with dissociative identity disorder (DID) is admitted to an inpatient psychiatric unit. A nurse-manager asked all staff to attend a meeting. Which reason for the meeting is the <u>most likely</u>?
1. To review the restraint protocol with the staff
2. To inform the staff that no one should refuse to work with the client
3. To warn the staff that this client may be difficult and challenging to work with
4. To allow staff members to discuss concerns about working with a client with DID

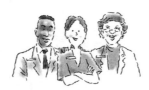

Know when to request a consultation from other medical professionals.

27. A 26-year-old man is reported missing after being the victim of a violent crime. Two months later, a family member finds him working in a city 100 miles from his home. The man doesn't recognize the family member or recall being the victim of a crime. Which condition is the client most likely exhibiting?
1. Depersonalization disorder
2. Dissociative amnesia
3. Dissociative fugue
4. Dissociative identity disorder

24. 1. In many cases, clients with DID have been subjected to child abuse. The social worker is the appropriate person to investigate the child's home setting. The client isn't at any more risk for elopement than the other adolescent clients. Until there has been an investigation into the client's home setting, confrontation wouldn't be appropriate or therapeutic. Clients with DID are always encouraged to interact with other clients on the unit.
CN: Safe, effective care environment; CNS: Management of care; CL: Application

25. 2. Because clients with DID often have sleep disorders, sleeping through the night is a sign of effective therapy. Forgetfulness, difficulty forming relationships, and hallucinations are signs of unsuccessful treatment.
CN: Psychosocial integrity; CNS: None; CL: Analysis

26. 4. Allowing all staff members to meet together may prevent the staff from splitting into groups of those who believe the validity of this diagnosis and those who don't. Unless this client shows behaviors harmful to himself or others, restraints aren't needed. Telling the staff no one should refuse to work with the client or this client will probably be very difficult and challenging sets a very negative tone as staff plan and provide care for the client.
CN: Safe, effective care environment; CNS: Management of care; CL: Application

27. 3. Dissociative fugue is sudden flight after a traumatic event. During the episode, the person may assume a new identity and not recognize people from his past. Depersonalization disorder is the sudden loss of the sense of one's own reality. Dissociative amnesia doesn't involve flight from work or home. Dissociative identity disorder is the coexistence of two or more personalities in one person.
CN: Psychosocial integrity; CNS: None; CL: Application

28. Which nursing intervention is <u>most appropriate</u> for a client who has just had an episode of dissociative fugue?
1. Let the client verbalize the fear and anxiety he feels.
2. Encourage the client to share his experiences during the episode.
3. Have the client sign a contract stating he won't leave the premises again.
4. Tell the client he won't resolve his problems by running away from them.

29. Which statement about dissociative disorders by a family member of a client with a dissociative disorder indicates that the nurse's teaching has been successful?
1. "They occur as a result of incest."
2. "They occur as a result of substance abuse."
3. "They occur in more than 40% of all people."
4. "They occur as a result of the brain trying to protect the person from severe stress."

30. Which nursing intervention would be <u>most appropriate</u> when working with a client who had a recent episode of dissociative fugue?
1. Place the client on elopement precautions.
2. Help the client identify resources to deal with stressful situations.
3. Allow the client to share his experiences about the dissociative fugue episode.
4. Confront the client about his running away from problems instead of dealing with them.

31. A 32-year-old client lost his home in a flood last month. When questioned about his feelings about the loss, he doesn't remember being in a flood or owning a home. Which of the following disorders is the client *most* likely exhibiting?
1. Depersonalization disorder
2. Dissociative amnesia
3. Dissociative fugue
4. Dissociative identity disorder

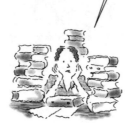

I'm feeling slightly overwhelmed—but it helps to tell someone.

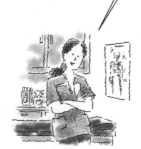

Helping the client help himself is an important aspect of teaching.

28. 1. An episode of dissociative fugue can be a very frightening experience. The client rarely remembers the events during the episode. Signing a contract would have little effect because a dissociative fugue episode isn't something the client consciously wanted to do. Because the client isn't conscious of "running away," this response isn't helpful.
CN: Psychosocial integrity; CNS: None; CL: Analysis

29. 4. Dissociative disorders are thought to be a form of coping with an extreme stressor or event that occurred in the client's life. Incest is only one of many reasons dissociative disorders occur. Typically, substance abuse isn't a cause (but may be an effect) of a dissociative disorder. Dissociative disorders are actually very rare.
CN: Psychosocial integrity; CNS: None; CL: Analysis

30. 2. Dissociative fugue is precipitated by stressful situations. Helping the client identify resources could prevent recurrences. Once the dissociative fugue episode is over, the client returns to normal functioning; he wouldn't be an elopement risk. The client usually has amnesia about the events during the dissociative fugue episode, which limits his ability to share the experience. The client doesn't realize that he's running away from his problems.
CN: Psychosocial integrity; CNS: None; CL: Analysis

31. 2. Dissociative amnesia commonly occurs after a person has been in a traumatic event. Depersonalization disorder is characterized by recurrent sensations of loss of one's own reality. Dissociative fugue is the sudden departure from one's home or work. Dissociative identity disorder is the coexistence of two or more personalities within the same individual.
CN: Psychosocial integrity; CNS: None; CL: Analysis

32. The nurse is assessing a client with dissociative amnesia. Which of the following circumstances would most likely result in this condition?
1. Binge drinking
2. A hostage situation
3. A closed-head injury
4. A fight with a family member

33. A client was the driver in an automobile accident in which a 3-year-old boy was killed. The client now has dissociative amnesia. He verbalizes understanding of his treatment plan when he makes which statement?
1. "I won't drive a car again for at least a year."
2. "I'll take my Ativan anytime I feel upset about this situation."
3. "I'll visit the child's grave as soon as I'm released from the hospital."
4. "I'll attend my hypnotic therapy sessions prescribed by my psychiatrist."

34. A client with dissociative amnesia shows understanding of her condition when she makes which statement?
1. "I'll probably never be able to regain my memories of the fire."
2. "I have problems with my memory due to my abuse of tranquilizers."
3. "If I concentrate hard enough, I'll be able to bring up memories of the car accident."
4. "To protect my mental well-being, my brain has temporarily hidden my memories of the rape from me."

35. Which intervention is <u>most appropriate</u> in the treatment of a client admitted for a diagnostic workup for possible dissociative amnesia?
1. Restrain the client if he attempts to wander off the unit.
2. Question the client every hour about orientation to time, place, and person.
3. Provide teaching on computed tomography scans and other imaging tests.
4. Encourage the client not to dwell on the traumatic event that lead to his memory loss.

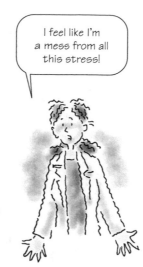

I feel like I'm a mess from all this stress!

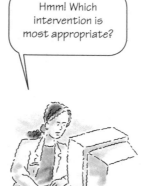

Hmm! Which intervention is most appropriate?

32. 2. Dissociative amnesia typically occurs after the person has experienced a very stressful, traumatic situation. Binge drinking doesn't cause dissociative amnesia. A closed-head injury could result in physiologic but not dissociative amnesia. Having a fight with a family member typically wouldn't be stressful enough to cause dissociative amnesia.
CN: Psychosocial integrity; CNS: None; CL: Application

33. 4. Hypnosis can be beneficial to this client because it allows repressed feelings and memories to surface. The client may be ready to drive again, and circumstances may dictate that he drives again before a year has passed. The client needs to learn other coping mechanisms besides taking a highly addictive drug such as lorazepam (Ativan). Visiting the child's grave on release from the hospital may be too traumatic and encourage continuation of the amnesia.
CN: Psychosocial integrity; CNS: None; CL: Application

34. 4. One of the cardinal features of dissociative amnesia is that the person has loss of memory of a traumatic event. With therapy and time, the person will probably be able to recall the traumatic event. This type of amnesia isn't related to substance abuse. With this disorder, the loss of memory is a protective function performed by the brain and isn't within the person's conscious control.
CN: Psychosocial integrity; CNS: None; CL: Analysis

35. 3. Clients with a type of memory problem commonly have a diagnostic workup to rule out any physical cause. Clients with dissociative amnesia typically don't have a problem with wandering. Frequent attempts to assess the client's orientation level could easily make the client more distressed and agitated. In many cases, the client doesn't have memories of the traumatic events before amnesia.
CN: Health promotion and maintenance; CNS: None; CL: Application

36. A client with dissociative amnesia indicates understanding about the use of amobarbital (Amytal) in his treatment when he makes which statement?
1. "This medication helps me sleep."
2. "This medication helps me control my anxiety."
3. "I must take this drug once a day after discharge if the drug is to be therapeutically beneficial."
4. "I'm given this medication during therapy sessions to increase my ability to remember forgotten events."

36. 4. This drug is given to the client with dissociative amnesia to help her remember forgotten events. It isn't prescribed as a sleep aid or antianxiety agent. Because the drug is given during therapy to recall forgotten events, there would be no therapeutic benefit to taking this drug at home.

CN: Physiological integrity; CNS: Pharmacological and parenteral therapies; CL: Analysis

37. A client with dissociative amnesia says, "You must think I'm really stupid because I have no recollection of the accident." Which response would be <u>most appropriate?</u>
1. "Why would I think you're stupid?"
2. "Have I acted like I think you're stupid?"
3. "What kind of grades did you get in school?"
4. "As a protective measure, the brain sometimes doesn't let us remember traumatic events."

37. 4. This provides a simple explanation for the client. The use of "why" can put someone on the defensive. The second option takes the focus off the client. The third option changes the topic.

CN: Psychosocial integrity; CNS: None; CL: Application

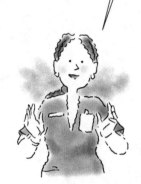

Sometimes a simple explanation is the best one.

38. Which nursing intervention is important in caring for the client with a dissociative disorder?
1. Encourage the client to participate in unit activities and meetings.
2. Question the client about the events triggering the dissociative disorder.
3. Allow the client to remain in his room anytime he's experiencing feelings of dissociation.
4. Encourage the client to form friendships with other clients in his therapy groups to decrease his feelings of isolation.

38. 1. Attending unit activities and meetings helps decrease the client's sense of isolation. Often, the client can't recall the events that triggered the dissociative disorder, so questioning him would not be helpful. The client would need to be isolated from others only if he's unable to interact appropriately. A client with a dissociative disorder has typically had few healthy relationships. Forming friendships with others in therapy could be setting the client up to continue in unhealthy relationships.

CN: Safe, effective care environment; CNS: Management of care; CL: Application

CN: Client needs category   CNS: Client needs subcategory   CL: Cognitive level

39. The nurse is performing an assessment on a client with depersonalization disorder. Which of the following characteristics would the nurse most likely assess with this client?
1. Disorientation to time, place, and person
2. Sensation of detachment from body or mind
3. Unexpected and sudden travel to another location
4. A feeling that one's environment will never change

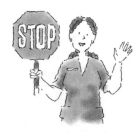

How can you tell when your client understands your instructions?

40. A client with depersonalization disorder verbalizes understanding of the ways to decrease his symptoms when he makes which statement?
1. "I'll avoid any stressful situation."
2. "Meditation will help control my symptoms."
3. "I'll need to practice relaxation exercises regularly."
4. "I may need to remain on antipsychotic medication for the rest of my life."

41. A client with depersonalization disorder spends much of his day in a dreamlike state during which he ignores personal care needs. Which nursing diagnosis is <u>most appropriate</u> for this client?
1. *Disturbed personal identity related to organic brain damage*
2. *Impaired memory related to frequently being in a dreamlike state*
3. *Dressing self-care deficit related to perceptual impairment*
4. *Deficient knowledge related to performance or personal care needs due to lack of information*

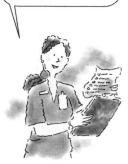

Making the right nursing diagnosis is critical for effective nursing care.

42. A client reports frequently feeling that he's floating above his body. During these times, he says he's aware of who he is and where he's located. Which of the following disorders is the client exhibiting?
1. Depersonalization disorder
2. Dissociative amnesia
3. Dissociative identity disorder
4. Dissociative fugue

39. 2. In depersonalization disorder, the person feels detached from his body and mental processes. The person is usually oriented to time, place, and person. Unexpected and sudden travel to another location is one of the characteristics of dissociative fugue. Clients with depersonalization disorder often feel the outside world has changed.
CN: Psychosocial integrity; CNS: None; CL: Application

40. 3. Relaxation can lead to a decrease in maladaptive responses. Although stress can be a predisposing factor in depersonalization disorder, it's impossible to avoid all stressful situations. Meditation is the voluntary induction of the sensation of depersonalization. This isn't a psychotic disorder, so antipsychotic medication wouldn't be therapeutic or beneficial.
CN: Psychosocial integrity; CNS: None; CL: Analysis

41. 3. Because of time spent in a dreamlike state, many clients with depersonalization disorder ignore self-care needs. There's no known organic brain damage with this disorder. Memory impairment is more of a problem with other dissociative disorders, such as dissociative identity disorder and dissociative amnesia. The dreamlike state can lead to problems meeting personal care needs, not a knowledge deficit.
CN: Safe, effective care environment; CNS: Safety and infection control; CL: Application

42. 1. One of the cardinal symptoms of depersonalization disorder is feeling detached from one's body or mental processes. During the feelings of detachment, the person doesn't become disoriented. Dissociative amnesia is defined as one or more episodes of being unable to recall important information. Dissociative identity disorder is the existence of two or more personalities that take control of the person's behavior. In a dissociative fugue, the person has no memory of his life before the flight.
CN: Psychosocial integrity; CNS: None; CL: Analysis

43. The nurse is teaching the family of a client with depersonalization disorder. The family wants to know which setting has the most success in treating this disorder. Which of the following responses would be the most accurate?
1. Inpatient psychiatric hospital
2. Community mental health clinic
3. Family practice physician's office
4. Support group for clients with depersonalization disorder

44. A client with depersonalization disorder tells the nurse, "I feel like such a freak when I have an out-of-body experience." Which response would be <u>most appropriate</u>?
1. "How often do you have these feelings?"
2. "I don't understand what you mean by a freak."
3. "Tell me more about these out-of-body experiences."
4. "How does your husband feel about you having these experiences?"

45. During an assessment on a client with dissociative disorder, which of the following characteristics would the nurse most likely assess?
1. A group of disorders with the common symptom of hallucinations
2. A group of disorders with a rapid disruption of the client's memory
3. A group of disorders with impairment of memory or identity due to the development of organic changes in the brain
4. A group of disorders with impairment of memory or identity due to an unconscious attempt to protect the person from emotional pain or traumatic experiences

46. A client with depersonalization disorder tells the nurse, "I feel like my arm isn't attached to my body." Which response would be most appropriate?
1. "Do you know where you are?"
2. "What makes you feel that way?"
3. "Don't worry because I can see your arm is attached to your body."
4. "This disorder causes people to feel that body parts may be unattached to the rest of the body."

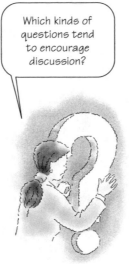

Which kinds of questions tend to encourage discussion?

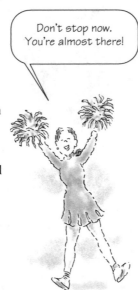

Don't stop now. You're almost there!

43. 2. Most clients with depersonalization disorder can be treated successfully on an outpatient basis. These clients only need to be hospitalized if they become suicidal or have severe depression or anxiety. Because no organic basis for the disorder usually exists, these clients aren't treated in a family practice physician's office. Because the disorder is rare, few support groups are composed only of clients with this disorder.
CN: Psychosocial integrity; CNS: None; CL: Application

44. 3. This open-ended response allows the client to focus and expand on this topic. Asking how often the experiences occur is a closed-ended question that doesn't encourage discussion of the experience. The second option could cause the client to focus too narrowly on only one aspect of the topic. Asking how the client's husband feels makes it appear that the nurse wants to change the topic.
CN: Psychosocial integrity; CNS: None; CL: Analysis

45. 4. A group of disorders in which there's impairment of memory or identity due to an unconscious attempt to protect the client from emotional pain or traumatic experiences describes dissociative disorders. Hallucinations are associated with schizophrenic disorders. The onset of dissociative disorders may be gradual, sudden, or chronic. There's no known organic cause for dissociative disorders.
CN: Psychosocial integrity; CNS: None; CL: Application

46. 4. Reinforcing that what the client feels is an expected result of the disease process would be most appropriate. Asking if the client knows where he is changes the topic. Asking why he feels that way could put the client on the defensive. Stating that his arm is attached to his body belittles the client's feelings.
CN: Psychosocial integrity; CNS: None; CL: Application

CN: Client needs category   CNS: Client needs subcategory   CL: Cognitive level

47. A client with a dissociative disorder suddenly wanders away from the facility. When the nurse finds him, he can't recall what happened. The nurse identifies this behavior as which dissociative disorder?
  1. Repression
  2. Depersonalization
  3. Derealization
  4. Dissociative fugue

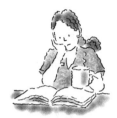

My mind keeps wandering to another place.

48. A nurse conducts an admission assessment on a client diagnosed with dissociative identity disorder. Which sign or symptom supports this diagnosis?
  1. A sense of being in a dream
  2. Inability to remember a particular event
  3. Having two or more personalities
  4. Ritualistic behavior

49. Which set of circumstances indicates the highest risk of suicide?
  1. Suicide plan, handy means of carrying out plan, and history of previous attempt
  2. Preoccupation with morbid thoughts and limited support system
  3. Suicidal ideation, active suicide planning, and family history of suicide
  4. Threats of suicide, recent job loss, and intact support system

50. A nurse finds a suicidal client trying to hang himself in his room. To preserve the client's self-esteem and safety, what should the nurse do?
  1. Place the client in seclusion with checks every 15 minutes.
  2. Assign a nursing staff member to remain with the client at all times.
  3. Make the client stay with the group at all times.
  4. Refuse to let the client in his room.

47. 4. Dissociative fugue is characterized by suddenly wandering away from one's usual place, accompanied by amnesia for all or part of the past. Repression is a defense mechanism in which thoughts and feelings are kept from consciousness. Depersonalization is a feeling of detachment or separation from one's self. Derealization is a feeling that the external world is unreal.
CN: Psychosocial integrity; CNS: None; CL: Application

48. 3. Dissociative identity disorder is characterized by having two or more distinct personalities, often in conflict with one another. A sense of being in a dream is common in depersonalization disorders. Selective amnesia refers to an inability to recall certain events that occurred during a specified period and is more common in traumatic stress disorders. Ritualistic behavior is seen in obsessive-compulsive disorders.
CN: Psychosocial integrity; CNS: None; CL: Application

49. 1. A lethal plan with a handy means of carrying it out poses the highest risk and requires immediate intervention. Although all of the remaining risk factors can lead to suicide, they aren't considered as high a risk as a formulated, lethal plan and the means at hand. However, a client exhibiting any of these risk factors should be taken seriously and considered at risk for suicide.
CN: Psychosocial integrity; CNS: None; CL: Application

50. 2. Implementing a one-on-one staff-to-client ratio is the nurse's highest priority. Doing so allows the client to maintain his self-esteem and keeps him safe. Seclusion would damage the client's self-esteem. Forcing the client to stay with the group and refusing to let him in his room don't guarantee his safety.
CN: Psychosocial integrity; CNS: None; CL: Application

51. A client with a dissociative identity disorder experiences amnesia. Which nursing diagnosis is most appropriate?
1. *Powerlessness*
2. *Ineffective coping*
3. *Disturbed sensory perception, visual*
4. *Risk for self-directed violence*

52. After taking a potentially lethal drug overdose, a client tells the nurse that his alter "did it." Which nursing diagnosis takes highest priority?
1. *Posttrauma syndrome*
2. *Anxiety*
3. *Risk for self-directed violence*
4. *Disturbed personal identity*

53. A severely depressed client who has made multiple suicide attempts matter-of-factly tells the nurse that her family life was normal and uneventful. Which behaviors would lead the nurse to suspect a diagnosis of a dissociative identity disorder (DID) in this client? Select all that apply:
1. Inability to recall important personal information too severe to be explained by ordinary forgetfulness
2. Absence of any physiological effects of a substance, such as alcohol or drugs
3. Ability to selectively and consciously choose to avoid certain painful topics
4. A sense of grandiosity, that she's special and has a particular mission for mankind
5. Posttraumatic symptoms, such as flashbacks, nightmares, and an exaggerated startle response

54. A client with dissociative identity disorder experiences frequent periods of memory loss. Which nursing intervention can help the client deal with the memory loss?
1. Orienting the client to time, place, person, and situation
2. Explaining to the client the circumstances surrounding the memory loss
3. Assessing for cues that the client is ready to discuss the memory loss
4. Telling the client not to worry because the memory loss has no physiologic base

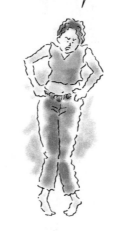

I know my highest priority at the moment.

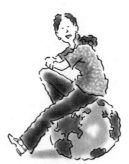

Congratulations! You should feel on top of the world!

51. 2. Amnesia may result from an inability to cope with anxiety. *Powerlessness, Disturbed sensory perception*, and *Risk for self-directed violence* aren't appropriate in this situation.
CN: Psychosocial integrity; CNS: None; CL: Analysis

52. 3. Taking a potentially lethal drug overdose indicates that the client poses a danger to himself. Because the alter may act again, the risk for self-directed violence persists. The other nursing diagnoses either aren't relevant or take lower priority.
CN: Psychosocial integrity; CNS: None; CL: Analysis

53. 1, 2, 5. A dissociative disorder is a persistent state of being disconnected from the totality of one's personhood, particularly painful emotions. With dissociative disorder, the inability to recall personal information is far more extensive than ordinary forgetfulness; the symptoms occur apart from any chemical inducement, and the individual doesn't have the ability to consciously make a decision to separate from painful emotions or topics. A sense of grandiosity isn't characteristic of this disorder. Posttraumatic symptoms, such as flashbacks, nightmares, and an exaggerated startle response, are also signs and symptoms of DID.
CN: Psychosocial integrity; CNS: None; CL: Analysis

54. 3. Memory loss serves as a protective mechanism for many clients with dissociative identity disorder; the nurse should wait until the client is ready to discuss the problem, as shown by certain cues. Orienting the client may force the client out of the protective mechanism of the memory loss (which the client may not be ready for and can result in further harm). Explaining the circumstances surrounding the memory loss and telling the client not to worry aren't therapeutic interventions.
CN: Psychosocial integrity; CNS: None; CL: Application

CN: Client needs category   CNS: Client needs subcategory   CL: Cognitive level

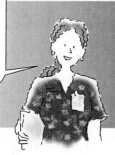

This chapter will test your knowledge of disorders of a highly sensitive nature. Remain professional at all times, and you'll do great. Good luck!

Chapter 21
Sexual disorders

1. A client has undergone surgery for the repair of an abdominal aortic aneurysm. Which response is <u>most appropriate</u> to the client's wife when she asks if her husband will be impotent?
   1. "Don't worry, he'll be all right."
   2. "He has other problems to worry about."
   3. "We'll cross that bridge when we come to it."
   4. "There is a chance of impotence after repair of an abdominal aortic aneurysm."

2. Which discharge instruction would be most accurate to provide to a female client who has suffered a spinal cord injury at the C4 level?
   1. After a spinal cord injury, women usually remain fertile; therefore, you may consider contraception if you don't want to become pregnant.
   2. After a spinal cord injury, women usually are unable to conceive a child.
   3. Sexual intercourse shouldn't be different for you.
   4. After a spinal cord injury, menstruation usually stops.

3. A nurse is caring for a 39-year-old male client who recently underwent surgery and is having difficulty accepting changes in his body image. Which nursing intervention is appropriate?
   1. Actively listening to the client as he expresses positive and negative feelings about his body image
   2. Restricting the client's opportunity to view the incision and dressing because it's upsetting
   3. Assisting the client to focus on future plans for recovery
   4. Assisting the client to repress anger while discussing the body image alteration

Therapeutic communication involves demonstrating sensitivity to your client's and his family's concerns.

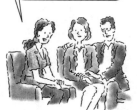

Note that question 3 is asking you which action is appropriate.

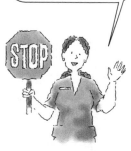

1. 4. Impotence and retrograde ejaculation are sexual dysfunctions commonly experienced by male clients after abdominal aortic aneurysm. Telling a family member that the client will be all right is offering false assurance. Stating that he has other problems isn't therapeutic and doesn't address the wife's concern. Telling the client's wife to "cross that bridge when we come to it" ignores her concerns and isn't therapeutic.
CN: Psychosocial integrity; CNS: None; CL: Application

2. 1. After a spinal cord injury, women remain fertile and can conceive and deliver a child. If a woman doesn't want to become pregnant, she *must* use contraception. Menstruation isn't affected by a spinal cord injury, but sexual functioning may be different.
CN: Physiological integrity; CNS: Physiological adaptation; CL: Application

3. 1. The nurse must observe for any indication that the client is ready to address his body image change. The client should be allowed to look at the incision and dressing if he wants to do so. It's too soon to focus on the future with this client. The nurse should allow the client to express his feelings and not repress them, because repression prolongs recovery.
CN: Psychosocial integrity; CNS: None; CL: Application

CN: Client needs category   CNS: Client needs subcategory   CL: Cognitive level

4. A female client with chronic obstructive pulmonary disease (COPD) tells a nurse, "I no longer have enough energy to make love to my husband." Which nursing intervention would be most appropriate?
1. Refer the couple to a sex therapist.
2. Advise the woman to seek a gynecologic consult.
3. Suggest methods and measures that facilitate sexual activity.
4. Tell the client, "If you talk this over with your husband, he'll understand."

5. A client with an ileostomy tells the nurse he can't have an erection. Which pertinent information should the nurse know?
1. The client will never regain functioning.
2. The client needs an abdominal X-ray.
3. The client has no problem with self-control.
4. Impotence is uncommon following an ileostomy.

6. A recently divorced 40-year-old client who has undergone radiation therapy for testicular cancer tells the nurse he is unable to achieve an erection. Which nursing diagnosis is most appropriate?
1. *Ineffective coping related to radiation therapy*
2. *Sexual dysfunction related to the effects of radiation therapy*
3. *Disturbed body image related to the effects of radiation therapy*
4. *Imbalanced nutrition: Less than body requirements related to radiation therapy*

7. Which action should a nurse include in the teaching plan of a newly married female client with a cervical spinal cord injury who doesn't wish to become pregnant at this time?
1. Provide the client with brochures on sexual practice.
2. Provide the client's husband with material on vasectomy.
3. Instruct the client on the rhythm method of contraception.
4. Instruct the client's husband on inserting a diaphragm with contraceptive jelly.

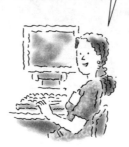

Several answers are possible. But which one is the most appropriate?

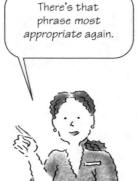

There's that phrase most appropriate again.

4. 3. Sexual dysfunction in COPD clients is the direct result of dyspnea and reduced energy levels. Measures to reduce physical exertion, enhance oxygenation, and accommodate decreased energy levels may aid sexual activity. If the problem persists, a consult with a sex therapist might be necessary. A gynecologic consult isn't necessary. Discussing this with her husband may not resolve the problem.
CN: Physiological integrity; CNS: Reduction of risk potential; CL: Application

5. 4. Sexual dysfunction is uncommon after an ileostomy. Psychological causes of impotence should be explored. An abdominal X-ray isn't indicated for sexual dysfunction. An ileostomy can change a person's self-control, making sexual functioning difficult.
CN: Physiological integrity; CNS: Physiological adaptation; CL: Analysis

6. 2. Radiation or chemotherapy may cause sexual dysfunction. Libido may only be temporarily affected, and the client should be provided with emotional support. The client may experience alopecia or skin changes as well as weight loss, but he isn't verbalizing concern in this area. The client hasn't verbalized fear or concern related to the cancer. Nutrition hasn't been mentioned.
CN: Psychosocial integrity; CNS: None; CL: Analysis

7. 4. Because the client experienced a cervical spinal cord injury, she won't be able to insert any form of contraception protection by herself; therefore, it's vital to provide her husband with instruction on insertion of a diaphragm. Providing the couple with literature on sexual practice doesn't address the client's concerns. During this time of crisis, the couple doesn't wish to have children, but they may reconsider, so providing information on vasectomy isn't appropriate. The rhythm method isn't the most effective way to prevent pregnancy.
CN: Psychosocial integrity; CNS: None; CL: Application

CN: Client needs category   CNS: Client needs subcategory   CL: Cognitive level

8. A female client tells the nurse she is having her menstrual period every 2 weeks and it lasts for 1 week. Which term *best* defines this menstrual pattern?
1. Amenorrhea
2. Dyspareunia
3. Menorrhagia
4. Metrorrhagia

9. Which aspect might be a major stressor for a couple being treated for infertility?
1. Examinations
2. Giving specimens
3. Scheduling intercourse
4. Finding out which partner is infertile

10. A 38-year-old female client must undergo a hysterectomy for uterine cancer. The nurse planning her care should include which action to meet the client's body image changes?
1. Ask her if she is having pain.
2. Refer her to a psychotherapist.
3. Don't discuss the subject with her.
4. Encourage her to verbalize her feelings.

11. A 50-year-old male client who had a myocardial infarction 8 weeks ago tells a nurse, "My wife wants to make love, but I don't think I can. I'm worried that it might kill me." Which response from the nurse would be most appropriate?
1. "Tell me about your feelings."
2. "Let's increase your rehabilitation schedule."
3. "Let me call the primary health care provider for you."
4. "Tell your wife when you're able you'll make love."

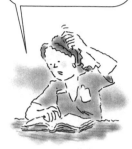

What's the difference between menorrhagia and metrorrhagia?

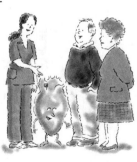

Let's put together a plan of care that will meet all of your needs.

8. 3. Menorrhagia is an excessive menstrual period. Amenorrhea is lack of menstruation. Dyspareunia is painful intercourse. Metrorrhagia is uterine bleeding from another cause other than menstruation.
CN: Physiological integrity; CNS: Reduction of risk potential; CL: Application

9. 3. The major cause of stress in infertile couples is planning sexual intercourse to correlate to fertility cycles. The inconvenience and discomfort of producing specimens and receiving examinations isn't a major stressor. Most couples undergoing fertility treatment understand that one partner is usually infertile.
CN: Health promotion and maintenance; CNS: None; CL: Application

10. 4. Encourage the client to verbalize her feelings because loss of one's reproductive organs may bring on feelings of loss of sexuality. Pain is a concern after surgery, but it has no bearing on body image. Referring her to a psychotherapist may be premature; the client should be given time to work through her feelings. Avoidance of the subject isn't a therapeutic nursing intervention.
CN: Psychosocial integrity; CNS: None; CL: Application

11. 1. The nurse should address the client's concerns. Asking the client to verbalize his feelings will permit the nurse to gain insight into the problem. The rehabilitation schedule shouldn't be increased until the nurse assesses the situation and is sure no harm will come to the client. Calling the primary health care provider before a complete assessment is made is inappropriate. Telling the wife that eventually the client will make love may place strain on the marriage.
CN: Psychosocial integrity; CNS: None; CL: Application

12. A 55-year-old female client who's in cardiac rehabilitation tells a nurse that she's unable to make love to her husband because she often feels fatigued and has a sense of doom. Which nursing intervention is most appropriate?
1. Instruct her not to have intercourse until she is ready.
2. Instruct her to take a nitroglycerin tablet prior to intercourse.
3. Encourage her to learn additional methods to use for sexual intercourse.
4. Encourage her to verbalize her feelings while you perform a physical examination on her.

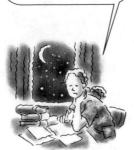

I know all about feeling fatigued.

12. 4. Because the client has a complaint of fatigue, she should be examined and her feelings should be explored. Instructing her not to have intercourse doesn't address her concerns. She shouldn't take nitroglycerin before intercourse until her fatigue is evaluated. Before recommending alternative methods for intercourse, the client should be assessed physically and psychologically.
CN: Psychosocial integrity; CNS: None; CL: Application

13. A 33-year-old female client tells the nurse she has never had an orgasm and that her partner is upset that he's unable to meet her needs. Which nursing intervention is most appropriate?
1. Ask the client if she desires intercourse.
2. Assess the couple's perception of the problem.
3. Tell the client that most women don't reach orgasm.
4. Refer the client to a therapist because she has sexual aversion disorder.

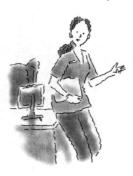

The NCLEX may include sexual identity questions for clients of different ages.

13. 2. Assessing the couple's perception of the problem will define the problem and assist the couple and the nurse in understanding it. When assessing the client, the nurse should be professional and matter of fact and shouldn't make the client feel inadequate or defensive by asking if she desires intercourse. Most individuals can be taught to reach orgasm if there is no underlying medical condition. A nurse can't make a medical diagnosis such as sexual aversion disorder.
CN: Psychosocial integrity; CNS: None; CL: Application

14. A 20-year-old female client is in the emergency department after being sexually assaulted by a stranger. Which nursing intervention has the <u>highest priority</u>?
1. Assisting the client in identifying which of her behaviors placed her at risk for the attack
2. Making an appointment for the client in 6 weeks at a local sexual assault crisis center
3. Encouraging discussion of the client's early childhood experiences
4. Assisting the client in identifying family or friends who could provide immediate support for her

14. 4. The client needs a lot of support to help her through this ordeal. Assisting the client in identifying behaviors that place her at risk for the attack places the blame on the client. Waiting 6 weeks to make an appointment is incorrect — the local crisis center must be called immediately. Some psychiatric disorders are related to early childhood experiences, but rape isn't.
CN: Psychosocial integrity; CNS: None; CL: Application

15. A 50-year-old client who is taking antihypertensive medication tells the office nurse who's monitoring his blood pressure that he can't have sexual intercourse with his wife anymore. Which problem is most likely the cause?
1. His advancing age
2. His blood pressure
3. His stressful lifestyle
4. His blood pressure medication

15. 4. Antihypertensive medication may cause impotence in men. Blood pressure itself doesn't cause impotence but its treatment does. Stress may cause erectile dysfunction, but there's no evidence that the client is under stress. Men are usually able to have an erection throughout their lives.
CN: Physiological integrity; CNS: Pharmacological and parenteral therapies; CL: Application

16. Adult victims of childhood sexual abuse need to be monitored for signs and symptoms of which disorder?
   1. Depression and substance abuse disorders
   2. Bipolar and somatization disorders
   3. Narcissistic disorders and bulimia nervosa
   4. Obsessive-compulsive and posttraumatic stress disorders

17. Which intervention is important for a client who engages in sexual acts with animals (zoophilia)?
   1. Place the client in the seclusion room.
   2. Assess triggers that stimulate the behaviors.
   3. Have the primary health care provider order antidepressant medication.
   4. Counsel the client not to discuss his sexual behaviors with anyone.

18. A 25-year-old client convicted of raping a female college student has completed his parole and has been attending a sex offenders group for 5 years. The client no longer wishes to participate in the group. Which action should the nurse take?
   1. Insist that the client remain in therapy.
   2. Perform a self-evaluation, and assess the discomfort level.
   3. Call the parole board, and tell them of the client's decision.
   4. Call the client's family, and tell them of his decision and progress.

19. A 32-year-old client who engages in voyeurism has come to the hospital for treatment so his family and friends don't find out. The nurse planning care for this client should include which intervention?
   1. Encourage the client to inform his family and friends so that he isn't living a lie.
   2. Suggest individual therapy to discuss socially unacceptable behavior.
   3. Develop the care plan without input from the client.
   4. Evaluate the client's defense mechanism.

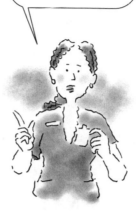

Don't despair over answering this question — focus on this disorder's symptoms.

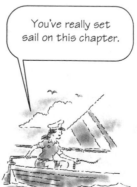

You've really set sail on this chapter.

16. 1. Childhood sexual abuse is closely linked to the development of depression and substance abuse disorders. It's also linked to the development of somatization and posttraumatic stress disorders and bulimia nervosa. Victims of childhood sexual abuse aren't predisposed to developing bipolar, narcissistic, or obsessive-compulsive disorders.
CN: Psychosocial integrity; CNS: None; CL: Analysis

17. 2. Assessing the triggers that stimulate inappropriate sexual behavior helps to prevent recurrence. The seclusion room should be used only to ensure the safety of the client and staff. Antidepressants aren't indicated for sexual disorders; hormonal therapy is the usual drug treatment. Clinical support and group therapy are used to teach sexually acceptable behavior.
CN: Psychosocial integrity; CNS: None; CL: Analysis

18. 2. If the client has successfully completed therapy, then the nurse must evaluate her own value system. Insisting that the client remain in therapy may not prove to be successful, as he must be motivated to undergo therapy. Calling the parole board may be an inappropriate decision, especially if the client has met all of his requirements. A nurse can't release confidential information to the client's family without his permission and consent.
CN: Psychosocial integrity; CNS: None; CL: Analysis

19. 2. Discussing inappropriate sexual behavior with the client increases compliance with treatment and decreases the risk of relapse. Informing family and friends isn't an initial intervention; disclosure to family and friends is usually delayed until the client acknowledges his behavior. All care planning should involve the client. An initial evaluation should focus on the antecedents to the inappropriate behavior.
CN: Psychosocial integrity; CNS: None; CL: Application

20. A client is admitted to the psychiatric unit for paraphiliac coercive disorder: rape. Which assessment question will provide the nurse with insight toward this client's cognitive distortion?
1. "Tell me what you're feeling."
2. "Do you have any lifestyle problems?"
3. "What brings you to the hospital for treatment?"
4. "Do you believe you're here for a sexual disorder?"

21. A 38-year-old female client was returning home from the store late one evening and was sexually assaulted. When she's brought to the emergency department, she's crying. Which concern for this client should be the nurse's first priority?
1. Filing a police report
2. Calling the client's family
3. Encouraging the client to enroll in a self-defense class
4. Remaining with the client and assisting her through the crisis

22. A client is admitted to the psychiatric unit as part of his probation period for exhibitionism and fetishism. The client seems to be adjusting well, but several clients report that their undergarments are missing. Which action would be most appropriate?
1. Notify the primary health care provider.
2. Search the client's room.
3. Call a community meeting, and let the clients settle the matter.
4. Privately assess whether the client is engaging in sexual activities on the unit.

23. A client is admitted to the hospital for scatophilia and tells the nurse that he doesn't want to talk to her about his sexual behaviors. Which response from the nurse is the most appropriate?
1. "I need to ask you the questions on the database."
2. "It's your right not to answer my questions."
3. "I know this must be difficult for you."
4. "OK, I'll just write 'no comment.'"

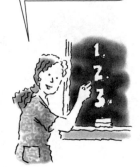

Prioritizing correctly is extremely important for question 21.

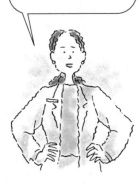

Clients with sexual disorders may be ashamed and unwilling to discuss the problem.

20. 4. If a client had a cognitive disorder, then he would be using denial as a defense mechanism and would deny having a sexual disorder. Asking what a client is feeling is important, but it doesn't provide information on the use of defense mechanisms. Asking about lifestyle problems will provide the nurse with information related to problems with relationships. Asking why the client is at the hospital will tell the nurse if the client has insight into his illness.
CN: Psychosocial integrity; CNS: None; CL: Application

21. 4. Sexual assault is treated as a medical emergency, and the client requires constant attention and assistance during the crisis. Filing a police report wouldn't take precedence over a medical emergency. Comforting the client by contacting family should be carried out after the client's injuries are treated. Encouraging the client to enroll in a self-defense class isn't appropriate during crisis.
CN: Psychosocial integrity; CNS: None; CL: Application

22. 4. Meeting with the client privately establishes trust. This client needs to be assessed for what triggers might be present to prompt this behavior. Notification of the primary health care provider shouldn't be done without assessment of the client. Searching the client's room without discussion is a violation of a trusting milieu. It isn't therapeutic to encourage the unit to confront one member of the community.
CN: Psychosocial integrity; CNS: None; CL: Application

23. 3. Stating "I know this must be difficult for you" acknowledges the client's feelings and opens communications. Insisting that the form needs to be completed doesn't open up communications or acknowledge the client's feelings. Clients have rights, but data collection is necessary so that help with the problem can be offered. Writing "no comment" alone would be inappropriate.
CN: Psychosocial integrity; CNS: None; CL: Application

CN: Client needs category   CNS: Client needs subcategory   CL: Cognitive level

24. Which therapy may be used with a client who admits to frottage?
 1. Electroconvulsive therapy
 2. Relaxation therapy
 3. Administration of psychotropic agents
 4. Positive reinforcement and group therapy

25. When treating a client admitted to the psychiatric unit for transvestic fetishism, the nurse should develop a care plan based on which diagnosis?
 1. *Ineffective health maintenance*
 2. *Ineffective sexuality patterns*
 3. *Complicated grieving*
 4. *Bathing self-care deficit*

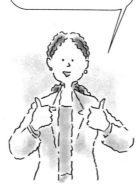

Keep going; you're doing great!

26. When working with a client with a paraphiliac disorder, which goal is appropriate for the client?
 1. To attend all meetings on the unit
 2. To use triggers to initiate sexual behaviors
 3. To inform his employer of the reason for hospitalization
 4. To verbalize appropriate methods to meet sexual needs upon discharge

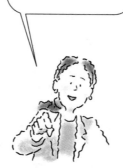

Effective care may involve managing interactions between clients.

27. A client admitted to the hospital with a diagnosis of pedophilia tells his roommate about his problems. His roommate runs down the hall yelling at the nurse, "I don't want to be in here with a child molester." Which response from the nurse is <u>most appropriate</u>?
 1. "Stop acting out."
 2. "Calm down, and go back to your room."
 3. "Your roommate isn't a child molester."
 4. "I can see you're upset. Sit down and we'll talk."

24. 4. Frottage involves rubbing against someone in a public place. Positive reinforcement and group therapy are used to assist a client with frottage to develop new sexual response patterns. Electroconvulsive therapy and relaxation therapy aren't indicated for this condition. Psychotropic medications are used for dangerous and compulsive practices and aren't indicated for this condition.
CN: Psychosocial integrity; CNS: None; CL: Analysis

25. 2. *Ineffective sexuality patterns* would be appropriate because transvestic fetishism refers to intense sexual arousal with cross-dressing. *Ineffective health maintenance* is an appropriate diagnosis for someone experiencing a health problem. *Complicated grieving* refers to the inability to recover from a loss. The client hasn't exhibited any problems with health, self-care, or loss. *Bathing self-care deficit* is a diagnosis for the inability to meet self-care needs.
CN: Psychosocial integrity; CNS: None; CL: Application

26. 4. Upon discharge, the client should verbalize an alternative appropriate method to meet his sexual needs and effective strategies to prevent relapse. It isn't imperative that the client attend all meetings on the unit, but it's important that he attend the prescribed group sessions. A client with a paraphiliac disorder should recognize triggers that initiate inappropriate sexual behaviors and learn ways to direct his impulses. The client may wish to discuss the disorder with his spouse but not necessarily his employer.
CN: Psychosocial integrity; CNS: None; CL: Analysis

27. 4. Acknowledging that the client is upset and sitting down and talking with him will allow the client to verbalize his feelings. If a client were agitated or anxious over his roommate, it wouldn't be therapeutic or safe to keep those clients together without intervention. Telling the client to stop acting out or to calm down isn't a therapeutic response. Stating that the pedophile isn't a child molester doesn't acknowledge the client's feelings.
CN: Psychosocial integrity; CNS: None; CL: Application

28. When assigning rooms for clients, a nurse should <u>not</u> place which of the following clients with a client who has a diagnosis of sexual sadism?
1. A client with a diagnosis of sexual masochism
2. A client with a diagnosis of voyeurism
3. A client who's an exhibitionist
4. A client who's a homosexual

28. 1. A client who's admitted with a diagnosis of sexual masochism is aroused through suffering and, therefore, shouldn't be placed with a client who's diagnosed with sexual sadism, who's aroused by inflicted pain. A voyeur is aroused by secretly observing someone who's naked or engaged in sexual activity. An exhibitionist is aroused through the exposure of one's genitals to an unsuspecting person. A homosexual enjoys relationships with someone of the same sex.
CN: Safe, effective care environment; CNS: Management of care; CL: Application

29. A nurse is obtaining a health history from a client when he states he has been diagnosed with voyeurism. Which of the following actions would the nurse expect to assess in this client?
1. Observing others while they disrobe
2. Wearing clothing of the opposite sex
3. Rubbing against a nonconsenting person
4. Using rubber sheeting for sexual arousal

29. 1. Voyeurism is sexual arousal from secretly observing someone who is disrobing. Transvestic fetishism describes someone who enjoys cross-dressing. Rubbing against someone who is nonconsenting is frottage. Using objects for sexual arousal is fetishism.
CN: Psychosocial integrity; CNS: None; CL: Application

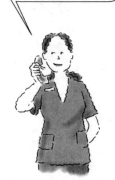

Hello, information? Do you know the answer to question 30?

30. The nurse is teaching the family of a client with scatophilia. Which response by the nurse is <u>most</u> accurate in teaching about the characteristics of this disorder?
1. The client uses the telephone for sexual arousal.
2. The client uses nonliving objects such as women's underwear for sexual gratification.
3. The client is aroused through contact with children.
4. The client is aroused by rubbing against a nonconsenting person.

30. 1. Telephone scatophilia is a paraphilia in which a person derives sexual arousal by engaging in lewd conversations on the telephone. Fetishism involves the use of nonliving objects whose presence are required or preferred for sexual excitement. Pedophiles engage in fondling or sexual activities with children under 13 years of age. Frottage is rubbing against a nonconsenting person for sexual arousal.
CN: Psychosocial integrity; CNS: None; CL: Application

31. A female being treated for infertility confides to the nurse that she hasn't told her partner she has been treated for a sexually transmitted disease in the past. What would be the most therapeutic response?
1. "Do you think withholding this information is the basis for a trusting relationship?"
2. "Don't you think your partner deserves to know?"
3. "What concerns do you have about sharing this information?"
4. "I can understand why you would want to keep this information from him."

31. 3. This response encourages the client to verbalize her concerns in a safe environment and begin to choose a course of action for how to deal with this issue now. Telling the client that she's withholding information that may cause distrust in her relationship or that her partner deserves to know conveys negative judgments. The fourth response doesn't encourage discussion or problem-solving.
CN: Psychosocial integrity; CNS: None; CL: Application

CN: Client needs category   CNS: Client needs subcategory   CL: Cognitive level

32. After learning that his gay roommate has tested positive for human immunodeficiency virus (HIV), a client asks the nurse about moving to another room on the psychiatric unit because the client doesn't feel "safe" now. What should the nurse do <u>first</u>?
1. Move the client to another room.
2. Ask the client to describe any fears.
3. Move the client's roommate to a private room.
4. Explain that such a move wouldn't be therapeutic for the client or his roommate.

33. A nurse lecturing on paraphilias informs her audience that recidivism is high for clients with paraphilias. Which definition best describes recidivism?
1. Insight into treatment
2. Aggressive sexual assault
3. Behaviors associated with sexual deviation
4. Continued inappropriate behavior after treatment

34. Which nursing diagnosis is most appropriate for a client with sexual masochism?
1. *Risk for self-mutilation*
2. *Ineffective role performance*
3. *Ineffective coping*
4. *Risk for other-directed violence*

35. Which statement made by a client with paraphilia indicates a potential for relapse?
1. "I am going to outpatient therapy."
2. "I am going to try to attend all therapy sessions."
3. "I don't need this, and I can't imagine why the judge sent me here."
4. "The physician wants me to take leuprolide acetate (Lupron). I think that will help."

36. A female client taking antidepressant medication complains to the nurse that she has a decreased desire for sex, which is causing significant marital stress. Which response by the nurse would be the <u>most appropriate</u>?
1. "Don't stop taking the medication."
2. "What are your thoughts on how you should handle this?"
3. "Doesn't your husband understand the importance of your medication?"
4. "Have you discussed this with your physician?"

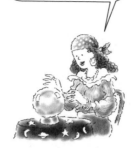

I predict you will be able to select which action should be performed first.

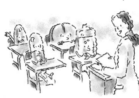

The NCLEX often tests your ability to educate accurately.

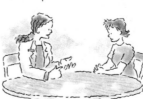

More than one answer may seen correct, but choose the most appropriate.

32. 2. To intervene effectively, the nurse must first understand the client's fears. After exploring the client's fears, the nurse may move the client or his roommate or explain why such a move wouldn't be therapeutic.
CN: Psychosocial integrity; CNS: None; CL: Application

33. 4. Recidivism is defined as continuing in an unacceptable behavior after completing treatment to correct that behavior. High level of insight isn't connected with any specific disorder. Aggressive sexual assault is a type of paraphilia. Sexually deviant behaviors are known as paraphilias.
CN: Psychosocial integrity; CNS: None; CL: Analysis

34. 1. A person with sexual masochism is sexually aroused by being the receiver of pain and, therefore, may injure himself. A person diagnosed with transvestic fetishism may have ineffective role performance. There is no evidence that this client isn't coping. A sexual sadist would be a danger to others.
CN: Psychosocial integrity; CNS: None; CL: Analysis

35. 3. A lack of insight to the problem may indicate a potential for relapse. Attending all therapy sessions and outpatient therapy demonstrates compliance with the treatment plan. Leuprolide acetate is an anti-androgenic that lowers testosterone levels and decreases the libido.
CN: Psychosocial integrity; CNS: None; CL: Analysis

36. 2. Encouraging the client to verbalize her thoughts will help the client to problem solve and identify feelings related to different choices. The first response is too directive and doesn't encourage exploration on the part of the client. The third response conveys negative judgment. The fourth response might be appropriate, but it also may give the impression that the nurse doesn't want to discuss this issue with the client.
CN: Psychosocial integrity; CNS: None; CL: Application

37. A mother brings her 14-year-old son to the psychiatric crisis room. The client's mother states, "He's always dressing in female clothing. There must be something wrong with him." Which response from the nurse would be most appropriate?

1. "Your son will be evaluated shortly."
2. "I'll tell your son that this isn't appropriate."
3. "I know you're upset. Would you like to talk?"
4. "I wouldn't want my son to dress in girl's clothing."

38. A 17-year-old female who enjoys playing ball with boys and is most comfortable in jeans tells her mother she doesn't want to go to the prom if she has to wear a frilly dress. Her mother asks, "What should I do with my daughter?" Which response from the nurse would be most appropriate?

1. Tell the client's mother, "She'll grow out of it."
2. Offer to speak to the client about her dressing habits.
3. Ask the client's mother to talk about her fears for her daughter.
4. Tell the client's mother to make her go to the prom but not wear a dress.

39. A 39-year-old male client wishes to undergo a sex-reassignment operation because he feels trapped in his male body. Which action is the next step the client should take if he wants to have the operation?

1. Tell his family and friends
2. Attend psychotherapy
3. Visit transsexual bars
4. See a surgeon

40. Which reason <u>best</u> explains the rationale for estrogen therapy for a male client who wishes to undergo sexual reassignment surgery?

1. To develop breasts
2. To cause menstruation
3. To assist with cross-dressing
4. To develop body hair and lack of menstruation

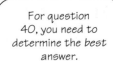

For question 40, you need to determine the best answer.

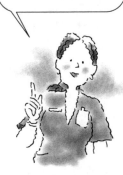

37. 3. Acknowledging the mother's feelings and offering her an opportunity to verbalize her concerns provides a forum for open communication. Telling the client's mother that he'll be evaluated shortly doesn't address her concerns. Telling the client that this behavior isn't appropriate doesn't assess his feelings nor does it analyze the behavior. The nurse shouldn't offer an opinion by stating she wouldn't want her son dressing in female clothing.
CN: Psychosocial integrity; CNS: None; CL: Application

38. 3. Asking the client's mother to verbalize her fears will permit the nurse to accurately assess the mother's distress. The client's mother may be upset over the behavior or the fact that her daughter doesn't wish to go to the prom. Telling the client's mother that her daughter will grow out of it may be offering the mother false reassurance. The nurse shouldn't speak to the client about her behavior as this implies a value judgment on the part of the nurse. Forcing her to go to the prom isn't therapeutic, and doesn't address the mother's fears.
CN: Psychosocial integrity; CNS: None; CL: Application

39. 2. Before having a sex-reassignment operation, the client should have several years of psychotherapy. The family, as well as friends, should be told of the client's plans. Visiting transsexual bars has no bearing on having a sex-reassignment operation. Seeing a surgeon isn't usually done on a regular basis until after the completion of psychotherapy.
CN: Psychosocial integrity; CNS: None; CL: Analysis

40. 1. A male who receives long-term estrogen therapy will develop female secondary sexual characteristics such as breasts. A male on estrogen won't menstruate because he doesn't have a uterus. Estrogen has no bearing on cross-dressing. Androgens would be taken by a female to develop body hair and stop menstruation.
CN: Psychosocial integrity; CNS: None; CL: Analysis

CN: Client needs category   CNS: Client needs subcategory   CL: Cognitive level

41. A nurse is caring for several clients with gender identity disorders. The nurse understands that which client is most at risk for anxiety related to transsexualism?

1. Elderly
2. Adolescent
3. Young adult
4. Prepubescent child

42. What is the gender identity disorder that results in the person believing he or she is really the opposite sex?

1. Exhibitionism
2. Homosexuality
3. Transsexualism
4. Transvestitism

43. A transsexual client wishes to have a sexual reassignment operation and tells the nurse he's ready to begin hormonal therapy. Which fact about the client must be true <u>before</u> estrogen therapy is administered?

1. He has cross-dressed and lived as the opposite sex for several years.
2. He has decided against undergoing the operation.
3. He has decided he needs more psychotherapy.
4. He has been functioning sexually as a female.

44. According to Erikson, an adolescent who is suffering from gender identity disorder is unable to progress through which developmental task?

1. Initiative versus guilt
2. Intimacy versus isolation
3. Industry versus inferiority
4. Identity versus role confusion

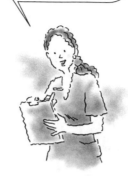

A client's age can affect his anxiety related to gender identity disorders.

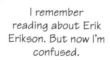

I remember reading about Erik Erikson. But now I'm confused.

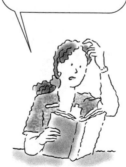

41. 2. Adolescents who are transsexuals are usually very distraught over the changes occurring within their body. Elderly persons, young adults, and young children aren't experiencing rapidly developing secondary sexual characteristics in their bodies; therefore, they aren't at high risk for anxiety.

CN: Psychosocial integrity; CNS: None; CL: Analysis

42. 3. Transsexuals believe they're really of the opposite sex. An exhibitionist is someone who's sexually aroused by displaying one's genitals in a public place. A homosexual enjoys sexual relations with a person of the same sexual orientation. A transvestite enjoys cross-dressing.

CN: Psychosocial integrity; CNS: None; CL: Application

43. 1. Before a sexual reassignment operation, the client should live as the opposite sex after undergoing several years of psychotherapy. A client wishing to take hormonal therapy is in the final step before receiving the operation and therefore hasn't decided against the surgery. Psychotherapy is an ongoing modality for someone requesting a sexual reassignment operation. A male doesn't have female reproductive organs, so he couldn't have been functioning sexually as a female.

CN: Psychosocial integrity; CNS: None; CL: Analysis

44. 4. According to developmentalist Erik Erikson, adolescence is a time when role identity is found as a result of independence and sexual maturity; role confusion would result from the inability to integrate all experiences. Initiative versus guilt is when a child begins to conceptualize and interpersonalize relationships. Intimacy versus isolation is a stage in which the adult meets other adults and establishes relationships. Industry versus inferiority is when a child incorporates and acquires social skills.

CN: Health promotion and maintenance; CNS: None; CL: Analysis

45. A 35-year-old client who has been married for 10 years arrives at the psychiatric clinic stating, "I can't live this lie any more. I wish I were a woman. I don't want my wife. I need a man." Which initial action would be most appropriate from the nurse?
1. Call the primary health care provider.
2. Encourage the client to speak to his wife.
3. Have the client admitted.
4. Sit down with the client, and talk about his feelings.

46. A 14-year-old female client admits to having transsexual feelings and states, "I would rather die than live in this body." Which is the <u>initial</u> action most appropriate for the nurse to take?
1. Explain to her that she is too young to have these feelings.
2. Call her parents, and let them know about her feelings.
3. Encourage her to verbalize her feelings.
4. Ask her if she plans to kill herself.

47. A female client enjoys wearing men's clothing. Her sister tells the nurse that the client wishes for a sexual reassignment operation. The client tells the nurse she just wants to be left alone. Which initial nursing intervention is most appropriate?
1. Tell the client she is repressing her true feelings.
2. Encourage the client to verbalize her feelings.
3. Tell the client's sister to mind her own business.
4. Encourage the client to avoid her sister.

48. A mother is concerned about her son and says he's 10 years old and has been playing with dolls since he was 2. Which initial strategy should be included in his care plan?
1. Providing counseling for his mother
2. Instructing the mother to throw away the dolls
3. Instructing the mother on play that's age-appropriate
4. Exploring with the child his feelings related to the dolls

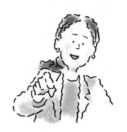

What should you do first?

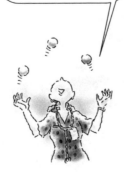

Keep going! Fewer than 10 questions to go!

45. 4. Sitting down with the client and exploring his feelings will allow the nurse to assess him. The primary health care provider shouldn't be notified until an assessment is made. The client shouldn't speak to his wife until he has processed his feelings. An assessment of the client should be made *before* admitting the client to the unit.
CN: Psychosocial integrity; CNS: None; CL: Application

46. 4. Whenever a client verbalizes feelings of preferring death to life, the nurse should always make sure that the client doesn't have a plan. Transsexual tendencies usually arise during the adolescent years, so it is appropriate for the client to have these feelings. Calling her parents wouldn't be a priority until after a psychological safety assessment is completed. Encouraging her to verbalize her feelings isn't an initial action for the nurse.
CN: Psychosocial integrity; CNS: None; CL: Application

47. 2. The client needs to verbalize her feelings regarding wearing male attire as well as her desire to be left alone. Telling the client she is repressing her true feelings is judgmental. It's inappropriate for a nurse to tell a family member to mind her own business or to tell the client to avoid her sister.
CN: Psychosocial integrity; CNS: None; CL: Application

48. 4. It's important to assess the child's feelings as well as to explore his preference for dolls rather than sports. The mother may need to be instructed on methods to cope with his behaviors but only after the child is permitted to verbalize. Until proper assessment is made, it's inappropriate to remove the dolls. There's no evidence of age-inappropriate play.
CN: Psychosocial integrity; CNS: None; CL: Application

49. A newly graduated nurse expresses concern to the nurse-manager about working with clients who want to discuss sexual problems. Which response by the nurse-manager is appropriate?
1. "It's part of the job. You'll get used to it."
2. "You can refer those types of questions to other health care professionals."
3. "If you've graduated from nursing school and passed the NCLEX, you qualify as a sex counselor."
4. "Tell me more about your concern."

50. A 57-year-old hypertensive male client expresses concern about his sexual functioning. Which question is <u>most</u> helpful in obtaining further assessment data?
1. Medication history
2. Sexual practices
3. Medical conditions
4. Family history

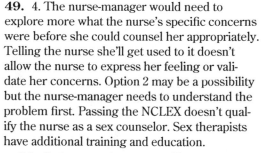

We have a history together.

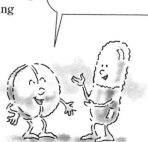

51. A male client brings a list of his prescribed medications to the clinic. During the initial assessment, he tells the nurse that he has been experiencing delayed ejaculation. Which of the following drug classes would <u>most likely</u> be associated with this condition?
1. Anticoagulants
2. Antibiotics
3. Antihypertensives
4. Steroids

52. After a myocardial infarction (MI), a client tells the nurse he's afraid he'll have another heart attack if he attempts sexual intercourse. Which nursing diagnosis is <u>most</u> appropriate?
1. *Deficient knowledge related to sexual dysfunction*
2. *Disturbed body image related to lifestyle changes*
3. *Sexual dysfunction related to disturbances in self-esteem*
4. *Disturbed body image related to effects of treatment*

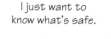

I just want to know what's safe.

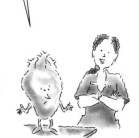

49. 4. The nurse-manager would need to explore more what the nurse's specific concerns were before she could counsel her appropriately. Telling the nurse she'll get used to it doesn't allow the nurse to express her feeling or validate her concerns. Option 2 may be a possibility but the nurse-manager needs to understand the problem first. Passing the NCLEX doesn't qualify the nurse as a sex counselor. Sex therapists have additional training and education.
CN: Safe effective care environment; CNS: Management of care; CL: Analysis

50. 1. Many antihypertensive medications can affect sexual functioning; the nurse must assess if the client is taking other medications that may also alter sexual functioning. Sexual practices are part of the nursing assessment, as are other medical conditions and family history. However, obtaining a thorough medication history and reviewing effects on the client may help alleviate misconceptions and easily identify the source of the problem.
CN: Physiological integrity; CNS: Pharmacological and parenteral therapies; CL: Application

51. 3. Antihypertensive agents can cause or contribute to sexual dysfunction. Anticoagulants, antibiotics, and steroids have no known effect on sexual function.
CN: Physiological integrity; CNS: Pharmacological and parenteral therapies; CL: Application

52. 1. After an MI, many clients fear that engaging in sex will trigger another one. The nurse should teach the client about when he can safely resume sexual activity and which positions to use during intercourse to conserve energy. The client's fears result from lack of knowledge, not disturbances in self-esteem or body image.
CN: Psychosocial integrity; CNS: None; CL: Application

53. A 42-year-old female client complains of painful intercourse. Which nursing <u>diagnosis</u> is most useful in planning this client's care?
1. *Ineffective coping*
2. *Disturbed body image*
3. *Ineffective sexuality patterns*
4. *Sexual dysfunction*

54. A 46-year-old female client is diagnosed with a problem in sexual functioning. When planning her care, which nursing action takes <u>highest</u> priority?
1. Assessing the client's sexual functioning
2. Assessing the client's role in her sexual relationship
3. Determining the nurse's own beliefs and feelings about this issue
4. Interviewing the client's sexual partner

55. A 35-year-old male client states he has little or no sexual desire. He also states that this is causing great distress in his marriage. What further information would be the <u>most useful</u> in assessing the situation? Select all that apply:
1. The client's age when he had his first girlfriend
2. When the problem first appeared and potential contributing factors
3. Medications and dosages
4. Report of recent bladder or prostate problems
5. Age of the client's wife

56. Pedophilia is diagnosed by the presence of specifically defined behaviors and characteristics. Which statements regarding pedophilia are true? Select all that apply:
1. A strong sexual attraction to prepubescent children exists.
2. Male children are more commonly the focus of attention than female children.
3. The pedophile is usually very attentive to a child's needs in order to gain the child's attention.
4. The disorder generally begins in early adulthood.
5. The pedophile must be age 16 or older or at least 5 years older than the child.

CN: Client needs category   CNS: Client needs subcategory   CL: Cognitive level

53. 4. *Sexual dysfunction* is the most useful nursing diagnosis for this client because she has identified painful intercourse as a physical problem, which can alter the giving and receiving of pleasure and satisfaction. *Ineffective coping* would apply if the client stated she avoids intercourse or expresses alternative coping mechanisms. *Disturbed body image* isn't appropriate because the client hasn't stated she feels uncomfortable in some way about herself. *Ineffective sexuality patterns* would apply if the client stated that she doesn't engage in intercourse or have the ability to relate to others sexually.
CN: Psychosocial integrity; CNS: None; CL: Application

54. 3. The nurse must first identify her own beliefs and feelings about the issue and remain nonjudgmental. The other actions may be relevant but take lower priority.
CN: Safe, effective care environment; CNS: Management of care; CL: Application

55. 2, 3. Option 2 is correct and provides opportunity to gather useful information in better understanding the client's current condition. Option 3 is correct because certain medications can have a profound effect on sexual desire. The client's age when he started dating has no bearing on the current problem. Reporting previous problems is useful but wouldn't provide a sufficient explanation for the lack of sexual desire. The age of the client's wife is irrelevant and doesn't provide assessment data.
CN: Psychosocial integrity; CNS: None; CL: Analysis

56. 1, 3, 5. Pedophilia is a disorder characterized by a strong sexual attraction to prepubescent children that generally begins to manifest itself in adolescence, not early adulthood. By definition, the pedophile must be age 16 or older or at least 5 years older than the child. The pedophile generally is attentive to the needs of children in order to gain their trust, loyalty, and attention. Female, not male, children are more commonly the focus of attention.
CN: Psychosocial integrity; CNS: None; CL: Application

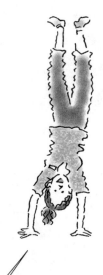

Time to celebrate! You finished chapter 20!

New information about eating disorders is released almost continuously. For the latest about disorders of critical importance for young people, check the Web site of the National Eating Disorders Association at **www.nationaleatingdisorders.org.**

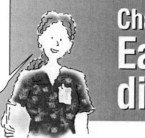

Chapter 22
Eating disorders

1. A parent with a daughter with bulimia nervosa asks a nurse, "How can my child have an eating disorder when she isn't underweight?" Which response is <u>best</u>?
   1. "A person with bulimia nervosa can maintain a normal weight."
   2. "It's hard to face this type of problem in a person you love."
   3. "At first there is no weight loss; it comes later in the disease."
   4. "This is a serious problem even though there is no weight loss."

2. A 15-year-old female is brought to the clinic by her parents because of a significant amount of weight loss in the past 4 months. Which accompanying conditions would indicate that the client is suffering from anorexia nervosa?
   1. Hypertension
   2. Amenorrhea
   3. Hyperthermia
   4. Diarrhea

3. Which statement made by the client about the binge-purge cycle that occurs with bulimia nervosa indicates understanding of the disorder?
   1. "There are emotional triggers connected to bingeing."
   2. "Over time, people usually grow out of bingeing behaviors."
   3. "Bingeing isn't the problem; purging is the issue to address."
   4. "When a person gets too hungry, there's a tendency to binge."

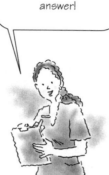

Choose the best answer!

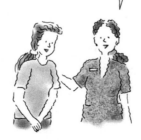

Help your client understand her behavior.

1. 1. A client with bulimia nervosa may be of normal weight, overweight, or underweight. Weight loss isn't a clinical criterion for bulimia nervosa. The second option doesn't address the need for information about the relationship between weight change and bulimia nervosa. The third option is incorrect because there may be little or no weight loss. The fourth option doesn't address the issue of weight change in a client with bulimia nervosa.
CN: Psychosocial integrity; CNS: None; CL: Application

2. 2. Anorexia nervosa is characterized by profound weight loss caused by severe restriction of food intake by the client. If severe enough, it causes amenorrhea in females, along with decreased—not increased—body temperature. It usually doesn't produce diarrhea, but it may produce constipation because decreased oral intake leads to decreased GI motility.
CN: Physiological integrity; CNS: Reduction of risk potential; CL: Application

3. 1. It's important for the client to understand the emotional triggers to bingeing, such as disappointment, depression, and anxiety. People don't outgrow eating behaviors. This leads a person to believe binge eating is a normal part of growth and development when it definitely isn't. The third option negates the seriousness of bingeing and leads the client to believe only vomiting is a problem, not overeating. Physiologic hunger doesn't predispose a client to binge behaviors.
CN: Physiological integrity; CNS: Reduction of risk potential; CL: Application

CN: Client needs category   CNS: Client needs subcategory   CL: Cognitive level

4. A client with bulimia and a history of purging by vomiting is hospitalized for further observation because she's at risk for which of the following?
  1. Diabetes mellitus
  2. Electrolyte imbalance
  3. GI obstruction
  4. Septicemia

5. A client with a diagnosis of bulimia nervosa is working on relationship issues. Which nursing intervention is the most important?
  1. Have the client work on developing social skills.
  2. Focus on how relationships cause bulimic behavior.
  3. Help the client identify feelings about relationships.
  4. Discuss how to prevent getting overinvolved in relationships.

6. A young female client with bulimia nervosa wants to lessen her feelings of powerlessness. Which short-term goal is most important <u>initially</u>?
  1. Learn problem-solving skills.
  2. Decrease symptoms of anxiety.
  3. Perform self-care activities daily.
  4. Verbalize how to set limits with others.

7. A female client with bulimia nervosa tells a nurse her parents don't know about her eating disorder. Which goal is appropriate for this client and her family?
  1. Decrease the chaos in the family unit.
  2. Learn effective communication skills.
  3. Spend time together in social situations.
  4. Discuss the client's need to be responsible.

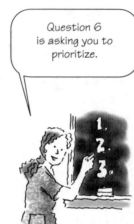

Question 6 is asking you to prioritize.

4. 2. Clients with bulimia who purge by vomiting are at greatest risk of electrolyte imbalances which can lead to cardiac arrhythmias. Purging by vomiting does not result in diabetes mellitus, GI obstruction, or septicemia.
CN: Physiological integrity; CNS: Physiological adaptation; CL: Application

5. 3. The client needs to address personal feelings, especially uncomfortable ones because they may trigger bingeing behavior. Social skills are important to a client's well-being, but they aren't typically a major problem for the client with bulimia nervosa. Relationships *don't cause* bulimic behaviors. It's the inability to handle stress or conflict that arises from interactions that causes the client to be distressed. The client isn't necessarily overinvolved in relationships; the issue may be the lack of satisfying relationships in the person's life.
CN: Psychosocial integrity; CNS: None; CL: Application

6. 1. If the client can learn effective problem-solving skills, she'll gain a sense of control and power over her life. Anxiety is commonly caused by feelings of powerlessness. Performing daily self-care activities won't reduce one's sense of powerlessness. Verbalizing how to set limits and protect self from the intrusive behavior of others is a necessary life skill, but problem-solving skills take priority.
CN: Psychosocial integrity; CNS: None; CL: Analysis

7. 2. A major goal for the client and her family is to learn to communicate directly and honestly. To change the chaotic environment, the family must first learn to communicate effectively. Families with a member who has an eating disorder are often enmeshed and don't need to spend more time together. Before discussing the client's level of responsibility, the family needs to establish effective ways to communicate with each other.
CN: Psychosocial integrity; CNS: None; CL: Application

CN: Client needs category   CNS: Client needs subcategory   CL: Cognitive level

8. When discussing self-esteem with a client with bulimia nervosa, which area is the <u>most important</u>?
1. Personal fears
2. Family strengths
3. Negative thinking
4. Environmental stimuli

9. Which complication of bulimia nervosa is <u>life-threatening</u>?
1. Serum calcium 10.1 mg/dl
2. Heart rate 56 beats/minute
3. Serum potassium 2.9 mEq/L
4. Respiratory rate 16 breaths/minute

10. A nurse is talking to a client with bulimia nervosa about the complications of laxative abuse. Which statement by the client indicates that she's beginning to understand the risks associated with laxative abuse?
1. "I don't really have much taste for food, so there's no loss in getting it out of my system more quickly."
2. "Laxatives help me get rid of extra calories before they're added to my body. I know I just shouldn't eat the extra calories to begin with."
3. "Laxatives are over-the-counter medications that have no harmful effect."
4. "Using laxatives prevents my body from absorbing essential nutrients, such as protein, fat, and calcium."

11. A female client with bulimia nervosa tells a nurse she and her parents don't agree on anything. Which method is best to address this problem when the family comes for a family meeting?
1. Focus on conflict resolution skills.
2. Establish an internal locus of control.
3. Construct a three-generation genogram.
4. Discuss age-specific developmental problems.

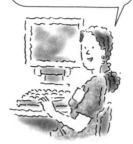

It is *most* important that you read question 8 carefully.

8. 3. Clients with bulimia nervosa need to work on identifying and changing their negative thinking and distortion of reality. Personal fears are related to negative thinking but isn't the most important. Exploring family strengths isn't a priority; it's more appropriate to explore the client's strengths. Environmental stimuli don't cause bulimic behaviors.
CN: Psychosocial integrity; CNS: None; CL: Application

9. 3. Electrolyte imbalance such as hypokalemia (normal serum potassium is 3.5 to 4.5 mEq/L) can be a life-threatening complication of bulimia nervosa due to purging behaviors. A serum calcium level of 10.1 mg/dl is within normal range. A heart rate of 56 beats/minute indicates bradycardia, but isn't life-threatening. A respiratory rate of 16 breaths/minute is within the normal range (16 to 20 breaths/minute) and not life-threatening.
CN: Physiological integrity; CNS: Reduction of risk potential; CL: Application

10. 4. A serious complication of laxative abuse is malabsorption of nutrients, such as proteins, fats, and calcium. Laxative abuse doesn't tend to affect the client's sense of taste. Clients with bulimia nervosa need to change their negative thinking with respect to calories and the use of laxatives.
CN: Physiological integrity; CNS: Reduction of risk potential; CL: Application

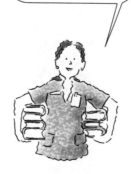

You're doing great! It looks like all your studying is paying off.

11. 1. To decrease conflict and promote family harmony, the nurse would teach the family conflict resolution skills. Establishing a plan to promote internal control or constructing a three-generation genogram won't help the family solve conflicts. Discussion of age-specific developmental problems won't promote conflict resolution or promote family harmony.
CN: Psychosocial integrity; CNS: None; CL: Application

12. A female client is talking to a nurse about her binge-purge cycle. Which question should the nurse ask about the cycle?
1. "Do you know how to stop the binge-purge cycle?"
2. "Does the binge-purge cycle help you lose weight?"
3. "Can the binge-purge cycle take away your anxiety?"
4. "How often do you go through the binge-purge cycle?"

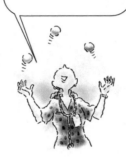

Consider all the answers. Then choose the best one.

13. A nurse is assessing a client with bulimia nervosa for possible substance abuse. Which question is best to obtain information about this possible problem?
1. "Have you ever used diet pills?"
2. "Where would you go to buy drugs?"
3. "At what age did you start drinking?"
4. "Do your peers ever offer you drugs?"

14. A female client with bulimia nervosa is discussing her abnormal eating behaviors. Which statement by the client indicates she's beginning to understand this eating disorder?
1. "When my loneliness gets to me, I start to binge."
2. "I know that when my life gets better I'll eat right."
3. "I know I waste food and waste my money on food."
4. "After my parents divorce, I'll talk about bingeing and purging."

15. A nurse is assessing a client with a history of recent binge eating. Which of the following symptoms would the nurse most likely observe in this client?
1. Ageusia
2. Headache
3. Pain
4. Sore throat

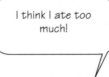

I think I ate too much!

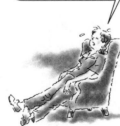

12. 4. This is an important question because there's often a range of frequencies, such as from a once-a-week pattern to multiple times per day. The frequency of binge-purge cycles may also alert the nurse to the degree of risk from fluid and electrolyte imbalances. Asking the client if she knows how to stop the binge-purge cycle isn't appropriate as it will generate feelings of self-blame and shame. It's common for clients to experience daily fluctuations in weight (some report variations of up to 10 lb). Although the binge-purge behavior may decrease anxiety initially; it tends to generate overall negative feelings about self.
CN: Psychosocial integrity; CNS: None; CL: Application

13. 1. Some clients with bulimia nervosa have a history of or actively use amphetamines to control weight. The use of alcohol and street drugs is also common. The second and fourth questions could be answered by the client without revealing drug use. The age the client started drinking may not show current substance use.
CN: Psychosocial integrity; CNS: None; CL: Application

14. 1. Binge eating is a way to handle the uncomfortable feelings of frustration, loneliness, anger, and fear. The second option indicates the client is experiencing denial of the eating disorder. The third option addresses the client's guilt feelings; it doesn't reflect knowledge of her eating disorder. The fourth option shows the client isn't ready to discuss her eating disorder.
CN: Psychosocial integrity; CNS: None; CL: Analysis

15. 3. After a binge episode, the client commonly has abdominal distention and stomach pain. A sore throat is associated with vomiting. Ageusia (loss of taste) or headache aren't associated with binge eating.
CN: Physiological integrity; CNS: Physiological adaptation; CL: Application

CN: Client needs category   CNS: Client needs subcategory   CL: Cognitive level

16. A mother of a female client with bulimia nervosa asks a nurse if bulimia nervosa will stop her daughter from menstruating. Which response is best?

1. "All women with anorexia nervosa or bulimia nervosa will have amenorrhea."
2. "When your daughter is bingeing and purging, she won't have normal periods."
3. "The eating disorder must be ongoing for your daughter's menstrual cycle to change."
4. "Women with bulimia nervosa may have a normal or abnormal menstrual cycle, depending on the severity of the problem."

17. Which nursing diagnosis should have the highest priority in the plan of care for a client with an eating disorder?

1. *Interrupted family processes*
2. *Imbalanced nutrition: Less than body requirements*
3. *Disturbed body image*
4. *Ineffective coping*

18. A female client with bulimia nervosa tells a nurse her major problem is eating too much food in a short period of time and then vomiting. Which short-term goal is the <u>most important</u>?

1. Help the client understand every person has a satiety level.
2. Encourage the client to verbalize fears and concerns about food.
3. Determine the amount of food the client will eat without purging.
4. Obtain a therapy appointment to look at the emotional causes of bulimia nervosa.

19. Which statement indicates a female client with bulimia nervosa is making progress in interrupting the binge-purge cycle?

1. "I called my friend the last two times I got upset."
2. "I know I'll have this problem with eating forever."
3. "I started asking my mother or sister to watch me eat each meal."
4. "I can have my boyfriend bring me home from parties if I want to purge."

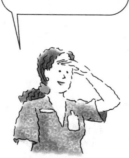

Help the client see the importance of reaching a short-term goal.

16. 4. Women with bulimia nervosa may have a normal or abnormal menstrual cycle, depending on the severity of the eating disorder. Not all women with eating disorders have amenorrhea. The eating disorder can disrupt the menstrual cycle at any point in the illness.
CN: Health promotion and maintenance; CNS: None; CL: Analysis

17. 2. The most immediate priority is to meet the nutritional needs of the client to prevent complications. The other nursing diagnoses are all important long-term goals that can be addressed once the client's immediate physiologic needs have been met.
CN: Safe, effective care environment; CNS: Management of care; CL: Analysis

18. 3. The client must meet her nutritional needs to prevent further complications, so she must identify the amount of food she can eat without purging as her first short-term goal. Binge eaters can't recognize their satiety level or their feelings of fullness. Obtaining knowledge or verbalizing her fears and feelings about food are *not* priority goals for this client. After meeting immediate physiological needs, therapy is an important part of dealing with this disorder.
CN: Physiological integrity; CNS: Reduction of risk potential; CL: Application

19. 1. A sign of progress is when the client begins to verbalize feelings and interact with people instead of going to food for comfort. The second option indicates the client needs more information on how to handle the disorder. Having another person watch the client eat isn't a helpful strategy as the client will depend on others to help control food intake. The last option indicates the client is in denial about the severity of the problem.
CN: Psychosocial integrity; CNS: None; CL: Analysis

20. A client with bulimia nervosa asks a nurse, "How can I ask for help from my family?" Which response is the <u>most appropriate</u>?
  1. "When you ask for help, make sure you really need it."
  2. "Have you ever asked for help before?"
  3. "Ask family members to spend time with you at mealtime."
  4. "Think about how you can handle this situation without help."

21. A female client with bulimia nervosa tells a nurse that she doesn't eat during the day, but after 5:00 p.m., she begins to binge and vomit. Which intervention should be the most useful to this client?
  1. Help the client stop eating the foods on which she binges.
  2. Discuss the effects of fasting on the client's pattern of eating.
  3. Encourage the client to become involved in food preparation.
  4. Teach the client to eat earlier in the day and decrease intake at night.

22. A female client with bulimia nervosa tells a nurse she was doing well until last week, when she had a fight with her father. Which nursing intervention should help most?
  1. Examine the relationship between feelings and eating.
  2. Discuss the importance of therapy for the entire family.
  3. Encourage the client to avoid certain family members.
  4. Identify daily stressors and learn stress management skills.

23. Which statement from a bulimic client shows that she understands the concept of <u>relapse</u>?
  1. "If I can't maintain control over things, I'll have problems."
  2. "If I have problems, then that says I haven't learned much."
  3. "If this illness becomes chronic, I won't be able to handle it."
  4. "If I have problems, I can start over again and not feel hopeless."

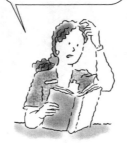

Is most appropriate the same as "prioritize?"

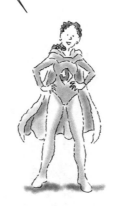

If at first you don't succeed. Try try again—to choose the correct answer.

20. 2. Determine whether the client has ever been successful in asking for help. Previous experiences affect the client's ability to ask for help now. The client needs to ask for help anytime without analyzing the level of need. Having other people around at mealtime isn't the only way to ask for help. Developing a support system is imperative for this client.
CN: Psychosocial integrity; CNS: None; CL: Analysis

21. 2. If a person fasts for most of the day, it's common to become extremely hungry, overeat by bingeing, and then feel the need to purge. Restricting food intake can actually trigger the binge-purge cycle. In treatment, the client is taught to identify foods that trigger eating, discuss the feelings associated with these foods, and work to eat them in normal amounts. Involvement in food preparation won't promote changes in the client's behaviors. The last option doesn't address how fasting can trigger the binge-purge cycle.
CN: Psychosocial integrity; CNS: None; CL: Application

22. 1. The client needs to understand her feelings and develop healthy coping skills to handle unpleasant situations. Family therapy may be indicated but shouldn't be an immediate intervention. Avoidance isn't a useful coping strategy; eventually the underlying issues need to be explored. All clients can benefit from stress management skills, but for this client, care must focus on the relationship between feelings and eating behaviors.
CN: Psychosocial integrity; CNS: None; CL: Application

23. 4. This statement indicates that the client knows a relapse is just a slip, and positive gains made from treatment haven't been lost. Negative self-statements can lead to relapse. Control issues relate to powerlessness, which contribute to relapse.
CN: Psychosocial integrity; CNS: None; CL: Application

CN: Client needs category   CNS: Client needs subcategory   CL: Cognitive level

24. What's the treatment team's priority in planning the care of a client with an eating disorder?
1. Preventing the client from performing any muscle-building exercises
2. Keeping the client on bedrest until she attains a specified weight
3. Meeting daily to discuss manipulation and countertransference
4. Monitoring the client's weight and vital signs daily

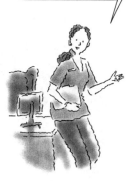
Remember to prioritize!

24. 3. Clients with eating disorders commonly use manipulative ploys and countertransference to resist weight gain (if they restrict food intake) or to maintain purging practices (if they're bulimic). Such clients commonly play staff members against one another. Muscle building is acceptable because it burns relatively few calories. Keeping the client on bedrest until a specified weight is reached may result in power struggles and prevent focusing on pertinent issues. Monitoring the client's weight and vital signs is important but not on a daily basis unless the client's condition warrants such scrutiny.
CN: Psychosocial integrity; CN: None; CL: Application

25. A nurse should be alert for which findings in a client with bulimia nervosa? Select all that apply:
1. Severe electrolyte imbalances
2. Damaged teeth due to the eroding effects of gastric acids on tooth enamel
3. Pneumonia from aspirated stomach contents
4. Cessation of menses
5. Esophageal tears and gastric rupture
6. Intestinal inflammation

25. 1, 2, 4, 5. Constant bingeing and purging behaviors can result in severe electrolyte imbalances, erosion of tooth enamel from constant exposure to gastric acids, menstrual irregularities, esophageal tears and, in severe cases, gastric rupture. Aspiration pneumonia is unlikely because the vomiting is controlled. Intestinal inflammation isn't typically associated with bulimia nervosa.
CN: Physiological integrity; CNS: Physiological adaptation; CL: Application

26. A client with anorexia nervosa attended psychoeducational sessions on principles of adequate nutrition. Which statement by the client indicates the teaching was effective?
1. "I eat while I'm doing things to distract myself."
2. "I eat all my food at night right before I go to bed."
3. "I eat small amounts of food slowly at every meal."
4. "I eat only when I'm with my family and trying to be social."

26. 3. Slowly eating small amounts of food facilitates adequate digestion and prevents distention. Healthy eating is best accomplished when a person isn't doing other things while eating. Eating right before bedtime isn't a healthy eating habit. If a client eats only when the family is present or when trying to be social, eating is tied to social or emotional cues rather than nutritional needs.
CN: Health promotion and maintenance; CNS: None; CL: Application

27. A client with anorexia nervosa tells a nurse, "I'll never have the slender body I want." Which intervention is best to handle this problem?
1. Call a family meeting to get help from the parents.
2. Help the client work on developing a realistic body image.
3. Make an appointment to see the dietitian on a weekly basis.
4. Develop an exercise program the client can do twice a week.

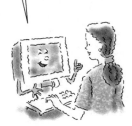
All options may be good, but choose the best one.

27. 2. With anorexia nervosa, the client pursues thinness and has a distorted view of self. A family meeting may not help the client develop a more realistic view of the body. Although meeting with a dietitian might be helpful, it isn't a priority. Clients with anorexia nervosa typically exercise excessively.
CN: Psychosocial integrity; CNS: None; CL: Application

28. A client with anorexia nervosa tells a nurse, "My parents never hug me or say I've done anything right." Which intervention is the <u>best</u> to use with this family?

1. Teach the family principles of assertive behavior.
2. Discuss the difficulties the family has in social situations.
3. Help the family convey a positive attitude toward the client.
4. Explore the family's ability to express affection appropriately.

29. Which communication strategy is best to use with a client with anorexia nervosa who is having problems with peer relationships?

1. Use concrete language and maintain a focus on reality.
2. Direct the client to talk about what is causing the anxiety.
3. Teach the client to communicate feelings and express self appropriately.
4. Confront the client about being depressed and self-absorbed.

30. A nurse plans to include the parents of a client with anorexia nervosa in therapy sessions along with the client. What fact should the nurse remember about parents of clients with anorexia?

1. They tend to overprotect their children.
2. They usually have a history of substance abuse.
3. They maintain emotional distance from their children.
4. They alternate between loving and rejecting their children.

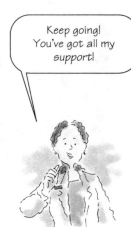

Keep going! You've got all my support!

28. 4. There's often a lack of affection and warmth in families who have a member with an eating disorder. Although assertiveness is an important skill, the family member needs to realize assertiveness isn't always rewarded. Difficulties in social situations are important to address, but the intervention must focus on how to express positive feelings and affection. A positive attitude helps a person become better able to handle the pressures of life, but it may not change the family's display of affection.

CN: Psychosocial integrity; CNS: None; CL: Application

29. 3. Clients with anorexia nervosa often communicate on a superficial level and avoid expressing feelings. Identifying feelings and learning to express them are initial steps in decreasing isolation. Clients with anorexia nervosa are usually able to discuss abstract and concrete issues. Discussions shouldn't be limited to the client's feelings of anxiety as the client may not be aware of the cause of the anxiety, which may result in misdirected self-reflection. Confrontation usually isn't an effective communication strategy as it may cause the client to withdraw and become more depressed.

CN: Psychosocial integrity; CNS: None; CL: Application

30. 1. Clients with anorexia nervosa typically come from a family with parents who are controlling and overprotective. These clients use eating to gain control of an aspect of their lives. Having a history of substance abuse, maintaining an emotional distance, and alternating between love and rejection aren't typical characteristics of parents of children with anorexia nervosa.

CN: Psychological integrity; CNS: None; CL: Application

CN: Client needs category   CNS: Client needs subcategory   CL: Cognitive level

31. A nurse is talking to a family of a client with anorexia nervosa. Which family behavior is most likely to be seen during the family's interaction?
1. Sibling rivalry
2. Rage reactions
3. Parental disagreement
4. Excessive independence

32. A nurse is working with a female client with anorexia nervosa who has acrocyanosis in her extremities. Which short-term goal is the most important for the client?
1. Do daily range-of-motion exercises.
2. Eat some fatty foods daily.
3. Check neurologic reflexes.
4. Promote adequate circulation.

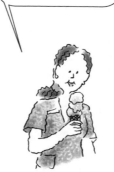

Fatty foods are almost never the right answer!

33. A female client with anorexia nervosa is discharged from the hospital after gaining 12 lb. Which statement by the client best indicates that the nurse's reinforcement of discharge teachings has been effective?
1. "I plan to eat two small meals a day."
2. "I feel that this is scary, but I'm not going to write about it in my journal."
3. "I have to diet because I've gained 12 pounds."
4. "I'll need to attend therapy for support to stay healthy."

34. A female client with anorexia nervosa tells a nurse she always feels fat. Which intervention is the best for this client?
1. Talk about how important the client is.
2. Encourage her to look at herself in a mirror.
3. Address the dynamics of the disorder.
4. Talk about how she's different from her peers.

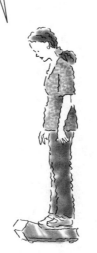

Clients with anorexia nervosa have an intense fear of gaining weight.

31. 3. In many families with a member with anorexia nervosa, there is marital conflict and parental disagreement. Sibling rivalry is a common occurrence and not specific to a family with a member with anorexia nervosa. Emotions are overcontrolled and there's difficulty appropriately expressing negative feelings. In these families, the members tend to be enmeshed and dependent on each other.
CN: Psychosocial integrity; CNS: None; CL: Application

32. 4. Circulation changes will cause extremities to be cold, numb, and have dry and flaky skin. Exercise may help prevent contractures and muscle atrophy, but it may have only a limited secondary effect on promoting circulation. Intake of fatty foods won't have an impact on the client's skin problems. Checking neurologic reflexes won't necessarily assist with handling skin problems.
CN: Physiological integrity; CNS: Reduction of risk potential; CL: Application

33. 4. The client is planning to attend therapy after discharge, which shows an understanding of the need for continued counseling. Eating only two small meals a day is an unrealistic plan for meeting nutritional needs. Feeling insecure when leaving a controlled environment is a common response to discharge. Gaining 12 pounds indicates that the client's nutritional needs are being met at the present caloric intake.
CN: Psychosocial integrity; CNS: None; CL: Analysis

34. 3. The client can benefit from understanding the underlying dynamics of the eating disorder. The client with anorexia nervosa has low self-esteem and won't believe the positive statements. Although the client may look at herself in the mirror, in her mind she'll still see herself as fat. Pointing out differences will only diminish her already low self-esteem.
CN: Psychosocial integrity; CNS: None; CL: Application

35. The grandparents of a client with anorexia nervosa want to support the client, but aren't sure what they should do. Which intervention is best?
1. Promote positive expressions of affection.
2. Encourage behaviors that enhance socialization.
3. Discuss how eating disorders create powerlessness.
4. Discuss the meaning of hunger and body sensations.

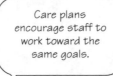

Care plans encourage staff to work toward the same goals.

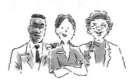

36. A nurse is analyzing the need for health teaching in a female client with anorexia nervosa who lives in a chaotic family situation. Which question is <u>most</u> important for the nurse to ask the client?
1. "How many months have your periods been irregular?"
2. "How often do you think about food in a 24-hour period?"
3. "What were the circumstances before your eating disorder?"
4. "How much and what kinds of exercise do you engage in every day?"

37. An adolescent female client with anorexia nervosa tells a nurse about her outstanding academic achievements and her thoughts about suicide. Which factor must the nurse consider when making a care plan for this client?
1. Self-esteem
2. Physical illnesses
3. Paranoid delusions
4. Relationship avoidance

38. In making a care plan for a family with a member who has anorexia nervosa, which information should be included?
1. Coping mechanisms used in the past
2. Concerns about changes in lifestyle and daily activities
3. Rejection of feedback from family and significant others
4. Appropriate eating habits and social behaviors centering on eating

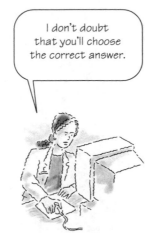

I don't doubt that you'll choose the correct answer.

35. 1. Clients with eating disorders need emotional support and expressions of affection from family members. It wouldn't be an appropriate strategy to have the grandparents promote socialization. Although clients with eating disorders feel powerless, it's better to have the grandparents focus on something positive. Talking about hunger and other sensations won't give the grandparents useful strategies.
CN: Psychosocial integrity; CNS: None; CL: Application

36. 3. This question lets the nurse get information about the family and background situations that influenced the client's needs and distorted eating. The other options deal with menstrual history, exercise patterns, and food obsessions. Although they're relevant, they don't provide information related to the family situation.
CN: Psychosocial integrity; CNS: None; CL: Analysis

37. 1. The client lacks self-esteem, which contributes to her level of depression and feelings of personal ineffectiveness, which in turn may lead to suicidal thoughts. Physical illnesses are common with clients with anorexia nervosa, but they don't relate to this situation. Paranoid delusions refer to false ideas that others want to harm you. No evidence exists that this client is socially isolated.
CN: Psychosocial integrity; CNS: None; CL: Analysis

38. 1. Examination of positive and negative coping mechanisms used by the family allows the nurse to build a care plan specific to the family's strengths and weaknesses. The way the family copes with concerns is more important than the concerns themselves. Feedback from the family and significant others is vital when building a care plan. Eating habits and behaviors are symptoms of the way people cope with problems.
CN: Psychosocial integrity; CNS: None; CL: Application

CN: Client needs category   CNS: Client needs subcategory   CL: Cognitive level

39. Which goal is best to help a client with anorexia nervosa recognize self-distortions?
1. Identify the client's misperceptions of self.
2. Acknowledge immature and childlike behaviors.
3. Determine the consequences of a faulty support system.
4. Recognize the age-appropriate tasks to be accomplished.

40. Parents of a client with anorexia nervosa ask about the risk factors for this disorder. After the parents receive reinforcement of the teaching plan from the nurse, which statement by the parents <u>best</u> indicates that the teaching has been effective?
1. "Risk factors include the inability to be still and emotional lability."
2. "Risk factors include a high level of anxiety and disorganized behavior."
3. "Risk factors include low self-esteem and problems with family relationships."
4. "Risk factors include a lack of life experience and no opportunities to learn skills."

41. A client with anorexia nervosa has started taking fluoxetine hydrochloride (Prozac). The nurse should closely monitor the client for which adverse reaction?
1. Drowsiness
2. Dry mouth
3. Light-headedness
4. Nausea

42. A client with anorexia nervosa is worried about rectal bleeding. Which question should be asked to obtain more information about this problem?
1. "How often do you use laxatives?"
2. "How many days ago did you stop vomiting?"
3. "Are you eating anything that causes irritation?"
4. "Do you have bleeding before or after exercise?"

43. A female client with anorexia nervosa tells a nurse that she has developed hair on most of her body. Which of the following disorders would the nurse most likely expect to be associated with anorexia nervosa?
1. Anemia
2. Osteoporosis
3. Dehydration
4. Electrolyte imbalance

Knowing adverse reactions to key drugs is important.

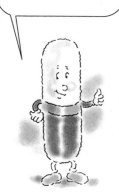

You're heading down the home stretch! Keep going!

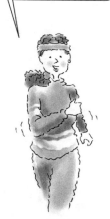

39. 1. Questioning the client's misperceptions and distortions will create doubt about how the client views himself. Acknowledging immature behaviors or determining the consequences of a faulty support system won't promote client recognition of self-distortions. Recognizing the age-appropriate tasks to be accomplished by the client won't help the client recognize distortions.
CN: Psychosocial integrity; CNS: None; CL: Analysis

40. 3. There are several risk factors for eating disorders, including low self-esteem, history of depression, substance abuse, and dysfunctional family relationships. Restlessness and emotional lability are symptoms of manic depressive illness. Anxiety and disorganized behavior could be signs of a psychotic disorder. A lack of life experiences and an absence of opportunities to learn life skills may be a result of anorexia nervosa.
CN: Psychosocial integrity; CNS: None; CL: Analysis

41. 4. Nausea is an adverse reaction to the drug that compounds the eating disorder problem, and the client must be closely monitored. Although the adverse reactions of drowsiness, dry mouth, or light-headedness may occur, they aren't likely to interfere with treatment.
CN: Physiological integrity; CNS: Pharmacological and parenteral therapies; CL: Application

42. 1. Excessive use of laxatives will cause GI irritation and rectal bleeding. If the client stopped vomiting but is still using laxatives, rectal bleeding can occur. Clients who are anorexic eat very little, and what they eat won't cause rectal bleeding. Exercise doesn't cause rectal bleeding.
CN: Health promotion and maintenance; CNS: None; CL: Application

43. 3. When a client with anorexia nervosa has fine hair all over her body (lanugo), the nurse would perform a more extensive assessment of the skin. Lanugo indicates dehydration due to starvation. Anemia is associated with hematologic complications. Osteoporosis is associated with the musculoskeletal system. Electrolyte imbalance is associated with body metabolism.
CN: Health promotion and maintenance; CNS: None; CL: Application

44. A female client with anorexia nervosa is talking to a nurse about her group therapy. Which statement shows the group experience has <u>helped</u> the client?

1. "I feel I'm different and I don't need a lot of friends."
2. "I'll tell my parents it's not just me who has problems."
3. "I can see how to do things better and become the best."
4. "I think I have some unrealistic expectations of myself."

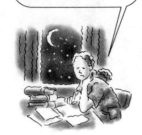

My plan to study all night is starting to seem unrealistic.

44. 4. A goal of group therapy is to provide methods to assess whether personal expectations are unrealistic. Other goals are to learn to handle problems; not to blame parents or others; decrease perfectionist tendencies; and decrease isolation and learn to have healthy peer relationships.

CN: Psychosocial integrity; CNS: None; CL: Application

45. A nurse and her female client who has anorexia nervosa are working on the goal of developing social relationships. Which action by the client is an indication the client is meeting her goal?

1. The client talks about the value of peer relationships.
2. The client decides to talk to her parents about her friends.
3. The client expresses the need to establish trust relationships.
4. The client attends an activity without prompting from others.

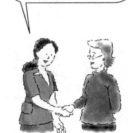

The client must agree to the goal or it won't work.

45. 4. When a client with anorexia nervosa attends an activity without prompting from others, it's a positive sign the client is working toward developing social relationships. Talking about the value of relationships is also beneficial but is only the first step in establishing them. Talking to parents about friends is a start but doesn't necessarily indicate that the client can establish relationships. Expressing the need to establish trust relationships is a first step, but an indication of success would be actually initiating such a relationship.

CN: Psychosocial integrity; CNS: None; CL: Application

46. What initial action should a nurse take when a young female client with anorexia nervosa says, "I'll try to eat something"?

1. Provide a small portion of a healthy food.
2. Weigh the client before and after eating.
3. Ask the client what she thinks she can eat.
4. Suggest the client drink something before eating.

46. 1. Small amounts of food won't overwhelm the client when given at frequent intervals. They also won't overtax the GI and cardiac systems. Weighing the client before and after meals is a useless, stress-provoking action. Asking the client questions may provoke anxiety. It's better to give the client food when she asks. Drinking something before eating isn't necessary; the fluid may prevent the client from being able to eat a sufficient amount of the food.

CN: Physiological integrity; CNS: Reduction of risk potential; CL: Application

47. A client with anorexia nervosa tells a nurse, "I feel so awful and inadequate." Which response is best?

1. "You're being too hard on yourself."
2. "Someday you'll feel better about things."
3. "Tell me something you like about yourself."
4. "Maybe relaxing by yourself will help you feel better."

47. 3. This statement redirects the client to talk about positive aspects of self. The other options minimize her feelings or don't address the client's concerns or encourage the client to change her self-image.

CN: Psychosocial integrity; CNS: None; CL: Application

CN: Client needs category   CNS: Client needs subcategory   CL: Cognitive level

48. Which of the following is the <u>priority</u> during assessment of a client with an eating disorder?
1. Cultural and gender needs
2. Substance abuse history
3. Academic achievement and performance
4. Level of danger to self or others

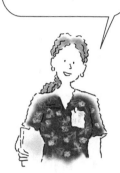

The term *priority* indicates that you should select the answer which would be of first concern during assessment.

49. An adolescent female client with anorexia nervosa starts outpatient treatment. Which client statement indicates that she has a basic understanding of her eating disorder?
1. "I'm not worried because no one ever dies from anorexia."
2. "I still feel fat even though I'm told that I'm not."
3. "My old school friends aren't important to me anymore."
4. "I don't feel right unless I do an intense workout every day."

50. Which question is <u>most</u> useful in assessing the self-esteem of a client with anorexia nervosa?
1. "How would you describe yourself to others?"
2. "What activities do you enjoy doing with your friends?"
3. "Do you play any sports at school or in your community?"
4. "How do you decide how to spend your free time?"

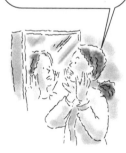

Do others see me as I see myself?

51. Which psychosocial finding should a nurse expect when assessing a client with anorexia nervosa?
1. Avoidant behavior
2. Antisocial behavior
3. Introverted behavior
4. Hypervigilant behavior

48. 4. The priority in assessment should be to determine if the client is a danger to herself or to others. Cultural and gender needs, substance abuse history, and academic performance are an important part of assessment but not the priority.
CN: Safe, effective care environment; CNS: Management of care; CL: Analysis

49. 2. A client with anorexia nervosa shows a basic understanding of the disorder if she can talk about feeling fat even though she's actually underweight, or if she expresses an intense fear of gaining weight. Anorexia nervosa has a mortality of approximately 10% to 15%. People with eating disorders tend to isolate themselves from friends and family members because of their intense focus on food, weight, and exercise. A client with anorexia nervosa may exercise compulsively to prevent weight gain; this behavior indicates continuing presence of the eating disorder.
CN: Psychosocial integrity; CNS: None; CL: Analysis

50. 1. Clients with anorexia nervosa tend to have low self-esteem even if they're high achievers in school, activities, and sports; asking for a self-description can uncover the client's distorted body image and low self-esteem. Questions about activities with friends, involvement in sports, or how the client decides to spend her free time don't necessarily elicit information about self-esteem.
CN: Psychosocial integrity; CNS: None; CL: Analysis

51. 3. Clients with anorexia nervosa typically demonstrate introverted behavior. Clients with bulimia, not anorexia nervosa, tend to show avoidant and dependent behaviors. Clients with eating disorders don't necessarily demonstrate antisocial behavior. Hypervigilant behavior is common in clients with posttraumatic stress disorder, not eating disorders.
CN: Psychosocial integrity; CNS: None; CL: Analysis

52. A nurse notes severe hypocalcemia in a client with anorexia nervosa. Which history finding supports a diagnosis of osteoporosis?
1. Eating a vegetarian diet
2. Drinking well water
3. Going scuba diving
4. Smoking cigarettes

53. A female client with anorexia nervosa is receiving care from her family after successfully completing the refeeding stage of treatment. Which nursing intervention takes priority at this time?
1. Providing a strong support system and opportunities to do reality testing
2. Teaching the family stress-reduction skills to help promote family harmony
3. Promoting anticipatory grieving over the loss each family member is experiencing
4. Assisting the family to work on the issues of autonomy and separation

54. A client with bulimia nervosa has a history of severe GI problems caused by excessive purging. Based on this finding, the nurse must stay alert for which physiologic problem?
1. Renal calculi
2. Esophageal tears
3. Focal seizures
4. Muscle atrophy

55. A nurse is caring for an anorexic client with a nursing diagnosis of *Imbalanced nutrition: Less than body requirements* related to dysfunctional eating patterns. Which interventions would be supportive for this client? Select all that apply:
1. Provide small, frequent meals.
2. Monitor weight gain.
3. Allow the client to skip meals until the anti-depressant levels are therapeutic.
4. Encourage the client to keep a journal.
5. Encourage the client to eat three substantial meals per day.

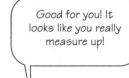

Good for you! It looks like you really measure up!

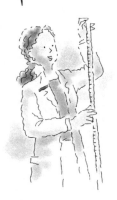

52. 4. Hypocalcemia and cigarette smoking increase the risk for osteoporosis. Eating a vegetarian diet, drinking well water, and going scuba diving don't predispose the client to osteoporosis.
CN: Physiological integrity; CNS: Reduction of risk potential; CL: Analysis

53. 4. When a client with anorexia nervosa successfully completes the refeeding stage of treatment, the family must work on separation and individuation of the client and on decreasing family rigidity and overprotectiveness. Although the client needs a strong support system, developing a sense of self is more important at this time; also, reality testing isn't a typical problem in clients with eating disorders. All families can benefit from learning stress-reduction skills; however, at this time, these skills take lower priority than developing client independence. Anticipatory grieving isn't particularly relevant for family members of a client with an eating disorder.
CN: Psychosocial integrity; CNS: None; CL: Application

54. 2. A bulimic client with severe GI problems from excessive purging is at increased risk for esophageal tears and irritation or esophagitis. Although clients with eating disorders may develop renal calculi, this client is at greater risk for developing esophageal tears. Focal seizures and muscle atrophy aren't related to severe GI problems.
CN: Physiological integrity; CNS: Reduction of risk potential; CL: Analysis

55. 1, 2, 4. Due to self-starvation, clients with anorexia can rarely tolerate large meals three times per day. Small, frequent meals may be tolerated better by the anorexic client and they provide a way to gradually increase daily caloric intake. The nurse should monitor the client's weight carefully because a client with anorexia may try to hide weight loss. The client may be emotionally restrained and afraid to express her feelings; therefore, keeping a journal can serve as an outlet for these feelings, which can assist recovery. An anorexic client is already underweight and shouldn't be permitted to skip meals.
CN: Health promotion and maintenance; CNS: None; CL: Analysis

Selected references

Anatomy & Physiology Made Incredibly Easy, 3rd ed. Philadelphia: Lippincott Williams & Wilkins, 2009.

Assessment Made Incredibly Easy, 4th ed. Philadelphia: Lippincott Williams & Wilkins, 2008.

Baranoski, S., and Ayello, E.A. *Wound Care Essentials: Practice Principles,* 2nd ed. Philadelphia: Lippincott Williams & Wilkins, 2008.

Bickley, L.S., and Szilagyi, P.G. *Bates' Guide to Physical Examination and History Taking,* 10th ed. Philadelphia: Lippincott Williams & Wilkins, 2009.

Bowden, V.R., and Greenberg, C.S. *Pediatric Nursing Procedures,* 2nd ed. Philadelphia: Lippincott Williams & Wilkins, 2008.

Boyd, M.A. *Psychiatric Nursing: Contemporary Practice,* 4th ed. Philadelphia: Lippincott Williams & Wilkins, 2008.

Cardiovascular Care Made Incredibly Easy, 2nd ed. Philadelphia: Lippincott Williams & Wilkins, 2009.

ECG Interpretation Made Incredibly Easy, 5th ed. Philadelphia: Lippincott Williams & Wilkins, 2011.

Fauci, A., et al. *Harrison's Principles of Internal Medicine,* 17th ed. New York: McGraw-Hill, 2009.

Fischbach, F., & Dunning, M.B., eds. *A Manual of Laboratory and Diagnostic Tests,* 8th ed. Philadelphia: Lippincott Williams & Wilkins, 2009.

Hockenberry, M.J., and Wilson, D. *Wong's Nursing Care of Infants and Children,* 8th ed. St. Louis: Mosby–Year Book, Inc., 2007.

Ignatavicius, D.D., and Workman, M.L. *Medical-Surgical Nursing: Patient-Centered Collaborative Care,* 6th ed. Philadelphia: Elsevier, 2010.

Judge, N.L. "Neurovascular Assessment," *Nursing Standard* 21(45):39-44, July 2007.

Karch, A.M. *Focus on Nursing Pharmacology,* 5th ed. Philadelphia: Lippincott Williams & Wilkins, 2010.

Kyle, T. *Essentials of Pediatric Nursing.* Philadelphia: Lippincott Williams & Wilkins, 2008.

Lippincott's Nursing Procedures, 5th ed. Philadelphia: Lippincott Williams & Wilkins, 2008.

Nettina, S.M. *Lippincott Manual of Nursing Practice,* 9th ed. Philadelphia: Lippincott Williams & Wilkins, 2010.

Nursing 2010 Drug Handbook. Philadelphia: Lippincott Williams & Wilkins, 2010.

Pillitteri, A. *Maternal & Child Health Nursing: Care of the Childbearing and Childrearing Family,* 6th ed. Philadelphia: Lippincott Williams & Wilkins, 2010.

Porth, C.M., and Matfin, G. *Pathophysiology: Concepts of Altered Health States,* 8th ed. Philadelphia: Lippincott Williams & Wilkins, 2009.

Professional Guide to Diseases, 9th ed. Philadelphia: Lippincott Williams & Wilkins, 2009.

Smeltzer, S.C., et al. *Brunner & Suddarth's Textbook of Medical-Surgical Nursing,* 12th ed. Philadelphia: Lippincott Williams & Wilkins, 2010.

Taylor, C.R., et al. *Fundamentals of Nursing: The Art and Science of Nursing Care,* 6th ed. Philadelphia: Lippincott Williams & Wilkins, 2008.

Townsend, M.C., and Pedersen, D.D. *Essentials of Psychiatric Mental Health Nursing: Concepts of Care in Evidence-Based Practice.* Philadelphia: F.A. Davis Company, 2008.

Wilson, D., and Hockenberry, M.J. *Wong's Clinical Manual of Pediatric Nursing,* 7th ed. St. Louis: Mosby–Year Book, Inc., 2008.

Index

t refers to table